PRACTICAL PALEO

A Customized Approach to Health and a Whole-Foods Lifestyle

Diane Sanfilippo, BS, NC

VB

Victory Belt Publishing Inc.
Las Vegas

First Published in 2012 by Victory Belt Publishing Inc.

ISBN 13: 978-1-936608-75-1

The information included in this book is for educational purposes only. It is not intended nor implied to be a substitute for professional medical advice. The reader should always consult his or her healthcare provider to determine the appropriateness of the information for their own situation or if they have any questions regarding a medical condition or treatment plan. Reading the information in this book does not create a physician-patient relationship.

Victory Belt ® is a registered trademark of Victory Belt Publishing Inc.

Book design by Joan Olkowski, Graphic D-Signs, Inc.
Illustrations by Alex Boake
Food photography (recipes) by Bill Staley
Photography (additional) by Kelty Luber

Cover Portrait:
Photography by Kelli Beavers
Hair styling by Samantha Gaiser
Make-up by Hayley Mason

Printed in the USA

RRD06-13

CONTENTS

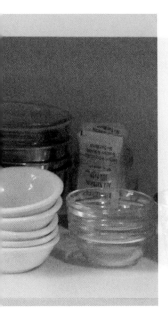

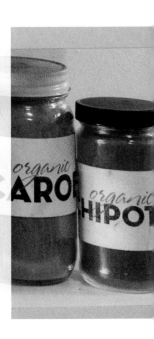

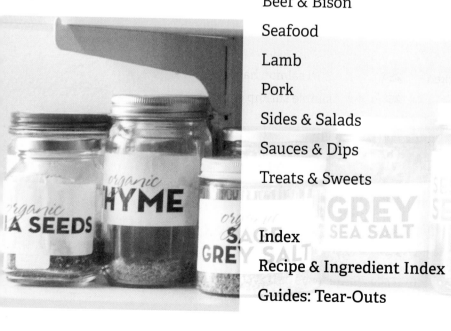

foreword

By Robb Wolf, *New York Times* best-selling author of *The Paleo Solution*

As I read through the review copy of *Practical Paleo* I had a number of thoughts: 1) Wow, this is going to be a really useful book for a lot of people! 2) DAMN! I wish I laid out some of the material in my book, *The Paleo Solution*, the way that Diane did in her book! She's making complex stuff, like poop and healing a leaky gut, easy to understand. 3) The food pictures make me hungry!

I've been researching and studying this Paleo concept for almost fifteen years and the evolution and reach of the information has been nothing short of re-markable. Years ago you had to hunt (and gather?) to find information on Paleo in general, to say nothing of how to alter your approach for specific problems such as gastrointestinal issues or autoimmunity.

People often come to me saying that Paleo worked for them, but they're un-sure of how to tread with loved ones—how to best help their Type 2 Diabetic mom, or their dad/friend/(insert other loved-one here) with a specific condi-tion. While I've personally answered these questions for thousands of people through my own website, blog, podcast, and book, **this** book takes all of the concepts that we know will help people and provides clear plans, laid out in an easy-to-understand way. It takes the guesswork out of how to move forward and take your health into your own hands—from lifestyle to diet to smart supplementation. All this with amazing-looking recipes to boot!

Once, it was tough to find this information, and if you were fortunate enough to find what you needed, it was in a dry, unaesthetic format. Those days are gone. My good friend, Diane Sanfilippo, has made a work of art in *Practical Paleo* that is as useful as it is beautiful. Are you an athlete? Suffer from digestive distress? Been diagnosed with an autoimmune condition? Maybe you just want to live a long life and look good naked? Whatever your goals, Diane has done the heavy lifting by condensing the science and a lot of practical how-tos into bite-sized pieces.

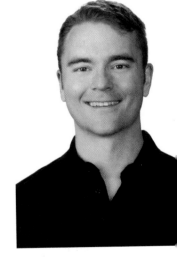

You don't need a pocket protector to read this book. In easy-to-understand language, you will learn the science behind the Original Human Diet and how it can unlock the door to better health. Science, recipes, customization, and beau-tiful, easy-to-read graphics—*Practical Paleo* has it all.

—Robb Wolf

dedication and gratitude

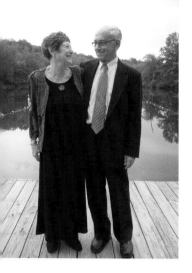

First and foremost, to my grandmother, Barbara Frank, who will be turning ninety when this book hits the shelf.

This book would not exist had you not been confused by the concept of an electronic book (eBook), and asked me, "what about a *real* book?" To which I replied, "I don't know, I never thought about it." A month or so later, I was slated to write this book. Your stories and support have been the number one motivation for me to get this project completed sooner rather than later, and now I feel so lucky that I can share my baby with you. And yes, this book will have to serve as a stand-in for a great grandchild...sorry Gram.

And to my grandfather, Bill, who passed away before ever knowing this book was in creation, for his confidence in me as a well-intentioned person and a businesswoman. His support through every phase of my life and career was unwavering. Whatever path I was on, he was confident that it was the right one for me... and if it wasn't the right path, he was confident that I'd blaze a trail for myself to make it that way.

To my parents, who raised me with the words: "do what makes you happy." Some may think those words will lead a child into an adult life that is hedonistic and irresponsible, but I have experienced first-hand how important that value has been in my life. After working several jobs along the way that I didn't wake up with a burning passion to tackle, their words to "do what makes you happy" still resonate. I feel lucky to wake up every day to a life I am choosing, and I thank them for their 100% support.

To my nutrition instructors at Bauman College, Nori Hudson and Laura Knoff, for not looking at me like I had a third eye when early in my nutritional education I showed up to classes with newfound passion for a grain and legume-free lifestyle; and for being supporters and promoters of the teachings of Dr. Weston Price, so that traditional and well-raised animal foods were consistently discussed as health-promoting options in a classroom where the curriculum was clearly created with a vegetarian slant.

To Robb Wolf, for igniting my vigor and passion for sharing the profoundly powerful message of Paleo nutrition. Eight hours of listening to you explain nutritional biochemistry and how it relates to all disease was enough to grip me, pull me in, make me never eat quinoa again, and to find the fire in my own belly to share this message with others in my own way. You gave me a boost when I needed it, but never a handout or help on a silver platter—I have a lot of respect for that. Your unrelenting motivation to just plain help people continues to motivate and inspire me. You are a gift to humanity.

To Chris Kresser, for being a levelheaded and trusted resource. When prescribing an approach to follow, you always provide factual information with the appropriate dose of common-sense. I can always trust your advice, and I don't take advice from many people.

To my trainer, Dave Engen, who was the first person to tell me that I should be eating coconut oil and *not* be eating gluten: I know I fought you tooth and nail on the concept of eating fat, swearing you didn't know what it was like to have to watch what you ate. You patiently waited while I figured out for myself that you were right. I still credit you every time I talk about my "resistance-to-change period" when teaching seminars.

To my friend, John Tsafos, who taught me how to find calm in a world of chaos. Though you may not realize it now, I was a much more anxious person before we became friends.

To my teaching partner, Liz Wolfe, for allowing me to drag you into this whole nutty world of being a nutrition "rockstar" and traveling the country to spread the word about real food. You have become a dear friend to me and the respect I hold for you and your work is enormous. I searched for over a year for a teaching partner, and I feel blessed that I found you.

To my old boss, Dan Antonelli at Graphic D-Signs, Inc. in New Jersey, for teaching me the skill to turn information into a piece of graphic art that people can use over and over to make their lives healthier.

To all of my friends, old and new, who have dealt with me being completely submerged in "work-mode" for the last several years, and with whom I need to spend more quality, relaxed, and fun time—thank you for always being there when I needed you.

To readers and followers of my work to-date... wow! The outpouring of support and gratitude you all provide is what makes this job worthwhile.

To my publisher, Erich Krauss; I can't imagine having worked with anyone else on this project. You treated my baby as if it were your own, and rallied to pull me through the immense effort it took to get it done.

Last, but certainly not least, to Bill Staley and Hayley Mason. Without the two of you, the recipes in this book would likely have been accompanied by iPhone photos tweaked with a 99-cent app. You opened your home up to me for six weeks, photographed and helped me test recipes, and supported me while I worked on the material for the rest of the book. Bill, I thank you for your tireless efforts in shooting with care and precision every recipe in this book with me, as if it were your own. Hayley, your constant reassurance that my recipes were on a good track was invaluable. And thanks to both of you for tasting every single recipe in the book—I know that was the toughest part! Your friendship has meant *the world* to me and this book would absolutely not be what it is without the two of you.

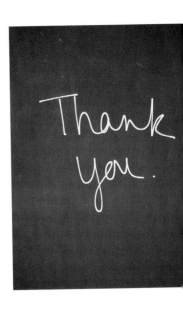

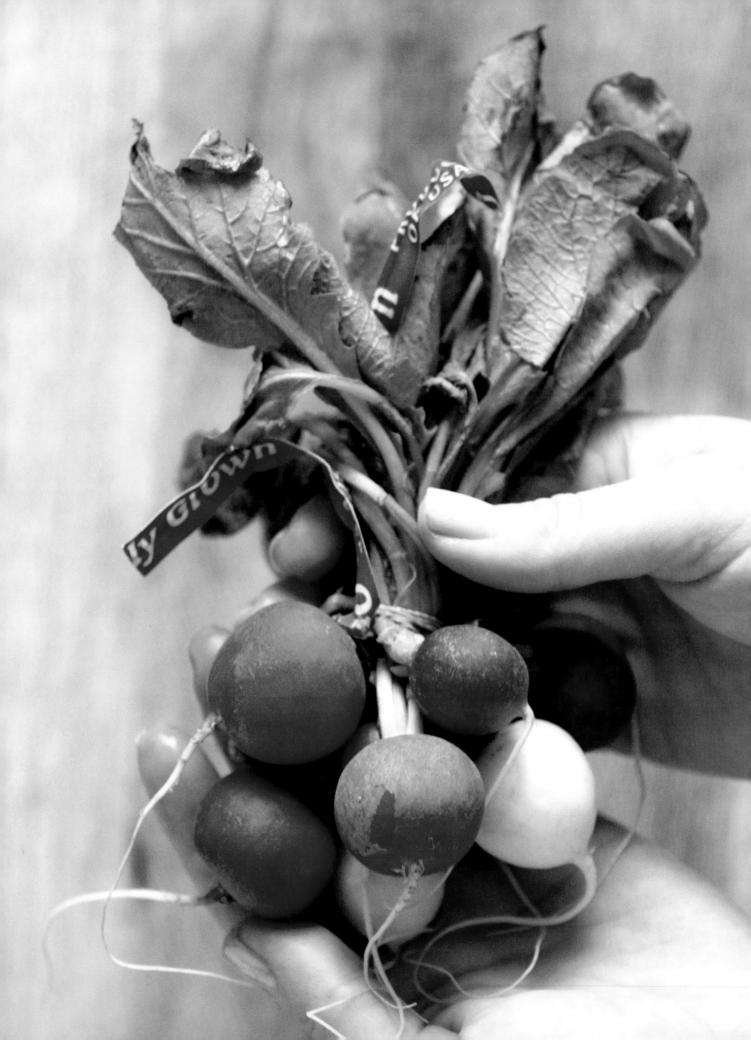

introduction

"Let food be thy medicine, and medicine be thy food."
    -Hippocrates

I grew up playing soccer, volleyball, and softball, but like most kids, I never focused on nutrition. In fact, while growing up, it never crossed my mind that I might need to change my eating habits. Whatever I liked, I ate. I was in pretty good shape, and I considered myself to be healthy and strong.

Then, during high school, I began to have disruptive bouts of digestive distress to the extent that I took Imodium A-D several times a week. I also suffered from repeated sinus infections throughout the year. The infections became so old hat that I simply demanded antibiotics when I visited the doctor. After all, I had been taught that pills were the best way to handle symptoms.

My close friends struggled with the same health issues. All of us had a range of chronic ailments like acne, pharyngitis, heartburn, headaches, dental cavities, and deteriorating vision, in addition to the sinus and digestive discomfort. It never occurred to any of us that we had the power to prevent these problems.

After eighteen years as an active youth, I became much less active in college, and my weight started to rise. My late nights with pizza and buffalo wings meant that "The Freshman 15" didn't end after freshman year. I continued to eat like an athlete even though I had all but abandoned that aspect of my life. By the time I finished college, I had put on thirty pounds. There is a photo from my graduation dinner that shows my bloated midsection—it's one I use as a "before" picture when I tell my story at seminars. At the time, I had no idea my body had fallen completely apart.

Like many people who gain weight during their college years, I thought, "This is just what happens when people get older." I learned later, of course, that it's what happens when people stop exercising and eat foods that do not support a healthy body. My symptoms may have been "common," but what I didn't realize until later is that common doesn't necessarily mean "normal."

After I had gained yet another ten pounds, a nurse practitioner brought up my weight during a routine check-up. She talked to me about food portion sizes and I suddenly realized how out of control my eating had become. Even though everyone around me ate the same way, I couldn't deny that I didn't feel or look good.

That winter, I joined a gym and tried to "watch

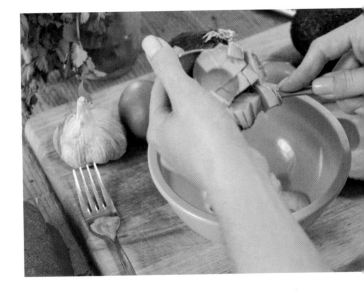

Diane Sanfilippo

11

what I ate," but I had no clue what that meant. I dined out on burgers and fries (on large seedy buns, of course), and washed it all down with Coke. I did know that soda wasn't healthy, so I sometimes substituted water instead. At home, I made dinners of pasta with red sauce and analyzed the meal in my head. "Well, that's just some pasta and tomato," I'd think, "so it's healthy." I gave myself a bit less than I served my boyfriend, and I sweated away on the cardio machines at the gym. You probably aren't surprised to hear that my weight *did not budge*.

Months later, I started a new job and found myself surrounded by middle-aged women on Weight Watchers. "Okay," I thought, "if they can do it, I can do it." So I started the diet and stayed on it ... until the end of each workday when I found myself still hungry with no points (how Weight Watchers evaluates and measures food intake) left. Still, in spite of my occasional cheating, the diet began to work.

What Weight Watchers taught me more than anything was to read food labels. Granted, I now teach people to read labels for entirely different reasons, but it was a start for me. For the first time, I paid attention to the number of calories, fat, and fiber contained in a serving. As a result, I lost my first twelve pounds from simply watching my diet and working out on the elliptical machine for thirty minutes several times a week. The initial weight loss gave me the confidence to exercise at the gym more often, and I started lifting weights again for the first time in four years.

Days turned into weeks and months, and before I knew it, I had lost thirty pounds. In many ways, I felt amazing. My body was finally getting back to a size that was more familiar to me, but the rest of my system was the same as it had always been—riddled with digestive distress, chronic sinus infections, and vision deterioration. I even had a new ailment to add to the mix: hypoglycemia (low blood sugar).

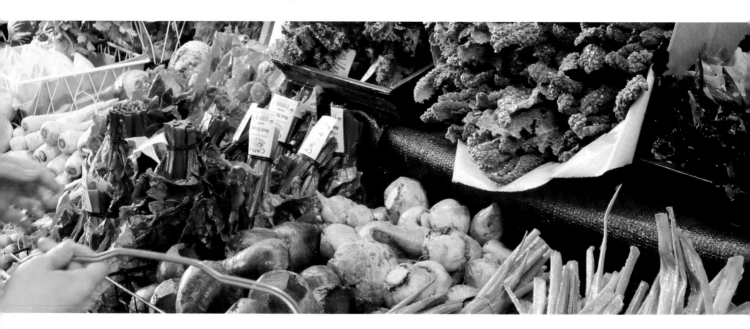

What was the problem? I continued to eat close to 300 grams of carbohydrates a day, reaching for bread with olive oil if my dinner wasn't "filling" enough. Low blood sugar attacks even caused me to nearly pass out at times. When I became shaky, sweaty, and lightheaded, a friend usually said, "Get her a granola bar!" Of course, that was the last thing I needed.

what I didn't know about grains was hurting me

It wasn't until several years later that I discovered the root cause of my chronic symptoms. At first, I thought it was preposterous that bread—innocent old bread—could be the source of such hefty problems. When I finally came to terms with the long list of conditions associated with gluten intolerance, it *still* took me a year to finally give it up. Then there was a big turning point for me.

Not long after converting to a 90% gluten-free way of eating I attended Robb Wolf's *Paleo Solution Seminar*. I had already studied nutrition for many years by then, but there were two big takeaways for me that day:

1. Avoid gluten like the plague, and
2. Managing blood sugar, insulin levels, and systemic inflammation are critical to health and can all be done fairly easily by removing grains and legumes from the diet.

I went home and gutted my house, cleaning it of every grain—quinoa, buckwheat, rice, millet, gluten-free oats, and more. I prepared meat and vegetables with some fat and spices, and I cooked eggs and bacon in the mornings, packing them in a glass container to take to work and eat at my desk. My coworkers were jealous as they gnawed on granola bars and downed bowls of cereal that were always well stocked in the office kitchen. When it was time for our lunch orders, mine was designed to provide me with as much protein and as many veggies as possible. When a work meeting over breakfast popped up at the last minute with only pastries and fruit as options, I took a ten-minute walk to the deli for hard-boiled eggs.

I brought foods with me to supplement my prepared lunches when I couldn't get enough healthy fare from a restaurant or deli. That took a bit of planning, of course, but it was actually easy to make it work.

The results were dramatic. I stopped suffering from all of the chronic ailments that had plagued me for most of my life. My digestion works predictably well now, I rarely get sinus infections, and the hypoglycemia is long gone. I no longer worry that I might pass out without a snack or that I might have to run to the bathroom when it isn't convenient. The vision deterioration I had experienced for years has halted, and I have not had a cavity in a long time. On the very rare occasion when I experience heartburn or a headache, I can quickly identify the food that caused it. At most, I get sick once or twice a year after air travel or too little rest. When that happens, I don't have to take antibiotics, and the bug passes through my system within three to five days. While my acne took a bit longer to alleviate, supplemental vitamins A and D in a concentrated, whole-food supplement eventually did the trick.

All of the ailments that haunted me for years were resolved by changing my diet. It was a matter of:

1. Healing my "gut" (digestive system), which, in turn, healed my entire body.
2. Balancing my blood sugar levels.

After these two main issues were addressed, it was simply a matter of fine-tuning my diet to optimize my health. I suffered needlessly for many years, but my new way of life is extraordinarily liberating.

your health requires that you help yourself

Not long after I discovered how to become and stay healthy, I found that I wanted to share my knowledge with others and help them feel the same liberation. So I decided to become a professional nutritionist. I started an organic meal delivery business, but after just a few months of providing meals to clients, I realized I was doing the work for them rather than actually transforming their lives. I had to teach them how to create new lifestyle habits.

Since making that decision and becoming a Certified Nutrition Consultant, it has been very rewarding to share my passion for nutritious food with others and help them create dietary plans that provide them with healthier, happier lives. The natural progression was then to extend my reach with a book.

I realize there is a lot of information out there about how and what to eat, but it's often difficult to understand. So whether you are totally new to the Paleo way of eating and living or have been on this path for a while, you can follow this book easily. My aim is to provide you with a resource that is practical and useful in your everyday life, explaining the basics of how food works in your body, as well as showing you examples of how to create a customized meal plan for your individual nutritional needs. When you finish the book, you will have the tools you need to easily shop for and create delicious meals that give your body what it requires to stay healthy and energized.

If you're looking for detailed scientific writing filled with jargon and citations that you can further explore online, however, you won't find it here. Hence, the word "practical" in the title. My goal is to distill my years of education and experience into a guide that's easy to understand and just plain useful.

this is not a diet

Practical Paleo is a way to change your lifestyle, leading to long-term health benefits far beyond the coming weeks or months. Remember that a "diet" is temporary. The book will show you how food works inside the body so that you can design a plan that works for *your* body.

If you're entirely new to this way of living, you may find it helpful to start by following one of the 30-Day Meal Plans in Part 2 of this book. If that feels too overwhelming for the way you live, simply follow the guides throughout the book on how to select real, whole foods. This will take you most of the way to a healthier you without ever following a specific plan.

Practical Paleo will serve not just the average person looking for improved health, but also those who have been diagnosed with a medical condition and perhaps told they'd suffer with those symptoms for life. If you fall into the latter group, this book was particularly created for *you*. I want you to know that there is a better way; pills and pain are not necessities for everyone in life. For many, it *is* possible to feel better, despite what you have been told, even perhaps by doctors. **You get to choose what you eat, and that is the most powerful medicine of all.**

finding health in a modern world

When I first told my 90-year-old grandmother that I was becoming a nutrition consultant, she had difficulty understanding how teaching people what to eat could be a job.

She was born in a different time when food was still real, whole, and made a short trip from the farm to the dinner table. She fondly recounts the days spent milking cows, collecting eggs, and feeding the animals.

When refined foods were introduced into our food supply, my grandmother and her peers strayed from their real food habits in favor of what was faster and more convenient. Grandma didn't need a lesson in how and what to eat when she was growing up, but *now* she does. Now, we *all* do.

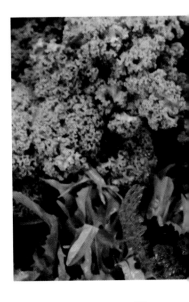

Modern grocery stores are enormous and filled with aisle after aisle of packaged, processed "foods" that your grandmother would not have seen in the kitchen of her youth. Those of us in subsequent generations were, by contrast, raised on pasteurized milk products, refined grains, and sugar-laden foods like boxed macaroni and cheese, bottled or canned sodas, and commercial cereals. Even health-conscious families scooped up boxes of instant oats, whole grain breads, and non-fat yogurts.

When we began to eat foods created in factories rather than grown on farms, we moved steadily away from health-promoting foundational nutrition and closer to building our bodies' tissues from edible, yet synthetic, nutrient-

your constitution

Your physical state of health and robustness—the foundation you may have, at varying levels, to maintain or achieve optimal health with more or less effort. For example, a person who was born to a healthy and robust mother, birthed naturally, breast-fed until self-weaned, and transitioned to whole, real food is likely to have a more robust constitution than someone without these advantages who was immediately fed an unhealthy diet of cereals and refined foods during his or her formative years.

poor, "food-like" substances. Isn't it obvious that problems would arise? It's pretty clearly seen in the declining health and vitality of the majority of people around us.

Today, medication keeps my grandmother alive as her body suffers the consequences of decades of eating processed foods and dealing with undiagnosed food allergies. It's sad that the majority of her severe health conditions could have been avoided by shunning factory foods when they began to appear on grocery store shelves. Still, my grandmother is lucky. A foundation of better childhood nutrition (pre-processed food, at the very least) allowed the development of a hearty survival mechanism. Her constitution is much sturdier than that of children today, who are not only born to mothers that were raised on modern processed foods, but are also fed commercially prepared infant formula that we are told is as safe and as healthy as breast milk, even though it is not. If Grandma had been raised on the foods that most people currently consume on a regular basis, she likely wouldn't have made it to age ninety.

I have explained to Grandma that most food today isn't produced the way it was when she was a kid, and therein lies the problem. I tell her that it's important to seek out and support the rare individuals who produce food with "old school" values in mind. After many decades of relying on processed food, much of these discussions fail to "stick." She remembers my "cookie monster" days and offers me some when I visit her, forgetting that I no longer eat such things. When I remind her that I feel better when I don't eat those foods, I always ask her: Do I look hungry? It's a cheeky question, but it proves the point that sufficient nourishment is found in foods that aren't derived from grains.

Grandma was intrigued when I told her that not only were people quite confused about what to eat, but that a change in nutrition—yes, a simple change in *food*—could actually help people feel better. Hence, the need for my profession.

Even people who have taken multiple medications for years to manage symptoms can resolve their health issues by changing their diets. This concept befuddled my grandmother partly because doctors, in her mind, are the final word, and they never offered dietary solutions. She lives with medical issues ranging from gallbladder disease to thyroid and other autoimmune complications, as well as diverticulitis and massive sciatic pain. I'm confident that she also has undiagnosed Celiac disease (a condition caused by gluten intolerance).

After a bout with colon cancer last year, I told my grandmother that she has an allergy to gluten. It seemed that she might more readily accept a dietary explanation for a disease of the digestive system. I sent her home with gluten-free bread and other options. Even though I don't recommend these for most people, this 90-year-old was hardly about to give up her morning toast or afternoon cookies. I simply hoped for at least a small change in her routine.

A few days after she got home from the hospital, I asked how she was feeling. She reported that she no longer had the pain in her abdomen that she had experienced every day for as long as she could remember. Other food-regulated issues aside, what appeared to be a lifelong food allergy—constantly aggravated by continuous exposure to gluten—subsided for reasons that escaped her. One cannot help but wonder if this long-term intolerance was modulating other aspects of her health as she aged. Hearing her say that she didn't feel the same pain was enough to solidify in my mind that she had suffered needlessly—likely for decades.

WHAT IS THIS THING CALLED GLUTEN?

The word gluten is often used as an umbrella term for the gliadin protein or a number of other constituents in grains to which people can react negatively. Gluten is found in grains and by-products of wheat, barley, rye, triticale, oats (typically from cross-contamination), and other grains, as well as in some other foods where these grains are used in processing.

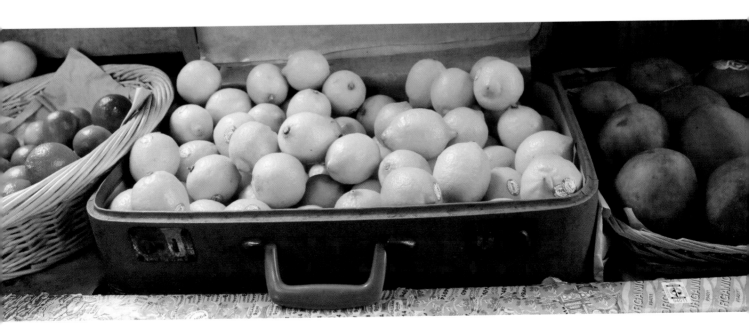

Diane Sanfilippo

why paleo is so powerful

FINDING GLUTEN

*Check out the Guide to:
Gluten on page 89 for
more information on
where gluten hides!*

I fully recognize that there are certain conditions for which a prescription or medical intervention may be lifesaving and necessary. Most chronic conditions, however, have their underpinnings in our overall level of immune health—the conditions that rest upon the aspects of our physiology that are directly affected by food. These conditions *can* and *will* be impacted by dietary and lifestyle changes if we're willing to make those changes. So how can we circle back toward the idea that health is a natural state for humans and that relying on medications to relieve symptoms is not usually a real solution?

While we've forgotten what "real food" is over the last few decades and have been left desperately seeking sustenance that will truly nourish our bodies, there is hope. The fact that we're disillusioned with the conventional wisdom—and for good reason—is a step in the right direction.

Still, many people are ready and willing to change but lack the information that will help them put their chronic symptoms in remission. Luckily, the health movement that has arisen from the disillusionment has gained extraordinary momentum for a reason: It has helped countless individuals overcome what were seemingly insurmountable, chronic, or even unrecognized health problems.

People are just beginning to realize that they are no longer destined to suffer from diseases—or even minor ailments—that are caused by modern food and

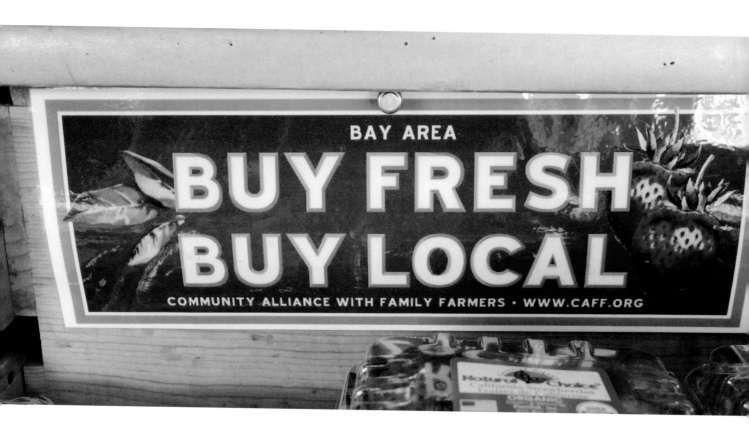

depleting lifestyles. We have found a better way. I want to share with you, as I've shared with my grandmother over the years, that we can indeed circle back to food that comes from properly raised animals and well-tended plants. You don't have to rely on factory-derived, packaged calories stamped with unfounded health claims that are nothing more than marketing spin. You can find extraordinary health in beautifully simple, unprocessed, whole foods.

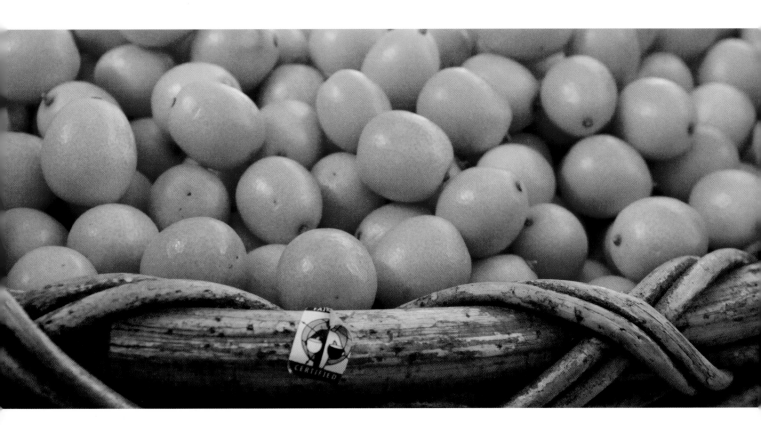

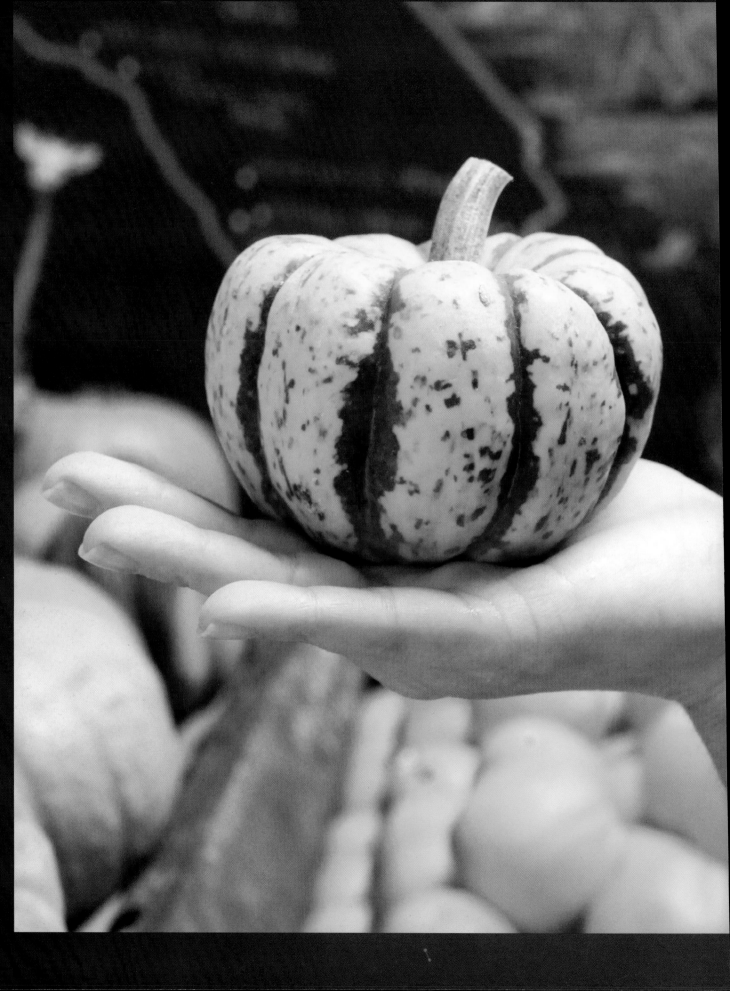

PART 1: THE WHY — FOOD AND YOUR BODY

what is paleo?

"Paleo" is short for Paleolithic, but the name is actually less important than the power of the overall approach.

While the term "Paleo" has gained traction in the mainstream media and on bookstore shelves everywhere due to the improved health of those who follow the lifestyle, you could call it "Primal," "Grain-Free," "Real Food," "Whole Food," "Nutrient-Dense," or "Ancestral." Whatever name you choose, the "Paleo" way of eating is simple: Mimic our ancestors, who suffered from fewer chronic diseases than modern populations. This doesn't mean that you'll recreate a caveman's food landscape, of course. Our food supply and our environment are different from our ancestors, so we must adapt as new information comes to light.

The lifestyle is simply about (1) eating whole foods that provide better fuel for your body and (2) avoiding processed, refined, nutrient-poor factory foods. This means avoiding grains, legumes (beans), refined sugar, and pasteurized dairy products. People believe eating whole foods is hard and limiting, but it isn't. It may be an adjustment at first, but it's simply a matter of eliminating foods that don't promote health in your body.

Still, applying such a way of eating to your life can be confusing. We must go a few steps further and create a plan that's customized for *your* body's needs to achieve *optimal* health. So after you've tackled basic food choices, it is critical to make sure you maintain proper digestive function and blood sugar regulation. You also need to understand what to do to reach your own personal health goals. Paleo is *not* a one-size-fits-all approach, but it's a way of eating that is appropriate for *all* human animals. In other words, you are a human animal, so there is a Paleo plan that is right for *you*.

This Paleo way of eating provides what I believe to be a fantastic framework upon which to build a solid nutritional plan. In fact, the quantity and quality of scientific research behind this movement is astounding, showing how an ancestral diet promotes excellent health. If you're interested in learning more about the science behind this way of eating, I recommend the research conducted by the leading experts listed below:

- Dr. Loren Cordain, author of *The Paleo Diet*
- Dr. Staffan Lindeberg, author of *Food and Western Disease: Health and Nutrition From an Evolutionary Perspective*
- Dr. Alessio Fasano, a leading researcher on the effects of gluten proteins on intestinal barrier function
- Robb Wolf, biochemist and *New York Times* bestselling author of *The Paleo Solution*
- Mathieu Lalonde, Ph. D., organic chemist
- Chris Kresser, LAc., Integrative Medicine Practitioner

didn't cavemen only live to be 30?

While the Paleo way of eating is not a replication of a caveman diet, let's shatter the myth about the life span of primitive humans. Their life span was based on several factors:

1. In the absence of modern medicine, infant mortality rates were high and estimated life span was based on an average of those who died at birth as well as those who lived long lives. It doesn't mean that every human alive in the Paleolithic era dropped dead at age thirty. In fact, those who lived to about age twenty went on to have an estimated life span closer to sixty years.
2. Deaths from infectious diseases were more common in the absence of modern medicine.
3. They were more vulnerable to predatory animals.
4. They were vulnerable to the elements due to inferior shelter.

making paleo work for you

Before you can land on the best nutritional plan for you, it's important to understand the basic principles behind this ancestral, real-food way of eating.

1. Eat whole foods.

If a food is not in its whole, natural form, chances are that it has been refined and is a less than optimal choice. When we intellectualize our diet and remove ourselves, as human animals, from the complex web that defines nature, we fight against our birthright of health. When you eat food as provided by nature, it actually promotes health, healing, and immunity against future ailments.

PALEO IS NOT AN RX
Paleo is a template, not a dietary prescription. There is no one cookie-cutter "Paleo diet." If you are eating solely chicken breasts, broccoli, and olive oil, you're missing the point entirely.

2. Avoid modern, processed, and refined foods.

These include grains, pasteurized dairy products, industrial seed oils (like corn, cottonseed, soybean, canola, or rapeseed), and artificial or refined sugar and sweeteners—especially high fructose corn syrup. If it has to pass through a factory before it is edible for you, reconsider whether or not it is actually food. More likely, it is an "edible product" or "food-like-substance."

3. Eat to maintain proper digestive function.

Your requirements for digestive function may be different from someone else depending on your constitution. Essentially, you must determine which foods your body cannot tolerate and stop eating them. For example, some people can tolerate dairy, or the occasional grain-based foods. When you experience symptoms of food intolerances, it is your body's way of telling you that you are disrupting your digestion.

Why is it so critical not to disrupt digestion? The ability to fight chronic, and even acute, disease states *begins* in the digestive system (the gut). Sixty to eighty percent of the immune system is within the gut. There is immune tissue that follows the entire length of your small intestine. You'll learn more than you ever thought you needed to know about this in the digestion and leaky gut sections of this book. If your body constantly suffers from digestive irritation, you set the stage for suppressed immune function in all other areas. This can result in a condition as innocuous as seasonal allergies or a problem that is much more aggressive like diverticulitis, eczema, psoriasis, or a number of inflammatory and autoimmune conditions.

4. Eat to maintain proper blood sugar regulation.

The amount of time it takes before your hunger kicks in again after a meal and how you feel (besides hungry) entering into your next meal are critical signs of how well your blood sugar levels are managed. If you're hungry and eating every two to three hours and feeling shaky, weak, or starving entering into each meal or snack, you are probably not eating the right balance of food for you. Figuring out how much protein, fat, and "good carbs" you should eat will help you to maintain well-balanced blood sugar throughout the day while comfortably eating roughly every four to six hours. Later in the book you will get filled in on the details and importance of blood sugar regulation.

5. Follow a plan that will help you reach your own personal health goals.

People often ask me if I think a Paleo diet is right for everyone. Since Paleo is about is eating healthy food and avoiding unhealthy food—i.e., eating whole foods as opposed to refined foods—then, yes, I think it's 100% right for everyone. Still, it would be a huge misstep to say that we can and should all eat exactly the same foods.

Does that mean you can try to create a nutritional plan based on what your specific ancestors ate? If your bloodline is 100% pure, you could try, but it would still be challenging to find the same foods that were eaten so long ago. Most of us, at least in the United States, are a mixture of different bloodlines from around the world, so it would be impossible to trace the diet of our ancestors. Instead, the Paleo concept is based on estimations of what humans of past generations would have eaten, as well as the nutritional and dietary history in many parts of the world. We can guess what different animal and plant foods would have been available in different climates on different terrain and with varied access to bodies of water. If we were to attempt to recreate early

BEYOND YOUR BELLY
Digestive disruption may appear in any form of chronic inflammatory condition; it does not always manifest as upper or lower GI upset like belching, burping, gas, bloating, diarrhea, or constipation, though all of those are surefire signs that your digestive process has gone awry.

Check out the Guide to Digestion on page 74 for a complete list of chronic inflammatory conditions associated with impaired digestive function.

natural diets with 100% accuracy, though, we would have to stretch to find the indigenous plants and animals that were available in the past.

While I propose that there are certain foods that should be considered optimal and included as part of your nutritional landscape, you may very well experience vibrant, long-term, and exemplary health eating foods outside of these recommendations. Someone who eats processed foods and maintains excellent health is hardly the norm, however. Unfortunately, in my experience, this kind of exemplary health is far from what most people are experiencing in the modern world.

ask yourself these questions

Beyond your ethnic heritage, you can evaluate your upbringing and foundational nutrition (or lack thereof), as well as your genetic predispositions to health or disease to the best of your ability. Then, answer these questions regarding your current health status:

- How do you feel most of the time?
- What is the status of your physical fitness or athletic performance?
- How is your body composition in terms of how much fat you have compared to muscle?
- How are your moods?
- Does your energy level fluctuate throughout the day?
- How is your appetite?
- Do you have food cravings? For sugar? For carbs? For salty or fatty foods?
- Does your skin look healthy, clear, and glowing?
- How is your vision?
- How is your dental health?
- Do you have regular bowel movements?
- Have you been diagnosed with a specific health condition?

If you answered all of these questions positively, congratulations! You're in a very small minority, and you can skip ahead to the recipes later in the book. If you're like most people, you probably didn't give a positive answer to all of the questions, which means you would benefit from evaluating your current approach to health and nutrition in short order. Read on to learn more about how food works in your body to either work with or against what will naturally keep you in a state of optimal health with regards to your digestive function and blood sugar regulation. These two components are the keys to long-term, optimal health and well-being as they can drive your body's systems either in the right or wrong direction.

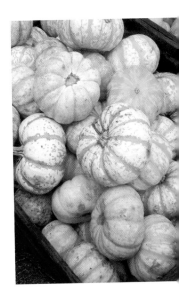

if you're ready to just get started with the food, jump right on in, the water's fine

If you simply want to improve your overall health, reviewing the one-page guides throughout the book and following the recipes will get you well on your way. If you have an existing health condition, set of symptoms, or a specific health goal, continue reading all of the chapters to learn how food operates in your body. Then, proceed to the 30-Day Meal Plans to find an approach that may be best for you.

You can identify which plan is right for you by reviewing the introductions to each meal plan, as well as the set of conditions and/or ill-health symptoms that each meal plan is designed to support. In the meantime, the chart that follows will give you a basic rundown of which foods to eat and which to eliminate for a Paleo lifestyle.

paleo eating basics: start here.

[+] eat whole foods

MEAT, SEAFOOD & EGGS

It is ideal to enjoy meat and seafood from grass-fed, pasture-raised, organic-fed animals or wild-caught and sustainable seafood sources. (Resources can be found in the guides on the following pages.)

VEGETABLES & FRUITS

Making a dietary change doesn't mean your food needs to be boring or repetitive! There are more than 50 kinds of vegetables in the guide on page 29. Use that guide regularly, as well as the recipes in the book, to discover new and interesting vegetables at your local farmers' market or grocery store. Better yet, grow your own outdoors or in an indoor vertical garden.

Fruit can be hard on your blood sugar if you overdo it, so I encourage you to limit your fruit intake. Avoid adding fruit to your meals; instead, eat it for dessert. If you exercise a great deal and want to maintain athletic performance, you can include more fruit in your nutritional plan.

NUTS & SEEDS

When you are new to a Paleo-type of diet, nuts are a great go-to snack item. That said, nut consumption can easily be overdone. If your goal is fat loss, I caution against eating too many nuts. Please refer to portion recommendations in the Meal Planning section.

FATS & OILS

When you're cooking or simply want to add healthy fats to a meal with very lean meats, choose the *best* quality fats you can find. Please refer to the "Fats and Oils Guide" later in the book for details as to which fats are recommended.

[-] eliminate refined foods

REFINED GRAINS

This includes, but is not limited to, cereals (yes, even rolled or steel-cut oatmeal), toast, muffins, scones, croissants, English muffins, sandwiches, burritos, tacos, pancakes, waffles, pasta, rice, pita bread, bagels, etc.

WHOLE GRAINS

Whole grains, including but not limited to wheat, barley, rye, oats, spelt, corn, rice, quinoa, millet, bulgur wheat, buckwheat, and amaranth.

PACKAGED SNACKS

Breakfast bars, granola bars, toaster pastries, snack bars, protein bars, prepackaged protein shakes, crackers, cookies, pretzels, chips, baked goods, snack pack items, etc.

DAIRY PRODUCTS

Eliminate processed and pasteurized milk, cheese, yogurt, cottage cheese, ice cream, frozen yogurt, etc. (See the Guide to: Food Quality on page 31 for information on dairy quality.) Raw dairy is a gray area.

CERTAIN BEVERAGES

Do not drink anything sweetened, especially with artificial sweeteners. This includes soda, diet soda, energy drinks, juice, sweetened teas, presweetened coffee drinks, shakes, or smoothies. Minimize your caffeine intake from coffee and tea. Avoid alcohol, especially gluten-containing forms. (See the FAQs on pages 119-120 for caffeine and alcohol recommendations).

SWEETENERS

These should only be used in small amounts, and manufactured foods with added sweeteners should be avoided. Refer to the Guide To: Sweeteners for the best and worst options on page 111.

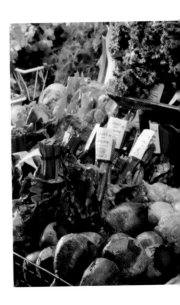

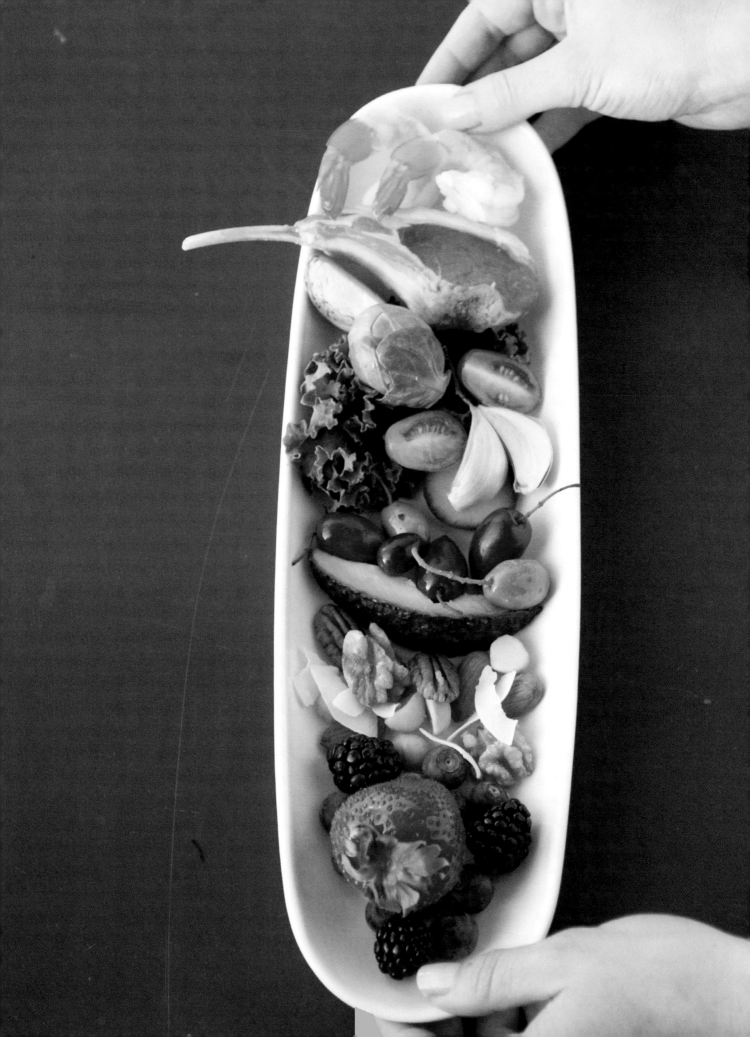

guide to: paleo foods

Eat whole foods. Avoid foods that are modern, processed, and refined. Eat as close to nature as possible, and avoid foods that cause stress for the body (blood sugar, digestion, etc.). Eat nutrient-dense foods to maintain energy levels. Enjoy your food, and hold positive thoughts while you consume it.

meat, seafood & eggs

INCLUDING BUT NOT LIMITED TO:

- Beef
- Bison
- Boar
- Buffalo
- Chicken
- Duck
- Eggs
- Game meats
- Goat
- Goose
- Lamb
- Mutton
- Ostrich
- Pork
- Quail
- Rabbit
- Squab
- Turkey
- Veal
- Venison
- Catfish
- Carp
- Clams
- Grouper
- Halibut
- Herring
- Lobster
- Mackerel
- Mahi mahi
- Mussels
- Oysters
- Salmon
- Sardines
- Scallops
- Shrimp
- Prawns
- Snails
- Snapper
- Sword-fish
- Trout
- Tuna

fats & oils

- Avocado oil
- Bacon fat/lard
- Butter
- Coconut milk
- Coconut oil
- Duck fat
- Ghee
- Macadamia oil
- Olive oil: CP
- Palm oil
- Schmaltz
- Sesame oil: CP
- Suet
- Tallow
- Walnut oil

nuts & seeds

- Almonds
- Brazil nuts
- Chestnuts
- Hazelnuts
- Macadamia
- Pecans
- Pine nuts
- Pistachios*
- Pumpkin seeds
- Sesame seeds
- Sunflower seeds
- Walnuts

liquids

- Almond Milk, fresh
- Coconut Milk
- Coconut water
- Herbal tea
- Mineral water
- Water

superfoods

GRASS-FED DAIRY:
- butter, ghee,

ORGAN MEATS:
- Liver, kidneys, heart, etc.

SEA VEGETABLES:
- Dulse, kelp, seaweed
- Herbs & spices

BONE BROTH:
- Homemade, not canned or boxed

FERMENTED FOODS:
- *Sauerkraut*, carrots, beets, high-quality yogurt, kefir, kombucha

NOTES
CP = cold-pressed
Bold = nightshades
Italics = goitrogenic

* = FODMAPs (p. 115)
^ = buy organic

vegetables

INCLUDING BUT NOT LIMITED TO:

- Artichokes*
- Asparagus*
- Arugula
- Bamboo shoots
- Beets*
- *Bok choy*
- *Broccoli*
- *Brussels sprouts*
- *Cabbage*
- Carrots
- Cassava
- *Cauliflower*
- Celery^
- Chard
- *Collard greens^*
- Cucumbers
- Daikon
- Dandelion greens*
- **Eggplant***
- Endive
- Fennel*
- Garlic*
- Green beans
- Green onions*
- Jicama*
- *Kale^*
- *Kohlrabi*
- Leeks*
- Lettuce^
- Lotus roots
- Mushrooms*
- Mustard greens*
- Okra*
- Onions*
- Parsley
- Parsnips
- **Peppers***^
- Purslane
- Radicchio
- *Radishes*
- *Rapini*
- Rutabagas
- Seaweed
- Shallots*
- Snap peas
- *Spinach^*
- Squash
- Sugar snaps
- Sunchokes*
- *Sweet potatoes*
- Taro
- **Tomatillos**
- **Tomatoes**
- Turnip greens
- Turnips
- *Watercress*
- Yams
- Yuccas

fruits

INCLUDING BUT NOT LIMITED TO

- Apples*^
- Apricots*
- Avocados*
- Bananas
- Blackberries*
- Blueberries^
- Cherries*
- Cranberries
- Figs*
- Grapefruit
- Grapes^
- Guavas
- Kiwis
- Lemons
- Limes
- Lychees*
- Mangoes*
- Melons
- Nectarines*^
- Oranges
- Papayas
- Passionfruit
- *Peaches*^
- *Pears*
- Persimmons*
- Pineapples
- Plantains
- Plums*
- Pome-granates
- Raspberries
- Rhubarb
- Star fruit
- *Strawberries^*
- Tangerines
- Watermelon*

herbs & spices

INCLUDING BUT NOT LIMITED TO

- Anise
- Annatto
- Basil
- Bay leaf
- Caraway
- Cardamom
- Carob
- **Cayenne pepper**
- Celery seed
- Chervil
- Chicory*
- **Chili pepper**
- **Chipotle powder**
- Chives
- Cilantro
- Cinnamon
- Clove
- Coriander
- Cumin
- Curry
- Dill
- Fennel*
- Fenugreek
- Galangal
- Garlic
- Ginger
- Horseradish*
- Juniper berry
- Kaffir lime leaves
- Lavender
- Lemongrass
- Lemon verbena
- Licorice
- Mace
- Marjoram
- Mint
- Mustard
- Oregano
- **Paprika**
- Parsley
- Pepper, black
- Peppermint
- Rosemary
- Saffron
- Spearmint
- Star anise
- Tarragon
- Thyme
- Turmeric
- Vanilla
- *Wasabi*
- Za'atar

The Why—Food & Your Body

29

guide to: stocking a paleo pantry

Fresh is best. Shopping the perimeter of the grocery store is ideal for the bulk of your foods, but you will want to add spices and some pantry items to your arsenal to cook up some tasty dishes and have some stand-by foods on-hand. Some of these foods are sold in cold sections of the store and need to be kept cold despite being packaged items.

herbs & spices

SOME HERBS CAN BE FOUND IN BOTH FRESH AND DRIED FORMS. INCLUDING BUT NOT LIMITED TO

- Anise
- Annatto
- Basil
- Bay leaf
- Caraway
- Cardamom
- **Cayenne**
- Celery seed
- Chervil
- Chicory*
- **Chili powder**
- **Chipotle**
- Chives
- Cilantro
- Cinnamon
- Clove
- Coriander
- Cumin
- Curry
- Dill
- Fennel
- Fenugreek
- Galangal
- Garlic
- Ginger
- *Horseradish*
- Juniper berry
- Kaffir lime leaves
- Lavender
- Lemongrass
- Lemon verbena
- Licorice
- Mace
- Marjoram
- Mint
- *Mustard*
- Nutmeg
- Onion powder*
- Oregano
- **Paprika**
- Parsley
- Pepper, black
- Peppercorns, whole black
- Peppermint
- Pumpkin pie spice
- Rosemary
- Saffron
- Sage
- Sea salt
- Spearmint
- Star anise
- Tarragon
- Thyme
- Turmeric
- Vanilla
- *Wasabi*
- Za'atar

canned & jarred

INCLUDING BUT NOT LIMITED TO

- Anchovy paste
- Applesauce*
- Capers
- Coconut milk*
- Coconut water/ Juice*
- Fish roe
- Herring - wild
- Olives
- Oysters
- Pickles
- Pumpkin
- Salmon - wild
- Sardines - wild
- **Sun-dried tomatoes**
- *Sweet potato*
- Tahini
- **Tomato paste**
- **Tomato sauce**
- Tuna - wild

nuts, seeds & dried fruit

- Almonds
- Almond butter
- Almond flour
- Banana chips (check ingredients)
- Brazil nuts
- Chestnuts
- Coconut butter*
- Coconut*: shredded, flakes
- Dates
- Dried apples*
- Dried apricots*
- Dried blueberries
- Dried cranberries
- Dried currants
- Dried figs*
- Dried mango*
- Dried pineapple
- Dried raspberries
- Hazelnuts
- Macadamia nuts
- Pecans
- Pine nuts
- Pistachios*
- Pumpkin seeds
- Sesame seeds
- Sunflower seeds
- Walnuts

add your own!

MAYBE YOU HAVE FAVORITE ITEMS NOT LISTED ABOVE THAT YOU KNOW ARE PALEO-FRIENDLY; WRITE THEM IN TO USE THIS AS A SHOPPING LIST

fats & oils

SEE THE FATS & OILS GUIDE FOR DETAILS

- Avocado oil: CP
- Bacon fat
- Ghee
- Coconut oil
- Macadamia oil: CP
- Extra-virgin olive oil
- Palm oil
- Palm shortening
- Sesame oil: CP
- Walnut oil: CP

sauces

- Coconut aminos* (soy-replacement)
- Fish sauce (Red Boat brand)
- **Hot sauce (gluten-free)**
- *Mustard (gluten-free)*
- Vinegars: apple cider*, red wine, distilled, rice and balsamic (avoid malt vinegar)

beverages

- Green tea
- Herbal tea
- Mineral water
- White tea
- Organic coffee

treats & sweets

FOR OCCASIONAL USE

- Carob powder
- Cocoa powder
- Honey
- Maple syrup
- Molasses
- Dark chocolate

NOTES
CP = cold-pressed
bold = nightshades
italics = goitrogenic
* = FODMAPs (p.115)

Buy as many of your pantry items as possible in organic form.

guide to: food quality

Seek out as much real, whole food as possible. This includes foods without health claims on the packages or, better yet, not in packages at all. Think produce and butcher counter meats and seafood. After you've mastered making proper food choices, it's important to begin looking at the quality of the items. While buying the best quality is ideal in a perfect world, don't let those "best" labels keep you from doing the best you can within your means.

meat, eggs & dairy

beef & lamb
Best! 100% grass-fed and finished, pasture-raised, local
Better: grass-fed, pasture-raised
Good: organic
Baseline: commercial (hormone/antibiotic-free)

pork
Best! pasture-raised, local
Better: free-range, organic
Good: organic
Baseline: commercial

eggs & poultry
Best! pasture-raised, local
Better: free range, organic
Good: cage-free, organic
Baseline: commercial

dairy
ALWAYS BUY FULL-FAT
Best! grass-fed, raw/unpasteurized
Better: raw/unpasteurized
Good: grass-fed
Baseline: commercial or organic —*not recommended*

seafood

Best! wild fish
Better: wild-caught
Good: humanely harvested, non-grain-fed
Baseline: farm-raised—*not recommended*

WILD FISH/ WILD-CAUGHT FISH
"Wild fish" indicates that the fish was spawned, lived in, and was caught in the wild. "Wild-caught fish" may have been spawned or lived some part of their lives in a fish farm before being returned to the wild and eventually caught. The Monterey Bay Aquarium maintains a free list of the most sustainable seafood choices on their website.

WHAT THE LABELS ON MEAT, EGGS & DAIRY MEAN

pasture-raised
Animals can roam freely in their natural environment where they are able to eat nutritious grasses and other plants or bugs/grubs that are part of their natural diet. There is no specific pasture-raised certification, though certified organic meat must come from animals that have continuous access to pasture regardless of use.

cage-free
"Cage-Free" means uncaged inside barns or warehouses, but they generally do not have access to the outdoors. Beak cutting is permitted. There is no third party auditing.

organic
Animals may not receive hormones/antibiotics unless in the case of illness. They consume organic feed and have outdoor access but may not use it. Animals are not necessarily grass-fed. Certification is costly and some reputable farms are forced to forego it. Compliance is verified through third party auditing.

natural
"Natural" means "minimally processed," and companies use this word deceivingly. All cuts are, by definition, minimally processed and free of flavorings and chemicals.

free-range/roaming
Poultry must have access to the outdoors at least 51% of the time, and ruminants may not be in feedlots. There are no restrictions regarding what the birds can be fed. Beak cutting and forced molting through starvation are permitted. There is no third party auditing.

naturally raised
"Naturally Raised," is a USDA verified term. It generally means raised without growth-promoters or unnecessary antibiotics. It does not indicate welfare or diet.

no added hormones
It is illegal to use hormones in raising poultry or pork; therefore, the use of this phrase on poultry or pork is a marketing ploy.

vegetarian-fed
"Vegetarian Fed" implies that the animal feed is free of animal by-products but isn't federally inspected. Chickens are not vegetarians, so this label on chicken or eggs only serves to indicate that the chickens were not eating their natural diet.

produce

Best! local, organic, and seasonal
Better: local and organic
Good: organic or local
Baseline: conventional

WHEN TO BUY ORGANIC:
Buy organic as often as possible, prioritize buying the Environmental Working Group's "The Dirty Dozen" as organic versus "The Clean Thirteen" - visit: www.ewg.org for details

PRODUCE SKUs:
Starts with 9 = organic - ideal
Starts with 3 or 4 = conventionally grown
Starts with 8 = genetically modified (GMO) or irradiated - avoid

fats & oils

SEE THE FATS & OILS GUIDE FOR DETAILS.
Best! organic, cold-pressed, and from well-raised animal sources
Better: organic, cold-pressed
Good: organic or conventional

nuts & seeds

KEEP NUTS & SEEDS COLD FOR FRESHNESS
Best! local, organic, kept cold
Better: local, organic
Good: organic
Baseline: conventional

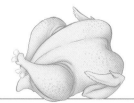

---

sources: www.humanesociety.org, www.ewg.org, www.sustainabletable.org

everything we've been taught about good nutrition is wrong

We live in a time when up is down and black is white. We have been taught to believe that the foods coming out of factories are safer and healthier than foods your great-grandmother ate.

✓ **Eat whole foods and avoid modern, processed, and refined foods.**

☐ Eat to maintain proper digestive function.

☐ Eat to maintain proper blood sugar regulation.

☐ Follow a plan that will help you reach your own personal health goals.

Think about it a minute. If "Food A" has gone through a factory and been processed from what it once was in nature into something else entirely, and "Food B" is identical to what it was in nature (with the exception of having been hunted, gathered, cooked, or some modern variation thereof), which food is healthier? It's a no-brainer, isn't it?

More "foods" are out there today touting health claims, yet we're less healthy with each passing generation. It just doesn't add up. Obesity is on the rise in children, who also frequently suffer from behavioral disorders, early-onset puberty, and autoimmune conditions diagnosed at younger and younger ages.

Unfortunately, the broad, sweeping claims about health and nutrition that we hear from so-called authorities originate from interests that have their hands deep in our pockets and are often not concerned with keeping us healthy.

Did you know that doctors are typically given less than a week of training in nutritional biochemistry? Yet people who are suffering as a result of long-term poor diet and lifestyle choices end up in their offices on a daily basis. Most dietitians are unable to help because they have been taught to promote and support the USDA recommendations, which have led us down a path of declining health for more than three decades.

The guidelines set forth by the USDA are not based on sound scientific theories or conclusive proof. They are based on illogical and potentially dangerous hypotheses and claims that simply don't hold water. So we're left to take dietary advice from the media, which inundate us with contradictions. We're barraged by recommendations that don't help, while people remain sick.

Know this:
We are not smarter than nature.
We cannot make better food than nature.
We need to eat real, whole food—period.

A responsible individual won't trust the status quo, the media, the government, or even a well-intentioned, but likely ill-informed, health care professional for information on how to achieve health. We must self-educate, never accept conventional wisdom at face value, and seek thorough information that we find sensible, helpful, and intuitive. Heck, if what I recommend in this book doesn't make sense to you based on your intuition and how it feels when you actually *follow* my advice, then try something else. Insanity is doing the same thing over and over again while expecting different results each time. Let's try to break this cycle. In order to do so, let me remind you what you've been fed.

what the government is feeding you

Let's look at how the United States government tells us to eat by way of its nutritional recommendations (known for many years as the USDA Food Guide Pyramid, before being re-branded as MyPlate and reprocessed every five years through Dietary Guidelines for Americans, a USDA-FDA joint venture.)

According to the most recent Dietary Guidelines for Americans:
"Individuals should meet the following recommendations as part of a healthy eating pattern while staying within their calorie needs:
- Increase vegetable and fruit intake.
- Eat a variety of vegetables, especially dark green and red and orange vegetables and beans and peas.
- Consume at least half of all grains as whole grains. Increase whole grain intake by replacing refined grains with whole grains.
- Increase intake of fat-free or low-fat milk and milk products, such as milk, yogurt, cheese, or fortified soy beverages.
- Choose a variety of protein foods, which include seafood, lean meat and poultry, eggs, beans and peas, soy products, and unsalted nuts and seeds.
- Increase the amount and variety of seafood consumed by choosing seafood in place of some meat and poultry.
- Replace protein foods that are higher in solid fats with choices that are lower in solid fats and calories and/or are sources of oils.
- Use oils to replace solid fats where possible.
- Choose foods that provide more potassium, dietary fiber, calcium, and vitamin D, which are nutrients of concern in American diets. These foods include vegetables, fruits, whole grains, and milk and milk products."*

*source: Dietary Guidelines for Americans 2010, www. dietaryguidelines.gov

At first-glance, it seems the USDA is trying to get people to eat more "real food," right? Not so fast! While a handful of their recommendations are intuitive—increasing vegetable intake, eating a variety of vegetables and protein foods, and increasing seafood consumption—four out of their nine overarching recommendations are extremely flawed from the standpoint of nutritional biochemistry and health. And, unfortunately, these are the biggest

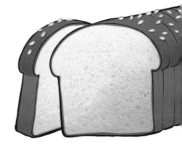

points of contention when trying to get people to open their minds up to a new possibility—that what we "think" we know about nutrition is wrong.

Let's take a closer look at these four questionable USDA recommendations.

what we've been fed: recommendation #1

This recommendation states: "Consume at least half of all grains as whole grains. Increase whole grain intake by replacing refined grains with whole grains." When people replace their "refined" grains with "whole" grains, how do you think this translates on their plates? Do you think it means they begin eating bulgur wheat and wheat berries instead of white bread, cereal, and pasta? (Not that I regard either bulgur or wheat berries as healthy, but they are more "whole" than standard supermarket fare.) No, it simply means that people will read packages of bread, cereal, and pasta for those shiny, happy words, "whole grain." They'll buy the same brands, albeit with different lettering. Nobody in the food production industry will lose money, and nothing on the business end will change. Only now you think that the bread you're buying is healthy, and you can't wait to tell your doctor/neighbor/friend that you've switched to whole grain bread.

Anything that has been popped, puffed, flaked, floured, shredded, or made into an instant form has been refined.* This includes gluten-free rolls, gluten-free oats, whole/sprouted grain breads, quinoa pasta, puffed cereals, and corn chips, to name a few. They are no longer in their natural state, no matter how "whole" the grains may have started out before the factory got hold of them.

Know this: Whole grain products are still refined foods.

The refinement process of whole grains simply includes more parts of the grain than are found in white bread, standard cereal, or pasta. Refined foods will never promote health more than whole foods, not even if the word "whole" is tacked onto them.

*source: Radhia Gleis, "popped, puffed ..."

**Dietary Guidelines for Americans 2010, www. dietaryguidelines.gov

Consumption of grains, specifically—even so-called "whole grains"—causes a host of problems for many people and we'll discuss the why and hows in great detail when we look at digestive function in the next section. For now, it is worthy to note that the basis for the USDA recommendation to eat "whole grains" is supported by what is termed "Moderate Evidence," which the USDA defines as a level of evidence that "... reflects somewhat less evidence or less consistent evidence. The body of evidence may include studies of weaker design and/or some inconsistency in results. The studies may be susceptible to some bias, but not enough to invalidate the results, or the body of evidence may not be as generalizable to the population of interest."**

In other words, the science on which they base their claims is not entirely sound nor can it be trusted. And they know it.

do umbrellas make it rain?

As we see repeatedly in nutritional research, most of the studies cited are epidemiological, which means they are based solely on the study of patterns and correlative information in populations. Discovering correlations does not provide evidence of any causation. It simply means that two factors seemed to be related, but it doesn't take into account every other possible variable involved. For example, you'd never say that the presence of the umbrellas you see people carrying outside on a rainy day *caused* the rain to fall, would you? These nutritional studies are not randomized controlled trials in metabolic wards (where food given to test subjects is carefully measured and recorded), which can be used to discover direct cause and effect. The latter would be the appropriate way to scientifically prove a basis for nutritional advice. When diet records are reported by the subjects in these epidemiological studies, they're based on what are known as "dietary recalls" that often date as far back as several years.

Let's get real! Do you remember what you ate last year? Last month? Last week? Even yesterday? Obviously, these claims are far from science.

When you see broad nutritional recommendations without actual biological explanations, you can assume they're derived from evidence reported in an epidemiological study using dietary recall as the source. Run the other way.

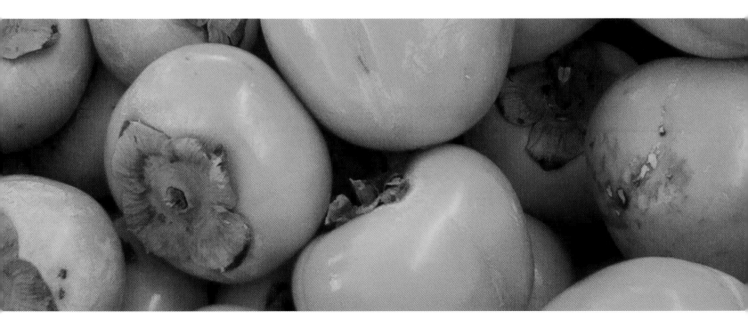

what about calcium on a paleo diet?

Fact #1: Calcium is abundantly present in more than just dairy foods. Did you know that bone broth, sardines, sesame seeds, and dark green leafy vegetables are sources of calcium? What's more, these whole, unprocessed foods are also fantastic sources of magnesium, a mineral required in order to help to assimilate calcium in your body. Boom. Right there you have a great way of getting calcium and magnesium into your diet.

Fact #2: To absorb and utilize calcium appropriately, we need to eat more than just the calcium. Simply consuming calcium as a mineral, whether it's from dairy or other food sources isn't enough to make stronger bones! We also need fat-soluble vitamins A, D, and K2 to help direct the show. At this time, vitamin K2 is emerging in research more and more for its value in orchestrating the placement of calcium in our bodies into our bones—where we want it—and not into our soft tissues. In other words: it's not just how much calcium you eat, but how much you absorb, and where it goes when you absorb it. If you want to build strong bone matrix with the calcium you're eating, be sure you're also eating foods rich in vitamin K2—primarily fermented cod liver oil or fermented grass-fed dairy (think

what we've been fed: recommendation #2

This one states: "Increase intake of fat-free or low-fat milk and milk products, such as milk, yogurt, cheese, or fortified soy beverages."

This could mean pasteurized, processed milk and dairy products from cows raised in circumstances like concentrated animal feeding operations (CAFOs) or an even more highly processed milk substitute made from legumes (soy). You will be hard pressed to find a raw, grass-fed milk producer selling low-fat or fat-free cows' milk. Why? Because vitamins A, D, and K2 are found in that nutritious, straight-from-the-farm beverage. Skimming and processing would be a waste of beautiful nutrients.

All of the products listed by the USDA are "fortified," which means that nutrients have been added to them. Why does this happen? To prevent nutrient deficiencies across populations—deficiencies that began to appear in the Western world when processed foods were introduced. As soon as we started pasteurizing, homogenizing, and stripping the fat from a formerly health-promoting food (raw/unpasteurized milk from grass-fed/pasture-raised cows), we destroyed and removed the naturally occurring vitamins—largely vitamins A and D—from the milk. We need these fat-soluble vitamins for proper growth,

REAL MILK INFO
Visit realmilk.com to find out where you can access raw milk.

kefir or 24-hour-fermented yogurt). Vitamin K2 will likely be indiscernible in pasteurized, grain-fed commercial (even organic) milk.

Fact #3: Grain consumption can actually inhibit calcium absorption. As you'll learn a bit later in this book, grain products all contain anti-nutrients called phytates. What phytates do is bind to minerals we are eating and keep them from being absorbed by our bodies. So, when people sit down to a bowl of cereal with milk, they're actually eating a food that blocks the absorption of any calcium in their meal right in the same meal!

Fact #4: Not all dairy is created equal. The dairy nature produces isn't the problem. The primary problem is that we think we have to process dairy to be "healthier" for us to consume, and we muck it all up! If you can find a great source of raw, grass-fed milk or other dairy products from a local producer and you feel good eating it, I say go right on ahead. Much of the research that is compiled on the problems with dairy are from studies examining either isolated dairy proteins like casein or whey, not the whole food wherein whey and casein come packaged together, or processed and reduced-fat forms of dairy foods.

strong immune systems, and the integrity of our bones (often referred to as bone density). It isn't just about how much calcium you consume.

Without vitamins A, D, and K2, in fact, your body doesn't have its "marching orders" for how to use the calcium you have ingested. Although most people ingest extra calcium from low-fat dairy products or supplements in the hope of building bone strength, they aren't getting enough of these vitamins for the calcium to be assimilated. In response to the problems of nutrient deficiency, the government mandated that vitamins be added back to milk after the natural nutrients are destroyed in processing, but this "fortification" adds synthetic (man-made) nutrients.

Yet, the USDA recommends that we eat fat-free or low-fat milk and milk products. Why? Do they mean that milk straight from the cow isn't recommended, and milk that has been processed and had its most traditionally valued constituents removed is actually healthier? Perhaps in addition to forgetting how real, nutritious milk should be produced and consumed, they have also misinterpreted epidemiological data yet again. Is the government smarter than Mother Nature?

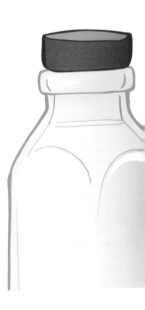

Know this: Real milk is raw (unpasteurized), comes from grass-fed/pasture-raised cows, and is not low-fat or fat-free.

If you are lactose-intolerant, you may be able to drink raw milk without a problem, as the lactase enzyme necessary for digestion of lactose is still present in raw milk. Real milk is a good dietary source of protein, fat, carbohydrates, calcium, and fat-soluble vitamins A, D and K2, all of which are important for bone density. If you find that you tolerate dairy well without sinus congestion, sneezing, digestive upset, or signs of chronic inflammation (see page 74), find a trustworthy source and enjoy your milk in its whole, full-fat, natural state.

If you don't tolerate dairy products well (after trying real milk/dairy as outlined above), you may still be well-served by the incorporation of grass-fed butter, which contains fewer of the commonly irritating dairy proteins. You could also use ghee, which is a product that contains virtually no dairy proteins (learn how to make it quite simply at home on page 236), or a butter-oil supplement (I recommend the Green Pasture brand), which has the lowest potential for containing any remaining traces of dairy proteins. Typically, an allergic or inflammatory response to dairy does not occur with pure butter-oil since the milk protein constituents such as casein and whey or sugars, like lactose, are the underlying problem. (See page 31 for more information about choosing dairy products responsibly.)

THE SKINNY ON FAT
Check out the Guide to:
Fats & Oils on page 44 for
more information.

what we've been fed: recommendations #3 & 4

These suggest that we: "Replace protein foods that are higher in solid fats with choices that are lower in solid fats and calories and/or are sources of oils."
And...
"Use oils to replace solid fats where possible."

These recommendations are based on the notion that cholesterol in the bloodstream is the *cause* of heart disease, and that by avoiding both dietary cholesterol and saturated fat that we can avoid heart disease. The problem is that these claims have never been supported by scientific literature. It should be noted that dietary cholesterol has only ever been shown to raise serum or blood levels of cholesterol by less than 1%. Additionally, naturally occurring saturated fat *can* raise both "good" (HDL) and "bad" (LDL) cholesterol, but this is not cause for alarm. Eating foods that support cholesterol production serves to support your body and gives it a break from having to manufacture cholesterol on its own.

Much of the research done on cholesterol metabolism was performed on rabbits, whose natural diet does not include cholesterol-containing foods! How would we expect human cholesterol metabolism to mimic that of a rabbit that isn't supposed to eat cholesterol in the first place?

Know this: The science has never existed to support the claims that have been made to demonize dietary cholesterol and saturated fat. The USDA is wrong, and their recommendations have made the refined seed oil industry lots of money while you've run scared from eggs, bacon, and butter.

The first report on Dietary Guidelines for Americans was created in the late 1970s, nearly twenty years after initial claims were made that dietary fat and cholesterol were harmful to our health. While these hypotheses were pushed as truth even as early as the 1950s in an effort to sell more factory-made vegetable oil products versus naturally occurring animal fats, it wasn't until more recently that we were inundated with fear-based information about the fat in real, whole foods. The corporate 'Food Giants' were presented with a way to replace animal fats and previously used tropical oils like coconut and palm with less expensive vegetable oils that were "partially hydrogenated." As we know now, these words indicate the presence of manmade trans fats. By 1978, an even more exciting development arose: The amount of fat used in many processed products could be *reduced* while still preserving flavor and palatability through the use of, you guessed it: high fructose corn syrup! Oh boy.

A *Time Magazine* article in 1984 entitled "Hold the Eggs and Butter" is among the most impactful propaganda that molded the modern food landscape that we know today. The article claimed that "Cholesterol is proved deadly, and our diet may never be the same."* Then, it went on to say: "For decades, researchers have been trying to prove conclusively that cholesterol is a major villain in this epidemic [of heart disease]. It has not been easy. Cholesterol is, after all, only one piece in a large puzzle that also includes obesity, high blood pressure, smoking, stress and lack of exercise. All of these play their part in heart disease 'like members of an orchestra,' explains Pathologist Richard Minick of the New York Hospital-Cornell Medical Center.... Despite its bad reputation, cholesterol is essential to life: it is a building block of the outer membrane of cells, and it is a principal ingredient in the digestive juice bile, in the fatty sheath that insulates nerves, and in sex hormones such as estrogen and androgen."*

Even within the article itself, the information contradicts the title and main claim. Unfortunately, more than the details, people remember headlines and cover images like the one used with the article—a sad looking plate of eggs and bacon arranged to form a frowning face. The biology and the science, or lack thereof, became secondary to the striking image, and the article created a massive fear of dietary fat (especially saturated fat) and cholesterol, claiming that heart disease risk was drastically increased when blood levels of cholesterol were high.

There is just one problem. According to Dr. Mike Eades, "... only about half the people who have heart attacks have elevated cholesterol levels."** Even

sources:
*Wallis, Caludia, et al. "Hold The Eggs and Bacon." TIME Magazine, March 26, 1984.

**Eades, Michael, MD. "You Bet Your Life: An Epilogue to the Cholesterol Story." www.proteinpower.com, October 11, 2010

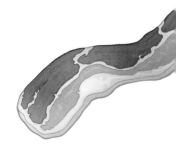

The Why—Food & Your Body   39

more contradictory information within the *Time* article states that: "The experts were still not quite able to pin the blame on cholesterol, however. Explains Fred Mattson, a leading researcher at the University of California at San Diego, 'We were missing a key piece of evidence: No one had ever shown that reducing the level of cholesterol in the blood did any good."

The entire country, for better or worse and in the wake of conflicting ideas, was thereafter encouraged to stop eating natural foods like butter, cream, egg yolks, and fatty meats—all based on science that didn't exist. And we bought it hook, line, and sinker. Egg substitutes appeared on the market (hardly whole foods), and eggs were made out to be bad for us, even though they are rich in essential nutrients, including choline, selenium, vitamin B2, and vitamin B12.

The boom of low-fat and fat-free profit-earning products began to snowball. Fat-free cookies, "light" yogurts loaded with sweeteners, fat-free puddings, and low-fat "buttery spreads" hit their stride, filling our cupboards and refrigerators and crowding out the natural foods that could be made from scratch in every kitchen in America.

We fell prey to the motivators of convenience, taste, and marketing without realizing it, and, as a nation, our waistlines and internal, biochemical, state-of-human-affairs became unbalanced.

Know this: Manmade trans fats and refined seed/vegetable oils (canola, soybean, and corn oil, to name a few) are not healthful and may even be considered food toxins.

IN FRAMINGHAM:
According to the Framingham Study, "the more saturated fat one ate, the more cholesterol one ate, the more calories one ate, the lower the person's serum cholesterol. We found that the people who ate the most cholesterol, ate the most saturated fat, and ate the most calories, weighed the least and were the most active."

source: "Cholesterol and Mortality: 30 Years of Follow-up From the Framingham Study." Journal of the AMA, April 1987. Vol 257, No 16

We know manmade trans fats are dangerous, but why must natural saturated fats like those in egg yolks, well-raised meats, coconut oil, and grass-fed dairy products take equal blame when their chemical structure and origin are entirely different? People all too often jump to the assumption that the naturally occurring forms of saturated fats are also harmful—quite possibly due to media reporting on the topic that continues to promote these notions. The reality is that the chemical structure of a short or medium chain "saturated" fat—from butter or coconut oil, for example—is actually easier for your body to break down and digest. Why? Because they place a lesser demand on bile salts, which the body uses to break down or "emulsify" and utilize fats.

we cannot improve what nature provides

Refining foods to "improve" them is oxymoronic at worst and nonsensical at best. We can only hope the government will step aside and allow greater quality of thought to prevail in the field of public health. If you're curious as to how governmental entities come to consensus on dietary guidelines, Marion Nestle's book, *Food Politics*, is an interesting resource. Though Nestle's overall dietary recommendations are, in my opinion, lacking, she is certainly respected as an authority on the complexities of how politics affect food policy in the United States and what's on your plate every day.

Regarding changes that were made to the Dietary Guidelines over the years, Nestle states that: "In an effort to achieve consensus on these innovations, the USDA invited leading nutrition authorities in government, research, the food industry, and agricultural commodity groups to review preliminary drafts because it 'felt that the food industry groups would have a vital interest in any food guide sponsored by the government.'" Indeed they did.

Of course, the "food industry" and "agricultural commodity groups" will be interested in the content of population-wide nutrition guidelines! It is their bottom line that takes a hit when a major government report indicates that their products are undesirable, or worse, pose a major public health risk.

Changes must be made, though, each time the guidelines are revisited, and as the food guide has shifted and changed (and certain food groups reduced to lower recommended quantities). Nestle says: "... the AMA (American Medical Association) noted that 'the recommendations carry with them the underlying potential for...discouraging the agricultural production of certain food products which may not in the view of the government be supportive of the dietary goals.... although opposition to the Dietary Goals often was expressed as skepticism about the quality of the underlying science, it derived more directly from the profound economic implications of the advice."*

Opposition to the "pyramid," "food guide," and "Dietary Goals" (one and the same, for our purposes) was *not* necessarily based on science or uplifting public health but on the economic implications of the advice.

The more you follow the USDA's recommendations, however, the more processed foods you'll have to buy. You can't possibly eat all of those servings of grains and low-fat dairy without eating breakfast cereal, low-fat milk, or low-fat yogurt, can you? In adhering to those suggestions, many large corporations make lots of money from your dietary "choices," and they don't have to spend much to produce the stuff. In fact, many USDA-compliant items are made with lowest common denominator commodities, such as corn, wheat, and soy. Sometimes, you're the one eating these commodities, while the dairy cow eats them the rest of the time. Either way, you're the end user.

Yes, this includes that innocent-looking light yogurt with the alluring ads describing fantastically indulgent flavors that include high fructose corn syrup in their ingredients. (I should know because I used to down those puppies like crazy.)

No wonder everyone is confused about what to eat, but don't worry. After you finish this book, your confusion will be gone and you'll have the tools you need at your fingertips to navigate the modern food landscape quite easily.

*source: Nestle, Marion. "Food Politics: how the food industry influences nutrition and health." Berkeley, CA. University of California Press. 2007.

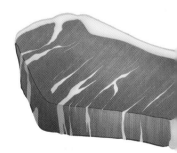

paleo at home: shopping for groceries

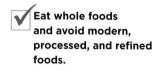

Eat whole foods and avoid modern, processed, and refined foods.

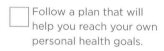

Eat to maintain proper digestive function.

Eat to maintain proper blood sugar regulation.

Follow a plan that will help you reach your own personal health goals.

Eating with a Paleo approach can seem daunting when you realize that you are no longer going to rely on the cheap, filler ingredients you may have been eating non-stop for decades.

No more rice and beans. No more bread, pasta, or cereal. These are all cheap foods, and rightfully so since they provide little nutritional value when you compare them to vegetables, meats, fruits, nuts, seeds, and quality fats and oils.

While much of the store is filled with items you could—and likely used to—buy, your mission now will be entirely different. Seek out as much whole food as possible. This means foods without health claims on the packages or, better yet, not even *in* packages. Instead, buy produce, butcher-counter meats, and seafood.

at the grocery store: walk the perimeter

If you are currently eating foods primarily from the center aisles of the grocery store, you are most likely purchasing refined, processed food. Instead, I suggest shopping the perimeter of the store. This is where you'll find produce, meat, seafood, and eggs. (It's also where you'll find the bakery, but avoid the bakery!) The outside sections of the store are where you'll find most fresh foods because it's where the store can easily supply power to the displays to keep food cool, damp, and unspoiled. Real food does not have a long shelf life and should spoil within a couple of weeks at most (except for frozen vegetables or meats).

Round out your grocery trip by cruising down just a few of the inner aisles. These can be useful for stocking up on items like cooking fats and oils, vinegars, mustards, "clean" sauces, spices, and selected canned or jarred items.

read before you eat

LABEL CRAZED?
Check out the Guide to: Food Quality on page 31 for more information.

When you purchase from the inner sections, *read the labels carefully!* If you aren't accustomed to checking ingredients, you'll be surprised how many seemingly innocent items are loaded with hidden sweeteners, preservatives, and artificial fats.

Become a label detective. If you don't know an ingredient, i.e. if it has a scientific name, this is an item to put back on the shelf, not in your cart. There are some very common additives even in a few so-called healthy items. Look for any of the sweeteners listed in the guide on page 111 or any of the forms of hidden gluten on page 89. Use the Paleo Pantry Guide on page 30 to navigate the aisles of the store.

If there is more packaging than product, it's probably not a great choice, so move on. If the packaging is trying *hard* to sell the product to you, it is almost certainly not healthy. This means claims like "Fat-Free!" "Low-Fat!" "Heart Healthy!" and "Whole Grain!" Real foods have no such labels and often have little to no packaging.

Buying anything labeled low-fat, non-fat, or fat-free is ill advised. Most dairy products found in grocery stores are produced from feedlot cows and are not real, whole foods. Fruity yogurts or yogurt drinks, sliced, string, or plastic wrapped blocks of cheese, and milk that has been enriched or fortified with vitamins A and D, are not in their whole form from nature, so avoid them. For more on dairy and how to choose it, see the guide on page 31.

budget priority #1: fats and oils

Fats comprise the most calorie-dense source of nutrition in your diet, so buy the highest quality fats and oils available to you. Fatty acids incorporate into the "phospholipid bilayer," a two-ply layer of cells that help to form your cell membranes. While all macronutrients incorporate into your cell tissues and contribute to the formation of new cells, fatty acids that incorporate into your cells can take longer to change over during natural progression of cell regeneration. For this reason, it is best to avoid poor quality or oxidized oils (damaged by light, heat, and/or air). Since battling cellular damage is one of your body's full-time jobs, the more you can run damage control by avoiding poor quality or damaged oils, the better.

Prioritizing your budget toward the highest quality fats is a very important first step. This means never eating trans fats and avoiding highly processed vegetable oils and rancid oils. It also means only choosing high quality, fresh nuts and seeds. If the nuts or seeds you buy smell off or rancid, toss them and buy new ones. The "Fats and Oils Guide" later in this book will help you make intelligent choices.

There are only a handful of healthy fats and oils you will need to buy at the grocery store as outlined in the next pages for both hot (cooking) and cold (salads and finishing) uses.

Keep coconut oil and ghee in a cool, dark cupboard, and keep butter and bacon fat in the refrigerator. Do not refrigerate coconut oil, as it will become extremely hard and difficult to use without re-melting. If you are concerned about the ghee, you can keep it in the refrigerator, but it should be shelf-stable for quite some time since it is pure fat with no dairy proteins.

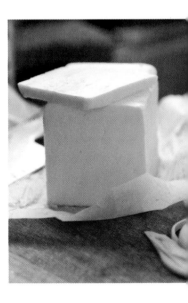

guide to: fats & oils

Cleaning up your diet by using the right fats and oils is essential to improving your health from the inside out. Changing the fats and oils you use at home is the first step toward creating dishes from nutrient-dense, whole foods based on what you have on hand. Avoid overly processed and refined forms of fats and oils. Opt for organic whenever possible. Refer to the "Guide to Cooking Fats" for more details.

eat these: HEALTHY, NATURALLY OCCURRING, MINIMALLY PROCESSED FATS

saturated: FOR HOT USES

BUY ORGANIC, UNREFINED FORMS

· Coconut oil
· Palm oil

IDEALLY FROM PASTURE-RAISED, GRASS-FED, ORGANIC SOURCES

· Butter
· Ghee, clarified butter
· Lard, bacon grease (pork fat)
· Tallow (beef fat)
· Duck fat
· Schmaltz (chicken fat)
· Lamb fat
· Full-fat dairy
· Eggs, meat, and seafood

unsaturated: FOR COLD USES

BUY ORGANIC, EXTRA-VIRGIN, AND COLD-PRESSED FORMS

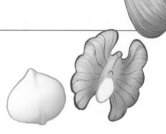

· Olive oil
· Sesame oil
· Macadamia nut oil
· Walnut oil
· Avocado oil
· Nuts & seeds (including nut & seed butters)
· Flaxseed oil**

NOTE: Unsaturated fats (typically liquid at 68 degrees room temperature) are easily damaged/oxidized when heat is applied to them. Do not consume damaged fats.

Cold-pressed flaxseed oil is okay for occasional use but supplementing with it or doses of 1-2 tablespoons per day is **not recommended as overall PUFA (polyunsaturated fatty acid) intake should remain minimal.

ditch these: UNHEALTHY, MAN-MADE FATS & REFINED SEED OILS ARE NOT RECOMMENDED

Hydrogenated or partially hydrogenated oils, as well as manmade trans-fats or "buttery spreads" like Earth Balance, Benecol, and I Can't Believe It's Not Butter are not healthy. These oils are highly processed and oxidize easily via one or more of the following: light, air, or heat.

· Margarine/buttery spreads
· Canola oil (also known as rapeseed oil)
· Corn oil
· Vegetable oil
· Soybean oil
· Grapeseed oil
· Sunflower oil
· Safflower oil
· Rice bran oil
· Shortening made from one or more of the above-listed "ditch" oils

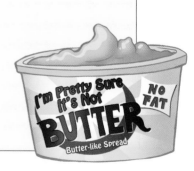

guide to: cooking fats

Choose fats and oils based on: 1. How they're made—choose naturally occurring, minimally processed options first; 2. Their fatty acid composition—the more saturated they are, the more stable/less likely to be damaged or oxidized; 3. Smoke point—this tells you how hot is too hot before you will damage the fats, though it should be considered a secondary factor to fatty acid profile.

culinary whizzes, listen up: COOK WITH GOOD FATS!

ITEM NAME	% SFA	%MUFA	% PUFA	SMOKE POINT UNREFINED/REFINED
best bets - recommended for high-heat cooking THE MOST STABLE FATS				
Coconut oil	86	6	2	350/450
Butter/ghee	63	26	.03	300/480
Cocoa butter	60	35	5	370
Tallow/suet (beef fat)	55	34	.03	400
Palm oil	54	42	.10	455
Lard/bacon fat (pork fat)	39	45	11	375
Duck fat	37	50	13	375
okay - for very low-heat cooking MODERATELY STABLE FATS				
Avocado oil*	20	70	10	520
Macadamia nut oil*	16	80	4	410
Olive oil*	14	73	11	375
Peanut oil**	17	46	32	320/450
Rice Bran Oil**	25	38	37	415
not recommended for cooking VERY UNSTABLE FATS				
Safflower oil**	8	76	13	225/510
Sesame seed oil*	14	40	46	450
Canola oil**	8	64	28	400
Sunflower oil**	10	45	40	225/440
Vegetable shortening**	34	11	52	330
Corn oil	15	30	55	445
Soybean oil	16	23	58	495
Walnut oil*	14	19	67	400
Grapeseed oil	12	17	71	420

SFA - saturated fatty acid   MUFA - monounsaturated fatty acid   PUFA - polyunsaturated fatty acid

* While not recommended for cooking, cold-pressed nut and seed oils that are stored in the refrigerator may be used to finish recipes or after cooking is completed—for flavor purposes.

** While the fatty acid profile of these oils may seem appropriate at first glance, the processing method by which they are made negates their healthfulness—they are not recommended for consumption, neither hot nor cold.

The Why—Food & Your Body

If dairy products are a problem for you, grass-fed ghee is the best choice since, again, the dairy proteins have been removed, leaving only the butter-oil behind.

Unsaturated oils like olive and cold-pressed sesame should preferably be stored in dark containers or bottles and kept in either cool, dark places or in the refrigerator.

budget priority #2: protein (meat/seafood/eggs)

Before going to the grocery store, it is best to be prepared with a list of the meats and seafood you want in order of priority. Understanding the levels of quality and the categories of environments in which animals have been raised, including what they have been fed, will help you choose the best quality. Watch for sales of these meats and seafood so that you can stock up. A small investment in an extra freezer will pay for itself in no time when you can buy meat in bulk at lower prices.

Of course, a better way to save on meat is to find a local farm from which you can purchase a whole animal or a portion of one. They are typically butchered to your order, and you may even be able to find someone else to share the meat with you if you don't want to buy an entire animal. Check out your local Weston A. Price Foundation chapter, CrossFit gym, Meetup.com group, or other communities centered around health and nutrition to find others looking for a "meat share."

Buy 100% grass-fed, pasture-raised meats whenever possible, and eat the cuts within your budget that appeal to you. Do not be concerned about the leanness of high quality meat. If your budget dictates lower quality meat, buy leaner cuts, as the fatty acid profile of conventional meats will hold a lower proportion of beneficial omega-3 fatty acids.

Meat from 100% pastured animals contains three to five times more CLA than products from animals fed conventional diets. CLA is an important antioxidant that has been shown in many studies to combat modern diseases like cancer, heart disease, and diabetes. People often take CLA supplements when they want to lose weight (fat), but eating it in whole foods is a better choice.

Just like humans, animals store toxins in their fat, so if you eat an animal that may have been exposed to poor quality/non-organic food, pesticides, herbicides, fungicides, antibiotics, and exogenous hormones (hormones from an outside source other than the animal's own production), most of the residue from those toxins will be in the animal's fat. Meat in the U.S. is graded based on "marbling," which refers to the amount of fat swirling through the meat. While that fat is tasty, and I welcome any amounts of it that end up in my grass-fed

EXTRA-VIRGIN

I highly recommend Kasandrinos Imports brand extra-virgin olive oil because it is 100% pure Greek olive oil without any additives or fillers, and it is pressed and bottled very quickly. Batches are imported and sold directly within the United States immediately, and it is the freshest, most delicious olive oil I have ever tasted.

You can find this high quality olive oil online at www.kasandrinos.com.

meat (which is naturally leaner than grain-fed meat and never thickly marbled it is the unhealthiest part of conventional meat. Conversely, whatever fat you can find on 100% grass-fed or pastured-animal meat will be healthy to eat because it will not contain toxins. Sadly, like humans, animals get fatter from the foods that are unnatural for them to eat.

budget priority #3: carbohydrates (veggies/fruit)

Buying produce that is in season allows you to get primarily locally grown items. You will also save money on these vegetables and fruits since shipping costs are less for your grocer. This is an environmentally conscious way to shop as well.

Vary the vegetables you eat so that you give your body a wider variety of nutrients. If you consistently reach for broccoli, try switching to Brussels sprouts. Instead of cabbage, try kale. Try sweet potatoes, beets, carrots, or turnips instead of potatoes.

Do you always have to buy organic? Here are some rules of thumb on that subject:

- If you are peeling off a thick skin or outer layer of the produce before eating it, you are safe to choose non-organic. This includes banana, pineapple, kiwi, melon, onion, avocado, and citrus fruit (unless you are using the zest or peel).
- If you are eating the item without peeling it, or it has a very thin, porous skin, organic is better. This includes apples, berries, stone fruits (peaches, nectarines, plums, and cherries), bell peppers, and leafy greens.
- Choose organic vegetables and fruits from The Environmental Working Group's "The Dirty Dozen" list whenever possible. Non-organic versions of their top 12 vegetables and fruits have been shown in tests to contain the highest levels of pesticide, herbicide, and fungicide residue. Visit the Environmental Working Group's website (www.ewg.org) regularly, as the list may change from year to year. You can also find a complete list that ranks more than 24 fruits and vegetables.

a few more dollar-stretching tips

Contrary to what some people believe, you will save money on whole foods if you shop at local farmers' markets, buying directly from the source. Each farmer's stand has its own prices, and these are often negotiable, especially if you are buying in larger quantities. The sellers are more likely to negotiate with you during the final operating hour of the market when they want to

THERE IS A SEASON
To find seasonal produce for your state or region, check out these websites, or simply search the web for "seasonal produce + your state's name."
www.simplesteps.org/ eat-local or www.fieldtoplate.com/ guide.php

empty their supplies. This may be even more likely at a Sunday market versus a Saturday market, since it's probably the last chance they have to sell their items for the week.

Another tip to stay within your budget is to rotate your produce and meat choices weekly, buying in bulk when prices are lowest.

You can also reduce your food budget by buying less desirable cuts of meat. I know this is counter-intuitive because most Americans are out there scarfing down boneless, skinless chicken breasts even though bone-in/skin-on chicken legs are tastier and less expensive. But if you're shopping for poultry at a farmers' market or from a local farm (which is ideal), they will often only sell you a whole chicken. Great! Roast the whole thing (recipe page 256), and after you've eaten it all, use the carcass to make broth (recipe page 234). Organ meats from local farmers are often less expensive since the general public is generally turned off by them. Making chicken liver pâté (recipe on page 384) can be very inexpensive if your farmer doesn't have a high demand for the livers.

Stews, soups, and ground meats are excellent ways to eat healthy if you are budget-conscious. Most of the recipes in this book are not expensive to make with the exception of those that call for wild salmon, other fish, scallops, or lamb chops. You can sometimes get great deals on lamb chops, however, if you buy directly from the farmer as I do.

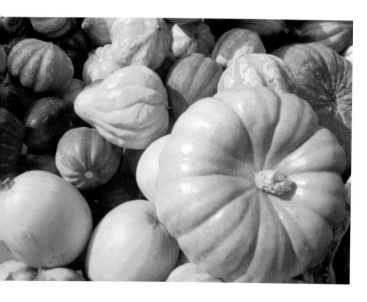

paleo in public: restaurants & parties

As a nutritionist, I have heard every reason under the sun why people can't keep their eating habits in check when they're away from the comforts of their coconut oil-stocked kitchen. I promise that you can still be social while maintaining a Paleo lifestyle.

✓ **Eat whole foods and avoid modern, processed, and refined foods.**

☐ Eat to maintain proper digestive function.

☐ Eat to maintain proper blood sugar regulation.

☐ Follow a plan that will help you reach your own personal health goals.

know before you go

When you are planning to eat at a restaurant, preview the menu to determine what will work for you (or choose a different restaurant if there are truly no healthy options). Most restaurants post their menus on their website for easy viewing or as a downloadable PDF file. An advantage of choosing what you'll order before you arrive is that it gives you more time to visit with your meal companions. Bear in mind, too, that many restaurants will accommodate you if you give them advance notice. Call the restaurant before you go to inquire about a gluten-free menu option, for example, or simply find out about the preparation of the dishes that sound good to you.

With a growing population of diners requesting gluten-free dishes, a lot of restaurants, such as Legal Seafood, P.F. Chang's, Outback Steakhouse, and Bonefish Grill, have now created separate gluten-free menus. This doesn't mean that your dining experience will be "perfectly Paleo," but you'll avoid digestive upset for the most part if you make gluten-free choices.

When you make reservations, use that opportunity to let the restaurant know about your special needs. If you are using an online reservation system, use the comments or notes section to share this information. If you prefer to be more discreet about your dietary requirements, take advantage of these quiet methods that avoid discomfort at the table while ordering.

Then, before you go, eat a small snack of some soy-free jerky, nuts, nut butter, a few bites of avocado, or leftover meat. If you aren't starving when you sit at the table, you will be much more likely to stay on track.

navigating the menu

Once you arrive and are seated at the restaurant, *pass on the breadbasket.* You may worry that you won't be able to resist the bread if it's right in front of you. Don't test yourself! If everyone in your party is agreeable, simply ask the waiter or waitress not to bring bread. It wouldn't hurt for your dining companions to pass on the bread as well. So instead of bread, ask for olives, cut celery, carrots, or cucumber if they're available.

While finger foods are often breaded, fried, or made with grains, dairy products, and seed oils, healthier entrées made from simple, clean ingredients are easy to find. Look for grilled, broiled, or baked meat options. These are less likely to be breaded. Skip the appetizers, or opt for a salad starter.

If a meal comes with French fries, bread, or pasta, simply ask that they either leave these off of your plate or substitute vegetables instead. Look on the menu for what vegetables might be available. If you see grilled squash as a side with another dish, chances are that you can ask for it with your entrée. Be an aware diner, however. Don't ask for mashed sweet potatoes if they aren't listed anywhere on the menu.

Some restaurants charge a bit extra for vegetables if you order them separately, but they will make the swap without blinking. You may even end up ahead of the game with a huge pile of veggies for no extra charge simply because the restaurant isn't accustomed to making substitutions and wants to accommodate you.

Of course, when making special requests, always be polite to your server. Nine times out of ten, he or she is trying to satisfy you without incident. Plus, many kitchen and wait staff members are being educated these days about food allergies. Simply understand the difference between a serious question and an off-putting demand. If you have overt Celiac disease or an extreme gluten sensitivity or food allergy, carry a detailed information card containing your dining requirements (a cutout card is included in The Guide To: Gluten on page 89). This will help the server understand that you are not just trying to be difficult.

ask the right questions

Even if your sensitivity is not severe, you can be firm in your requests while also remaining polite. Don't make assumptions about the contents of the food.

Ask the server for details; they're used to it. It's the only way to feel confident that the meal you'll be served will leave you feeling full and satisfied, not sick and disappointed. Some of the most important questions to ask include:

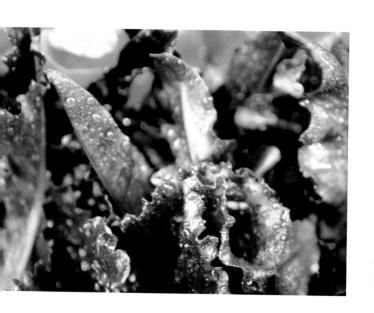

• **"Is any part of what I'm ordering breaded or dusted with flour of any kind?"** Often, protein sources are breaded or even lightly dusted with flour before sautéing, baking, broiling, or roasting. At nicer restaurants, this step can usually be left out when the chef prepares your meal to order.

- "I'm allergic to gluten, can you find out if there is gluten or flour in the sauce or any other part of this dish? If there is any uncertainty, please let me know, and I will order something else that you would recommend as a safe option for me."
- "What kind of frying oil do you use?" Most restaurants use vegetable oil for frying and, therefore, fried foods are not a good option when dining out. That includes sweet potato fries. It's the oil that is the problem, not the potatoes. Note that sweet potato fries are typically dusted or coated in flour before frying to create a crispy result!

but what are the best choices at, say, an italian restaurant versus a chinese restaurant?

italian food

Don't skimp on your protein source. Choose broiled, baked, or grilled chicken, fish, shrimp, or red meat. You can even order meatballs with red sauce, but be sure to ask if they contain flour or breadcrumbs, as some do. Order vegetables or salad on the side. Obviously, avoid bread, pasta, or breaded meats like Parmesan and Francese dishes. Protein sources at Italian restaurants are often dusted with flour before cooking even if they're not breaded and fried, so be sure to ask about this, as most of these dishes can be prepared without the flour. Other healthy options include the antipasto platter with meat and vegetables or grilled vegetables with olive oil and balsamic vinegar.

If you are dying for pasta, the restaurant may have a gluten-free option. While I don't recommend this as a regular practice, ordering it in a restaurant is better than buying these refined products to prepare at home. Pay attention to how *you* feel after eating gluten-free pasta, however. Many people are as sensitive to these products as those containing gluten. All refined grain products can leave you feeling lethargic and tired after a meal, which is not a sign that you have eaten healthful food. At home, you can make noodles from zucchini (see page 374 for a recipe) as a nutritious substitute.

mexican food

Choose primarily meat, salsa, and guacamole when at a Mexican restaurant. If you're having an appetizer, ask the server for jicama, cucumbers, raw celery, or carrots to dip into guacamole. If it's a more upscale Mexican restaurant, ask about a side of vegetables to add to your entrée. Skip the tortilla shells, wraps, and chips (which contain both corn and flour), as well as the beans and rice. Ask if there is flour in any sauces, and opt for grilled meats, if possible. At fast food restaurants like Chipotle, you can even find some meat that is not cooked in vegetable or soybean oil.

SONO CELIACO
Celiac disease is actually very common in Italy, the place where wheat pasta was "born." As a result, most restaurants there cater to the gluten-free diner, making it easy to navigate an Italian vacation and avoid wheat products. Carry a Celiac dining card with you in Italian (see p. 89), or simply say, "Sono celiaco," which means "I have Celiac disease."

japanese food and sushi

Sashimi is an easy option; or you can simply ask that the rolls you order be made without rice. I do this every time I eat sushi. Most sushi chefs will roll them any way you order them, even if the server thinks at first that it may not be possible. Ask for extra daikon radish (the white shredded stuff you thought was just a garnish), and eat that as filler along with your sashimi or rolls. Avoid fried/tempura rolls, as well as rolls that add tempura flakes for crunch, or simply ask that the flakes be left out. While some sushi restaurants don't allow for modifications, most will gladly accommodate your requests if you ask politely.

If you order rolls that come with sauces, be sure to let them know you cannot have anything with soy in it. In addition to soy sauce, this includes eel sauce and ponzu. If you are sure you are not sensitive to soy, bring your own wheat-free organic tamari (available in natural food stores or online) with you. Commercially prepared soy sauces are fermented with the use of wheat, and the vast majority of people find that avoiding even trace amounts of wheat helps them feel better. Historically, soy sauce was created as a fermented product that took much longer time to make without the use of wheat. As with most commercialized foods today, speed and cost-cutting prevail; and the common practice now involves the addition of wheat, making soy sauce a source of gluten.

If you're like me—sensitive to both gluten *and* soy—try a product called coconut aminos. This is a fermented coconut product that has an almost identical taste and texture to soy sauce. You can dip your sushi in it, as well as use it in recipes that call for soy sauce. It is one of the best substitutes I have found in years, and I now actually prefer the taste of it to soy sauce.

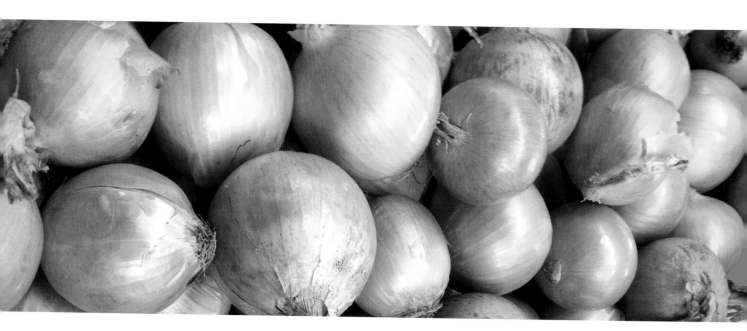

Avoid teriyaki dishes, gyoza, dumplings, edamame, and most other appetizers. As much as I love seaweed salad and think that sea vegetables are an excellent food choice, they are typically prepared commercially (not on location at each restaurant) and are loaded with soy sauce and often monosodium glutamate (MSG), which is a neurotoxic food additive.

indian food

At an Indian restaurant, Tandoori meats and grilled or roasted vegetables that are not drowning in sauces are best. Skip the naan and the rice, of course. If you would like to enjoy a curry dish, ask your server about the use of flour in the sauce. Traditionally, Indian food was cooked in ghee, but most modern Indian restaurants have moved on to less expensive vegetable oils. Request that ghee is used if it is available.

thai food

Opt for a curry dish or other coconut milk-based dish without the rice. Ask the server if the dish includes soy sauce, as this is often the problem with many Thai dishes. Many Thai restaurants now have gluten-free dishes, so this is one of the easiest ways to avoid grains while enjoying their food. Most Thai food is otherwise naturally gluten-free, and the main grain used is rice. While I don't recommend rice consumption as a regular practice for most people, if you feel that you can tolerate a small amount of white rice or rice noodles without digestive upset, you can indulge while dining out on Thai food as long as it is a rare occurrence. This means once a month at most. Again, pay attention to how *you* feel after eating these foods. Many people experience lethargy or bloating after meals containing rice.

pizza

There is simply no great way to enjoy a healthy version of pizza while dining out. If you want pizza, make one at home instead using almond meal or coconut flour. If you search online for "meatza recipe" or "Paleo pizza crust recipe," you will find instructions. After you have followed the Paleo dietary guidelines for a while, you may discover that you can handle gluten-free items sporadically. Then, you may be safe to order a gluten-free pizza. Understand also, however, that the cheese used is usually the lowest quality possible, as restaurants often source ingredients based on price.

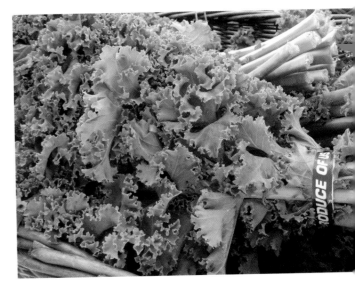

chinese food.

Unless you know the restaurant well enough to make special requests for no MSG and sauces without added sugar or soy sauce, I recommend that you avoid Chinese food altogether. If you're in a pinch, ordering steamed dishes is generally safe, but Chinese food is safer to cook at home, such as a stir-fry using coconut oil and coconut aminos (recipe on page 286). If you are sensitive to coconut, you can stir fry with ghee or another animal fat and use a sauce made from tahini (see page 386) to drizzle as a finisher.

paleo party prowess

If you're headed to a party, ask the host or hostess what they plan to serve so that you know what to expect. Of course, don't make a fuss about your dietary needs unless they're open and friendly about accommodating you. If you do feel comfortable explaining your way of eating to them, let them know that simply preparing grilled, baked, or roasted meats and vegetables with herbs and spices are all perfectly fine. Be sure to explain that some sauces can be problematic, so if it's possible, leaving them on the side is ideal.

Assuming there will be food you can eat is a surefire way to be disappointed and hungry. After all, most people use parties as an excuse to indulge in treats or unhealthy food. So consider taking a dish or two with you that you know will satisfy your hunger. The host or hostess will be happy to have the contribution, and you'll be relieved to know that you won't be hungry all night or suffering later. There are plenty of party-friendly recipes in the back of this book that will surely please a crowd!

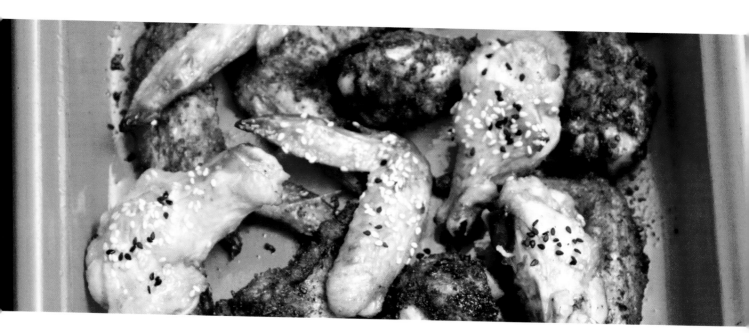

paleo on-the-go:
on the road or in the air

I know first-hand how tricky it can be to find good food while traveling away from home, but it's certainly not impossible with just a little bit of forethought and planning.

travel tips

- Use a cooler bag with a reliable/leak-proof ice pack to keep foods fresh in your hotel room.
- Request a mini-fridge in your hotel room. If necessary, claim you have severe food allergies.
- Pack foods in tall/narrow containers that stay upright and won't spill.
- Make good use of small and large zip-lock bags.
- Prior to your departure date, scout online for a Whole Foods Market, Trader Joe's, or other organic grocer or natural food co-op at your destination.
- If you're traveling by air, keep small, 2-3-ounce spill-proof containers around for liquids, and be sure the volume size of the container is stamped on it so that the TSA can see it easily. I highly recommend carrying extra-virgin olive oil this way for use on salads, etc.
- Use clear liquid containers for items like guacamole so that they can be viewed easily.
- Dry foods are perfectly acceptable in carry-on bags.
- Keep extra protein and fat sources on hand like jerky and nuts in the event of a flight delay. They're lightweight, so it's easy to pack extra.
- You can usually find salads with meat at airport food vendors. Simply remove the unwanted ingredients, and ask for lemons to use for dressing with the olive oil you have brought with you.
- Bunless burgers can often be made to order.
- In a pinch, very dark chocolate, nuts, and/or trail mix can work as healthy snacks.

carry these items with you:

- A small can opener.
- A small but sharp knife (only in your checked bag, not your carry-on, as the TSA will confiscate it).
- Small empty food storage containers and zip-lock bags for leftovers or ice.

☑ **Eat whole foods and avoid modern, processed, and refined foods.**

☐ Eat to maintain proper digestive function.

☐ Eat to maintain proper blood sugar regulation.

☐ Follow a plan that will help you reach your own personal health goals.

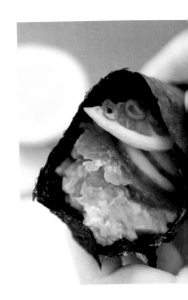

- Plastic utensils or a set of reusable utensils.
- A few paper or reusable lightweight plates.
- A small salt shaker (Redmond Real Salt makes one).
- Travel-sized jars of spices/herbs, such as black pepper, cinnamon, garlic powder, rosemary, or oregano.
- A small sponge and dish soap (if you have reusable items). This is especially helpful during a road trip.

When you travel, you may need to take some foods with you in order to continue to eat healthy. Here is a list of possible protein, carbohydrate, and fat options for traveling.

easy protein

- Applegate Farms deli meats (avoid any with carrageenan).
- Canned wild salmon or tuna. Wild Planet, Whole Foods, and Trader Joe's are good brands.
- Wild smoked salmon or precooked wild shrimp.
- Imported meats like chorizo often only have pork, spices, and salt as ingredients.
- Whole roasted chickens (either plain/salt and pepper, or with only ingredients you can recognize, as *most* contain undesirable ingredients).
- Jerky or kits from companies like Steve's Original, Sophia's Survival Food, or US Wellness Meats. Avoid brands with soy or additives you don't recognize.
- Hard-boiled eggs.
- Nuts (though more fat than protein) are good in a pinch.

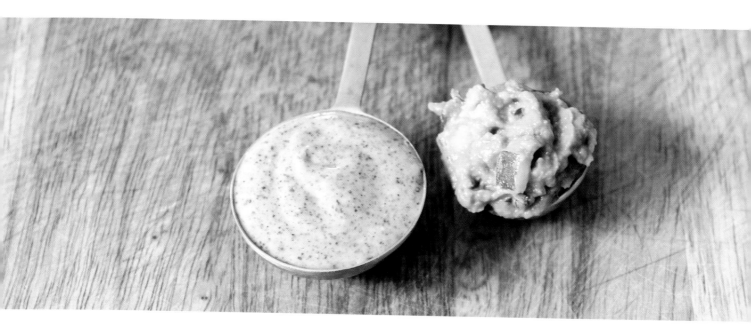

easy fats

- Extra-virgin olive oil in a portable, spill-proof container.
- Coconut oil sold in packets (Artisana brand), or use a spill-proof container.
- Nut butter, coconut butter packets (Artisana brand), or even a jar if you pack it in your checked suitcase.
- Macadamia nuts, walnuts, hazelnuts, coconut flakes.
- Guacamole is easy to find and easily portable.
- 80%+ dark chocolate—good quality, low sugar.

easy carbohydrates

- Vegetables like carrots, celery, and bell peppers travel well.
- Salads are easy to find most anywhere. Just keep them "naked" and with lots of veggies.
- Romaine lettuce hearts are perfect for wrapping proteins.
- Canned sweet potato or butternut squash. Don't forget the can opener!
- Fruits like apples, oranges, other citrus fruits, grapes, and bananas travel well. Berries are easy if you have a cooler bag. Fruit salad is easy to find in most places, even at the airport.
- Fruit/nut bars (Larabar is a good brand) or trail mix without additives.

your digestive system: the parts, the process, and the poop!

Your digestive system involves a series of steps that include several organs working in concert with one another.

In this chapter, you will learn about these various body parts, the process of assimilating/integrating food matter, and, yes, your poop.

Think of digestion as a North-to-South process. You may think it starts in your mouth and ends you know where, but digestion actually begins before the food enters your mouth. In fact, it begins in your brain.

the part: your brain

Remember when you were a kid, and your mother made you wait thirty minutes after lunch before swimming or running around to play?

There's a good reason to leave a window between eating and heightened activity: Your body can't focus on digesting food when you ask it to perform other actions like active play or exercise. Physical activity—or any activity that's stressful, including a dreaded work meeting or life event—occurs in a different *physical* and *mental* state than what you need for digestion. This stressful state is called the "sympathetic dominant" state or "fight or flight mode." In fact, your thoughts can impair or improve salivary response, stomach acid production, enzyme secretion, and the release of gastrointestinal (digestive) hormones.

It's your brain's job to decide for your body whether to divert attention to stress responses, such as when you exercise, or to nourishing functions like resting and digesting. If you're in fight or flight mode because of a mental or physical stressor, your body will divert energy and blood flow away from the digestive process and toward other priorities like managing and responding to the stressful stimuli.

If your body senses that it needs to be on alert or handling stressors, the natural cycle of "rest and digest" is switched off, which means that autonomic (automatic or subconscious) body functions are down-regulated. Therefore, if you want to digest your food *optimally*, allow a mental break or "chill-out" period when switching from a stressed (fight or flight) state into a state where you are ready to rest and digest food (known as the "parasympathetic" state).

This goes against most things you've been told about post-workout nutrition, doesn't it? You have likely been told to make sure you eat within thirty minutes of working out when you actually should wait until thirty minutes *after* your workout. What you've been taught is ideal for professional

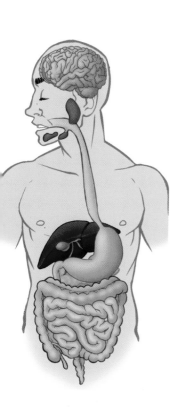

Eat whole foods and avoid modern, processed, and refined foods.

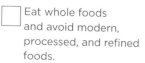 **Eat to maintain proper digestive function.**

Eat to maintain proper blood sugar regulation.

Follow a plan that will help you reach your own personal health goals.

athletes and bodybuilders, but not for the average person. Unless you're extremely active and need extra calories as a result, such as in the case of a coach who trains people all day or someone with a very active day job, the directive to eat within thirty minutes of a workout doesn't apply to you.

If your activity level is high, and you want to eat immediately after a workout, liquid forms are easier to digest, as they don't require the same digestive function.

The reason we have been told to eat within thirty minutes of working out is that we may gain a metabolic advantage from calories taken in during this window of time. The problem is that it's nearly impossible to gain this advantage from whole foods when your digestive system is still in fight or flight mode.

The average person who simply exercises regularly and does not perform any hard training as a competitive athlete takes in sufficient food each day to replace the nutrients depleted by exercise. In fact, many of my clients have found that dropping their post-workout shake allows them to finally lose the fat they've been battling for months. Instead, they wait at least thirty minutes and continue with solid whole foods at mealtime.

SYMPATHETIC VS. PARASYMPATHETIC
The sympathetic nervous system is dominantly activated when you are in fight or flight mode, and the parasympathetic nervous system is activated when you are in rest and digest mode. In order to optimize all digestive function, you need to be in a parasympathetic-dominant state, as you can only be dominantly in one state or the other.

what can go wrong?

Without calming down into rest and digest mode, your digestive function won't work optimally, which means decreased stomach acid production, as well as impaired (either too fast or too slow) overall digestion.

how to fix it

Whether you're in fight or flight mode acutely from an intense workout or chronically from a stressful life, the fix is the same. Take a few moments—as many as you can—to relax and breathe when you sit down to eat. (Yes, I said sit down, and I don't mean in the car while driving!) Making a conscious effort to activate the rest and digest mode so that you can eat in a calm, mindful state will help your entire digestive process run smoothly—literally.

So, relax, decompress, reset your mind, and take a few deep breaths before sitting down at the table to eat. Do your best not to eat on the run, in your car, or immediately before or after exercise.

the part: mouth, salivary glands, and esophagus

There are three pairs of enzyme-releasing salivary glands that begin a chemical breakdown process of your food while you chew. The enzyme, salivary amylase, begins the breakdown of carbohydrates, and lingual lipase starts to break down fats. The next time you eat a starchy food, chew it for a while, and notice that it tastes sweeter as the complex carbohydrates are broken down into simple sugars. This is the enzyme at work.

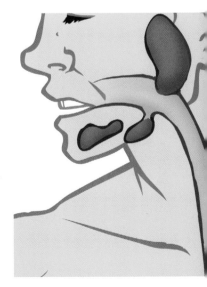

Saliva helps to moisten your food before it is sent on its way down your esophagus and into your stomach. The importance of chewing doesn't stop there, though. The action of chewing begins the mechanical breakdown of food. It also sends signals to your brain to initiate downstream digestive enzyme production so that your entire system is primed for food. Ever feel a rumble in your stomach while chewing gum? That's because your body has been tricked into thinking you're about to send food down the pipe. Chewing gum can stimulate your appetite for this reason.

what can go wrong?

If you don't chew properly, some of the symptoms you'll experience are bloating, belching, and undigested food particles in your stool like corn or leafy greens. These symptoms may also be a sign that you're eating foods your body doesn't tolerate.

how to fix it

Chew your food well, of course! Beyond that, be sure to eat whole foods that your body tolerates well. Foods high in anti-nutrients, such as grains and legumes, have built-in defenses against digestive enzymes and the digestive process. It's their job to survive that process so that they may go on to be planted and grow.

If you urgently run to the bathroom shortly after a meal, it's a surefire sign that your body has not tolerated something you have eaten. Corn, for example, is hard for people to chew completely due to its resilient outer coating. Any time you see something in your stool that looks the same as it did on your plate, you have a problem. Your digestive tract is a place where food should be broken down completely into molecules only visible with a microscope. What you eliminate is 80% bacteria, *not* mostly food.

There is a test called the Transit-Time Test (see page 74), which uses whole sesame seeds to mark how long it takes for food to move through your system. This test is a perfect example of why a grain or a seed of a plant may be hard for us to break down entirely. Even on a molecular level, some proteins may not be fully digested or assimilated by your body. As I said, this is common with grains and legumes because they fight your digestive system.

KIDS AND VEGGIES
Toddlers that have just begun to use their gums and teeth to chew foods typically have less amylase to mix with carbohydrate-rich food. This is why your young one may like sweeter foods. Continue to offer less sweet foods because the enzyme secretion will develop and increase as the child's chewing and gumming of foods becomes more consistent.

what's wrong with legumes?

Well, you already know that beans are famous for causing gas. This is due to the presence of carbohydrates that we can't properly break down in our bodies. The bottom line is: If you're experiencing gas symptoms, you have eaten a food you don't digest well.

It's possible to make beans more digestible by soaking, sprouting, and fermenting them, typically overnight. Many people take this approach to traditional food preparation and find that the beans are easier to digest. To assume this is a great protein source is misguided, however, as beans are primarily a source of carbohydrates, not protein. So this method may help you consume beans without digestive distress, but it isn't recommended as a regular practice. More nutrient-dense foods are always a better choice!

the part: stomach

Your stomach is a pouch that holds roughly 1-3 liters of food and liquid. A healthy stomach has a thick mucosal lining and is an extremely acidic environment. Yes, you read that correctly! The acidic environment serves several important purposes. It's your first line of defense against "bad bugs" or other pathogens that try to hitch a ride into your body by way of food; and it's where the breakdown of proteins begins.

Your stomach acid is necessary. After you swallow, food passes through your esophagus and enters your stomach, where it's the job of stomach acid (hydrochloric acid, HCl) to kill any microscopic, pathogenic material (bad bugs) in your food before it passes through to the small intestine. When your HCl level is adequate, pathogens are killed.

You probably swallow more pathogens than you think, but we only hear about one of these pathogens when stomach acid fails to destroy it, leading to food poisoning or an infection.

An entire array of digestive reactions occurs when food arrives in the stomach, as digestive-signaling hormones and enzymes "read" the contents of your stomach and begin to make secretions in response. The breakdown (or "denaturing") of food begins in the stomach by the actions of these enzymes.

Proteins are broken down by enzymes called proteases and peptidases, while fats are broken down by gastric lipase. While the majority of nutrients and substances you consume won't begin to be absorbed until they continue on through your small and large intestine, the absorption of water, some minerals, aspirin, and alcohol occurs at the stomach lining.

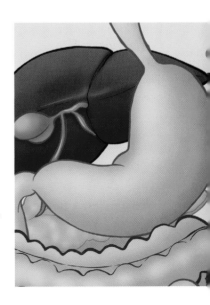

Gastric (stomach) secretions, including HCl and the aforementioned digestive enzymes and hormones, help to break down food while maintaining adequate stomach lining integrity and cell growth. Last, but not least, your stomach is responsible for the further mechanical digestion of food through "churning and burning," which breaks food down physically while mixing it with the gastric secretions. The resulting mix of denatured food plus gastric secretions is called "chyme."

what can go wrong?

When your stomach's lining is sufficient and allows the proper breakdown of food, you don't *feel* the high level of acidity. When you have *low* stomach acid, you end up with—you guessed it: bad bugs. That leads, as you may suspect, to heartburn and acid reflux. Most people reach for an antacid when they feel heartburn or acid reflux, but the actual cause of the problem is usually too *little* stomach acid.

According to Chris Kresser, L.Ac, acid reflux "is caused by increased pressure in the stomach resulting in a malfunction of the lower esophageal sphincter (LES). The increase in pressure is caused by bacterial overgrowth and malabsorption of carbohydrates, both of which are precipitated by low stomach acid. Reducing bacteria loads and limiting carbohydrate intake have both been shown to greatly improve, and in some cases completely cure, acid reflux and GERD (gastroesophageal reflux disease)."*

To reiterate, when you feel acid reflux or heartburn, you're actually feeling the effects of pressure and backup caused by poorly digested food and bacterial overgrowth—a result of low stomach acid, not too much. Low or inadequate stomach acid means "bad bugs" thrive, and certain foods aren't broken down, which causes the pressure and allows acidic HCl to creep back up your esophagus where it doesn't belong. The acid then causes a burning sensation in the sensitive lining of the esophagus.

source: Kresser, Chris. "The hidden causes of heartburn and GERD." April 1, 2010. http://chriskresser.com/the-hidden-causes-of-heartburn-and-gerd

digestive enzymes decoded!

The first portion of the name of an enzyme tells you what type of molecule it will break down, while the second part, the "-ase," tells you it's an enzyme.

lipase = lipid (fat) breakdown enzyme

protease = protein breakdown enzyme

amylase = amylopectin (a carbohydrate) breakdown enzyme

When stomach acid remains *in* your stomach where it belongs—provided you don't have a medical condition like a gastric ulcer—you don't feel it. Once again, your stomach is designed to have a thick, intact mucosal lining which enables the acid to do its job without your feeling anything at all.

Beyond simply keeping you comfortable while digesting foods, stomach acid is essential to not only the downstream signaling of appropriate enzyme secretions from other digestive organs, but also to the assimilation of minerals (like iron and calcium) and B vitamins (especially B12) into your cells from your food. Many conditions that are the result of nutrient deficiencies—including anemia, depression, anxiety, and fatigue-like symptoms from an iron or B12 deficiency, osteoporosis, or osteopenia—are rooted in low stomach acid. Without appropriate levels of stomach acid, you may suffer from vitamin or mineral deficiencies, frequent bouts of food poisoning, gas, belching, or bloating after a meal despite chewing your food very well.

how to fix it

Following the advice from the first two steps of the digestive process—getting into rest and digest mode and chewing foods well—will take you very far along the path to keeping your stomach acid at good levels. If, after taking those steps, you still feel symptoms of low stomach acid, you can take digestive bitters (a liquid tincture available at most health food stores), or you can take a small amount of fresh lemon juice or apple cider vinegar. Any of these strong bitter or sour liquids in just a small shot of water about fifteen minutes before meals can be helpful in stimulating HCl production. If your symptoms are severe, you may find that supplementing with HCl directly is most effective.

If you experience symptoms of low stomach acid like reflux, heartburn, or excessive fullness immediately after eating even though you have eliminated grains, legumes, sugar, and refined foods from your diet, it could be that your body needs more time to adjust before you will see the results of your dietary adjustments. If you have been on acid-blocking drugs, such as a PPI (Proton Pump Inhibitor), for an extended period of time, you will need to take further steps beyond simply increasing stomach acid to ensure you properly absorb and utilize nutrients from your food.

If symptoms of low stomach acid persist for longer than thirty days, there may be a more serious issue, such as a persistent gut pathogen (bad bug). In this case, I recommend working with a practitioner who understands your desire to maintain a whole foods diet and who will conduct a stool test to rule out H. Pylori, SIBO (Small Intestine Bacterial Overgrowth), or other problems. It is critical to resolve these issues in order to have full success with a nutrient-dense, whole-foods diet.

TRYING TO 'SOAK UP' BOOZE WITH BREAD? *While this seems logical enough, it's not actually helping your body to slow the absorption of alcohol from your stomach to your blood stream. A better approach would be to eat a meal or snack with some fat in it to lower the rate of gastric emptying.*

ways to support digestion, naturally

- **Reduce intake of carbohydrates, fiber, and sugar/sweeteners in all forms (including artificial), especially fructose.** All of these promote dysbiosis, which is imbalanced gut flora. This means you are feeding the bad bacteria in your digestive system and allowing them to increase in numbers.

- **Lemon juice or apple cider vinegar.** Try about 1 tablespoon in 1 ounce of water 10-20 minutes before a meal.

- **Digestive bitters.** You can find these in tincture form (liquid in a dropper) in many health food stores. Dosage will vary and will be marked on the bottle.

- **You can find HCl supplements at any health food shop—usually as betaine HCl or as part of a combination of digestive enzyme support.** I recommend only taking these supplements as part of a multi-pronged approach, understanding that rest and digest mode while eating, as well as chewing, are critical. You may take a low-dose of HCl per the instructions on the bottle and monitor your own symptoms thereafter. If you notice any "heat" or burning sensations in your upper gastric region, it means you have taken more than you need. If you take more HCl than you need but never feel a burning sensation, it may simply be a good sign of an intact mucosal lining.

- **In combination with supplemental HCl to combat feelings of acid reflux, I highly recommend adding mucosal lining support as well.** Chewable deglycerized licorice (sold as DGL in most places), marshmallow root, slippery elm, and/or peppermint herbal tea are helpful. (See the "Repair" step in the Guide to Leaky Gut on page 88 for more information.)

- **Here is an important caution, however, from integrative medicine practitioner Chris Kresser on HCl supplementation:** "HCl should never be taken by anyone who is also using any kind of anti-inflammatory medication such as corticosteroids (e.g. Prednisone), aspirin, Indocin, ibuprofen (e.g. Motrin, Advil, etc.) or other NSAIDS. These drugs can damage the GI lining that supplementary HCl might aggravate, increasing the risk of gastric bleeding or ulcer."*

source: Kresser, Chris. "Get rid of heartburn and GERD forever in three simple steps." April 16, 2010. http://chriskresser.com/the-hidden-causes-of-heartburn-and-gerd

the part: liver and gallbladder

The liver is a reddish-brown organ that weighs about 3.5 pounds and sits in the upper right quadrant of the abdominal cavity, just below the diaphragm. The gallbladder is a much smaller (8cm x 4cm) pouch-like organ that sits below the liver and connects to the duodenum (part of the small intestine) via the common bile duct. The common bile duct also connects the gallbladder and the pancreas.

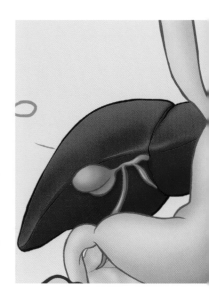

The liver is responsible for a lot of critical life functions like detoxification and protein synthesis, but it also plays a very large role in the digestive process. It produces bile, a soap-like substance that emulsifies dietary fats like butter, olive oil, and coconut oil—the way dish soap breaks up grease on a dirty pan—in order for you to digest and assimilate them into your body's cells and tissues. Your gallbladder stores the bile and releases it based on signals from the brain that communicate the timing and quantity of bile needed to properly break down dietary fats. You couldn't appropriately assimilate dietary fats, as well as fat-soluble vitamins A, D, E, and K, without your liver and gallbladder.

what can go wrong?

The primary issue you may experience with your liver and gallbladder involves the signaling hormone cholecystokinin (CCK), which enables your brain to communicate with your gallbladder. If this process goes awry, you may feel pain or discomfort after a fatty meal in the area under your sternum (the large hard bone in your upper chest). This may indicate a chronic disruption in the normal flow of bile from your gallbladder or that gallstones have developed and are beginning to block the normal release of bile from the gallbladder. This blockage may occur within the gallbladder itself or in the common bile duct (the set of tubes that allow the liver, gallbladder, and pancreas to secrete into the small intestine).

Often, people attempt to eat a low-fat diet when these symptoms develop since they understand that the gallbladder is working in response to dietary fats. This approach only tends to make matters worse because, in an effort to eat less fat, they usually increase their intake of grains. Due to the introduction of this anti-nutrient food and the lower demand for bile secretion, the CCK hormone signals are only disrupted further. Then, the gallbladder fails to secrete enough bile, which begins to back up.

Another—and possibly earlier—sign of a malfunctioning gallbladder or gallbladder signaling problem is green, yellowish, or light-colored stool. This color pattern suggests that dietary fats have not been properly broken down before elimination, which may indicate that your bile production or secretion is impaired. If all is working smoothly, you won't feel any discomfort after a fatty meal, and your stool color will be normal. (Read more on page 75 about

NO GALLBLADDER?
If your gallbladder has been removed, you may find that a more moderate or even a low-ish fat intake helps you feel better. Focus on fats that are easier for your body to break down without the need for bile. Contrary to popular belief, saturated fats are easier to digest than unsaturated fats! This is because the actual chemical structure of saturated fats like butter and coconut oil is much shorter, and our bodies can disassemble them/break them down much easier than those made from longer chains like mono or polyunsaturated fats (such as olive or walnut oil).

identifying healthy stool.)

Bear in mind, too, that your liver serves many critical functions beyond digestion. It is also responsible for the uptake of fatty acids once they're broken down in the small intestine. It is your liver that screens all incoming toxins to determine the proper immune response against possible invaders. Poor liver function can mean you won't be able to fight infections with full strength. So, overwhelming your liver with antigens (compounds against which your body needs to launch an immune response), whether from environmental or dietary toxins, is not a good idea!

how to fix it

Eliminating all grain products from your diet is step one in supporting the digestive functions of your liver and gallbladder. This will ensure that you are doing your best to keep the signaling from your brain to your gallbladder working properly. Also, since your liver is taxed heavily by alcohol and excess fructose intake, I recommend limiting or even curbing your intake of booze and fruit (especially juices).

Eat the majority of your dietary fats in the form of short and medium-chain fatty acids (butter, ghee, and coconut oil) versus longer chain fats (olive oil or other nut oils), and your body will use the bile it secretes more efficiently.

You may also find that supplementing with some bile salts and digestive enzymes—lipase specifically—helps your digestive process. This is particularly helpful for people who have had their gallbladder removed.

the part: pancreas

The pancreas is an organ that is part of your endocrine system, which means that it produces hormones. It sits with its "head" nestled adjacent the duodenum (part of your small intestine) and its "body" underneath your stomach. Your pancreas is responsible for the production and secretion of the hormones insulin and glucagon, as well as the digestive enzymes trypsin and chymotrypsin, which serve to break down peptide bonds in the proteins you eat.

Remember that there were digestive enzymes secreted in your stomach as well, so the pancreas is adding more into the mix now that food is moving toward your small intestine.

What do the pancreatic hormones do? Insulin is a storage hormone produced by the beta cells of the pancreas. It signals your body to carry glucose (sugar) and

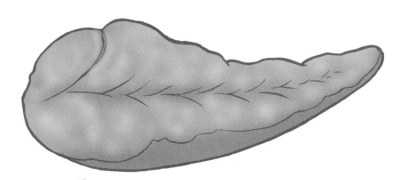

other nutrients from the bloodstream into the liver, muscles, and brain. Insulin release is triggered primarily by the intake of dietary carbohydrates and secondarily in response to dietary protein.

Glucagon is produced by the alpha cells of the pancreas and is the counter-regulatory hormone to insulin. It is released in response to the intake of dense sources of animal protein and in response to drops in blood glucose levels due to hunger or exercise. In other words, it signals your body to release glucose from storage in your liver in order to raise your blood sugar when necessary.

what can go wrong?

The river of hormones and enzymes should flow smoothly, but if you have a grain intolerance or very low intake of dietary fats, you end up with an excess of bile which then backs up. As a result, you might eventually develop gallbladder disease or gall stones, which "block up the works" of the common bile duct. In some serious cases, this back up can lead to pancreatitis, which is inflammation of the pancreas.

Pancreatitis or gallbladder disease can cause a disruption in the production and secretion of digestive enzymes and hormones from the pancreas. Any of these disorders may have serious downstream negative effects on digestive function and overall health.

Diabetes is a disease of the pancreas as well. In the case of Type 1 Diabetes, the beta cells of the pancreas are destroyed by your immune system, partly in an autoimmune response to the consumption of gluten-containing grain proteins (read more about this on page 89). This reaction leaves the pancreas unable to produce adequate insulin, and in many cases, it stops producing insulin entirely. This is why a Type 1 Diabetic usually needs to inject insulin in order to properly assimilate nutrients.

Remember that insulin is a nutrient storage hormone. For this reason, impaired pancreatic and insulin function can mean malnutrition and dangerous weight loss called "wasting." These are common symptoms for a Type 1 Diabetic. Without the action of insulin, even if an individual eats plenty of food, the body can't access, store, and pull the nutrients from the bloodstream and into the body's cells. Until insulin is injected and cellular nutrient storage occurs, a Type 1 Diabetic will continue to waste away. While most Type 1 Diabetics cannot regain any beta cell function, if detected early enough and a strictly grain-free diet is adopted, some *may* be able to reverse the condition.

While Type 1 and Type 2 Diabetes both involve problems with nutrient storage, they're very different. A Type 2 Diabetic still has beta cell function, but the signaling is disrupted due to diet and lifestyle. Unfortunately, some Type 2 Diabetics may experience beta cell burnout or destruction, which means that

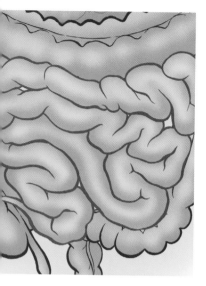

not all beta cell function will be regained when they change their diet. Those people may need to inject insulin, although they usually need it to a lesser degree than people with Type 1 Diabetes.

how to fix it

Pancreatic malfunction is often a downstream result of gallbladder malfunction, so address your gallbladder first, as previously outlined. If you have Type 1 Diabetes, it's critical that you eliminate gluten from your diet 100%. This means looking for hidden gluten in foods and being diligent about your food choices/requests when dining out. (See page 89 for a guide to finding hidden gluten in foods.)

the part: small intestine

The small intestine is seven feet of complex, hard-working, tube-like tissue that holds the key to much of your immune capability. There are three parts to the small intestine: the duodenum, the jejunum, and the ileum. Just on the other side of the cell walls that line your small intestine is an immune layer and your bloodstream.

Your small intestine is where most of your food is either broken into its end-usable forms of amino acids (from proteins), fatty acids (from fats), or glucose (from carbohydrates)—*or not*. If not, what you get is digestive or stomach irritation, malfunction, and malabsorption. Food particles, combined with stomach acid, bile, digestive hormones, and enzymes, interact with a brush-border lining in the jejunum as they move through. This is where your body decides if it recognizes food as particles it knows how to use (such as amino

signs & symptoms of disrupted digestion

- Burning feeling in your gut after meals (heartburn)
- Frequent belching after meals
- Indigestion
- Feeling of fullness after meals
- Frequent stomach upset
- Gas, flatulence after meals
- Constipation
- Diarrhea
- Chronic intestinal infections: bacterial, yeast, parasites

- Chronic candida infections (candidiasis), which can cause a host of symptoms such as skin rashes and vaginal yeast infections in women
- Undigested food in stool
- Known food sensitivities

acids, fatty acids, glucose, vitamins, and minerals) or as an enemy. It's truly the make or break stage in the game of digestion and absorption.

what can go wrong?

Before broken-down food particles are assimilated into your bloodstream, your immune system assesses whether they're safe or if they appear to be invading pathogens like bacteria or a virus. When the peace of your digestive tract is disturbed by food proteins that are hard to digest (mainly from grains or beans), an immune response is launched on the offending proteins because they're seen as invaders. You may feel this response in the form of digestive distress, or you may not feel any gastrointestinal upset at all. That's the kicker! The immune response in your body may be *entirely* different from the way the same irritants affect someone else. One man's diarrhea is another man's eczema, tendonitis, or migraine, for example. In fact, this irritation can lead to an inflammatory response *anywhere in your body.*

The problem starts upstream. Down-regulated, low, or slow digestive enzyme signaling or hormone signaling may cause the release of inadequate digestive secretions from the liver, gallbladder, and pancreas. Decreased stomach acid (HCl) or disrupted cholecystokinin (CCK), for example—all "upstream" problems that occur before food reaches the small intestine—set the stage for these issues. If your upstream processes of digestion are "broken," you run a greater risk of downstream malfunction as well.

Bacteria, which are found in smaller proportion in the stomach and most abundantly in the large intestine, can creep into the small intestine, promoting Small Intestinal Bacterial Overgrowth (SIBO). This can also cause an imbalance in stomach flora (good vs. bad bacteria) that can lead to food intolerances and digestive upset.

The largest issue, however, is leaky gut, a condition that occurs within the small intestine and is 100% diet-related. The leaky gut chapter is devoted entirely to that problem.

how to fix it

You guessed it! Avoid foods that are hard to digest: grains and legumes. Also avoid foods that withdraw nutrients for their processing, yet leave few nutrients behind. These include refined foods, sugar, and alcohol. Your best bet is to follow the advice in the leaky gut chapter.

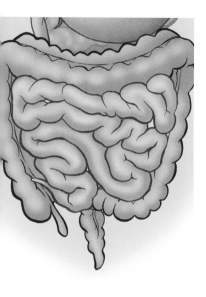

the part: large intestine and rectum

Stretching roughly five feet in length and comprised of two "parts," the cecum and the colon, your large intestine wraps around your small intestine and begins in the right lower portion of your abdomen roughly at or below your belly button. It makes up about 20% of the entire length of your intestinal canal. Your rectum is the final portion of your large intestine after your colon and measures about 4.5-5 inches in length.

The large intestine is the site for water absorption and the uptake of any remaining nutrients—specifically micronutrients (vitamins and minerals)—still left after the small intestine completes the bulk of the hard work. The large intestine's work takes place over roughly 12-18 hours and concludes with the creation and compaction of fecal matter. Proper gut flora is essential to good digestive function. The large intestine is where the majority of the gut flora (ideally, "good bugs" or "probiotics") live, and bacteria composes approximately 80% of the dry weight of the stool.

what can go wrong?

Inadequate or imbalanced gut flora is one of the primary issues behind poor large intestine function. If your eliminations are small, dense, difficult to pass, and foul-smelling, it can indicate extended "transit time." This means that your large intestine is taking far too long to pass waste. Food can be in your large intestine for anywhere from ten hours, which is ideal, to three days, which is far too long.

how to fix It

First of all, make sure that you drink enough water to be well hydrated. You need sufficient lubrication for your food to pass through your system. Don't overload on water, though. Contrary to popular belief, you can drink too much. This is because too much water can dilute your stomach acid if you drink it with meals. So, enjoy your water between meals, and drink extra before and after exercise to replace what you lose in your sweat.

Next, add fermented foods to your diet:
- Raw sauerkraut (see page 238 for a recipe)
- Kimchi (buy without sugar, or make it yourself)
- Fermented vegetables like shredded carrots (can be made with the sauerkraut recipe)
- Plain full fat yogurt made (preferably at home with a 24-hour fermentation process) from raw grass-fed milk (cow, goat, or sheep)
- Homemade kombucha (a fermented tea drink that is easy to make)

These fermented foods have moderate levels of probiotic content, which means they provide your digestive system with good bacteria when eaten in varying amounts and types on a daily basis. Making these items at-home is a more cost-effective way to balance the flora in your digestive system.

You can also take a supplement of probiotics in pill or powder form, however. There is not one brand or strain of probiotic bacteria that will work best for everyone, so your best bet is to try one out and see how you feel after taking it for a week. If your digestion improves, you have found a good one for you. If not, try another one with different bacterial strains or more potent quantities of bacteria. (Just compare the ingredients lists.)

Probiotic supplementation is also a good idea if you suffer from frequent diarrhea. When your digestive system rejects a food quickly, it often throws the baby out with the bathwater, so to speak. Your system flushes out the irritant it has decided was harmful while also flushing out the other contents of your small and large intestines. This may result in an imbalance in your gut flora that leaves your bowel movements feeling "off" for several days. "Re-inoculating" with probiotics can help you along and get your bathroom habits back on track.

Often, probiotic supplements are sold in the refrigerated section of a health food or grocery store, while others are sold right from the shelves. Which is better? It depends. While the refrigerated options are better protected and potentially fresher, some practitioners believe that if the probiotic needs to be refrigerated before you consume it, it stands little chance of remaining intact

is your appendix really useless?

Connected to your large intestine, your appendix was once believed to be a "vestigial" organ, meaning that it doesn't have a function in the body and is expendable. But is that true? It is now believed that your appendix may enhance your immunity by holding a blueprint for your beneficial gut flora (intestinal bacteria).

If you've had to take antibiotics, for example, you have wiped out all of your good intestinal bacteria. How does your body then repopulate the flora it needs? It initializes a re-colonization of gut flora, and your appendix may play a part in this initialization, as well as determining the type of flora your body needs. With the proper balance of gut flora, your body is better able to fight off infections.

So, what happens if your appendix has been removed? It becomes even more important to eat probiotic-rich foods and reinoculate with fermented foods and probiotic supplements.

until it arrives where it's needed in your digestive system. I believe finding the right probiotic for you is more a matter of trial and error. The proof is in the poop! And there's a good chance you won't need to try more than three at the most to find a supplement that works for you.

Be sure to eat good sources of soluble fiber as well, which "feed" the good bacteria and allow them to improve your digestion. These include sweet potatoes, plantains, taro root, cassava, butternut squash, or any vegetable, root, or tuber with starchy flesh. Be sure to peel or remove any skin on these vegetables because they contain insoluble fiber, which is quite difficult to digest.

Diet isn't the only thing you need to address for optimal large intestine function. If you're stressed, your body will not be able to maintain its normal peristaltic (digestive muscle) motions, which move your food particles through your digestive system. Stress can cause these muscle contractions to speed up or slow down. This happens frequently with travelers whose bodies are just "off" due to time changes, air pressure changes during airplane flights, or changes in the types of foods they eat.

Even changing your position during a bowel movement can help. Sitting on a toilet actually works against the way we were designed to defecate naturally because it causes the rectum to maintain a bent shape. On the other hand, squatting allows the rectum to achieve a straightened shape for easy stool passage.

quick tips: optimizing digestion

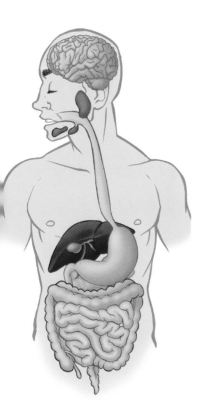

brain

Your brain talks to your stomach and to the rest of your digestive system. The best thing that you can do is sit down and relax before eating any food, whether it's a snack or a full meal. Take the time to decompress and get into the right state of mind for slow, mindful eating. The rest and digest mode is the first step in digesting food properly.

mouth, salivary glands, and esophagus

First, avoid foods high in anti-nutrients (grains and legumes) that resist digestive processing. Then, chew thoroughly until solid food feels almost like liquid in your mouth, and eliminate digestion-resistant insoluble fiber from your diet, such as whole grains, corn, and the skins of starchy tubers. If you experience gas, bloating, or undigested food in your stool, it is also best to limit insoluble fiber, such as in leafy greens like kale, as well as other produce like cauliflower, apples, and pears.

stomach

Remember that heartburn, acid reflux, belching, bloating after meals, and undigested food in your stool are all signs that your stomach acid is too low, not too high. Alter your diet, and take lemon juice, apple cider vinegar, or digestive bitters to increase your body's natural production of HCl, as well as improve the integrity of your stomach's mucosal lining. This will help to ensure that you have adequate stomach acid to properly digest your food.

liver and gallbladder

Pay close attention to how you feel after fatty meals, and check the color of your stools. Any pain or discomfort may indicate that you're not digesting fats well and that your liver and gallbladder need support. Be very strict about eliminating all grain products from your diet, and take supplemental digestive enzymes and ox bile if dietary changes don't bring enough improvement. There are times when the long-term damage takes more time and support to heal, but eliminating grains and reducing overall stress are the first critical steps.

pancreas

Remember the entire downstream effect of the digestive process and that adequate levels of HCl (stomach acid) are critical to signaling secretion of the appropriate amount of digestive enzymes from the pancreas. Your pancreas is smart, and it essentially "reads" the chyme to determine its secretions before food moves on through your small intestine. If you have symptoms of poor digestion, or if you know that you have compromised pancreatic function, supplementing with digestive enzymes may be a good idea for you.

small intestine

Any inflammatory condition is likely rooted in your ability to properly digest and absorb your food. If you struggle with acne, psoriasis, joint pain, or even an advanced autoimmune condition, you can largely resolve these issues by healing your small intestine and getting it to function in a calm state rather than a chronic state of immune-response (leaky gut).

large intestine and rectum

If you're constipated, it should be your first order-of-business to get to the root of the problem and resolve it. If that means some short-term supplementation of probiotics until you can either buy or make your own fermented foods, that's what you should do. Constipation can be quite painful, as well as toxic. Food should move through your body in a timely fashion (about 18-24 hours in total).

guide to: digestion

Since 60-80% of your immune system is *in your gut*, improving digestive function is the first step to calming systemic inflammation. When digestion is working smoothly without irritation and with a healthy transit time, your body's ability to maintain health will be optimized, and your immunity to infections will improve.

improving digestive function

1. Relax and get yourself into the "Rest-and-Digest" parasympathetic dominant mode.

2. Chew your food slowly and completely to begin digestive signaling between your brain and your mouth and to prepare food for initial breakdown in the stomach.

3. Minimize water intake with meals to maintain stomach acid concentration. Drink water in between meals when thirsty to promote healthy transit time and ensure food doesn't linger in the large intestine.

4. Avoid foods that are irritating to the system (primarily refined foods, grain products, legumes, and processed dairy) to allow for the best possible function of the small intestinal lining.

5. Avoid other dietary and lifestyle practices that promote leaky gut (as outlined on the Guide to: Healing a Leaky Gut).

6. Eat probiotic foods regularly: sauerkraut, kimchi, other fermented vegetables, kombucha, yogurt, or kefir from grass-fed and reputable raw milk sources.

7. Use a box or platform to elevate your feet when eliminating; moving from a seated position to the more natural squatting position may help stool pass more easily.

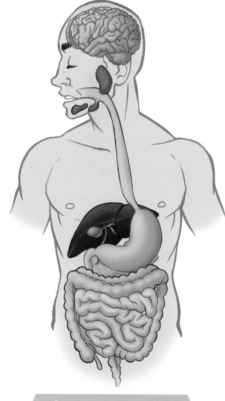

signs & symptoms of DISRUPTED DIGESTION

- Belching
- Bloating
- Gas
- Diarrhea
- Gurgling
- Any elimination other than "ideal"
- Chronic inflammation

test your transit time

A healthy transit time is between 18 and 24 hours.

1. Swallow 2 tablespoons of white sesame seeds following a meal.

2. Note the time and date when the seeds are swallowed.

3. Watch your eliminations for when the bulk of the seeds appear. While a few may be visible here or there, watch for when most of them appear together. They will be intact.

4. Note the time and date when the seeds are eliminated.

too FAST?

Your current diet may include foods that irritate your digestive system, and your body is attempting to move these foods through more quickly.

too SLOW?

Your current diet may need more soluble fiber and good bacteria ("probiotic") content. Additionally, be sure that you are well hydrated (drinking plenty of water in between meals) and that you are finding enough time during the day to relax.

chronic inflammatory conditions CAN ALL BE RELATED TO POOR DIGESTIVE FUNCTION

- Acne
- Allergies
- Alopecia
- Alzheimer's Disease
- Amenorrhea
- Anemia
- Anxiety
- Arthritis and Rheumatoid Arthritis
- Asthma
- Atherosclerosis
- Attention Deficit Disorder (ADD)
- Autoimmunity

- Bloating
- Bone Diseases
- Calcium Deficiency
- Cancer
- Canker Sores
- Celiac Disease
- Chronic Fatigue Syndrome
- Crohn's Disease
- Dermatitis
- Depression
- Diverticulitis
- Dyslexia
- Eczema
- Edema

- Endometriosis
- Epilepsy
- Fatigue, Lethargy
- Fibromyalgia
- Fibrosis
- Gallbladder Disease
- Gastric Ulcers
- Heart Disease
- Hepatitis
- Irritable Bowel Syndrome and Inflammatory Bowel Disease
- Infertility
- Joint Pain and

- Disease
- Kidney Disease
- Lactose Intolerance
- Liver Disease
- Lupus
- Migraines
- Mood Disorders
- Multiple Sclerosis
- Nephritis
- Pancreatitis
- Parkinson's Disease
- PCOS, Hormonal Imbalances
- Pre-and post-natal difficulties

- including difficulty with breast-feeding, infertility, miscarriages, and various obstetrical disorders
- Psoriasis
- Thyroid Disorders
- Diabetes (type 1 & 2)
- Ulcerative Colitis
- Vitamin or Mineral Deficiencies
- Vitiligo
- Weight Gain
- Weight Loss

guide to: your poop!

Understanding your eliminations will help you to figure out exactly what's going on with your digestive system. Track whether your toilet sees Ms. Ideal most often, or if some of her less than beautiful competitors are creeping onto the stage more than once in a while.

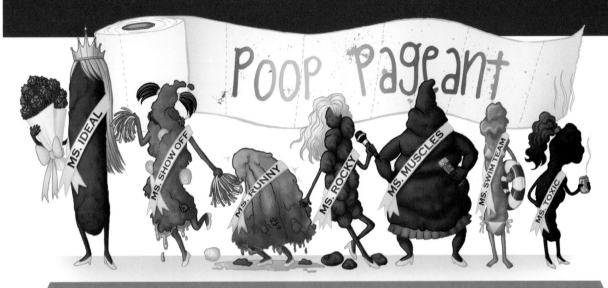

know your poop IT CAN TEACH YOU A LOT

FROM LEFT TO RIGHT, LET'S MEET OUR CONTESTANTS!

ms. ideal
Medium brown in color and solidly formed in the shape of an S or a C, passing easily and regularly one to two times per day.

ms. show off
Varying in color and generally solidly formed, she shows you pieces of foods you recently ate in their semi-whole, visibly identifiable form. She's what you'll see if you are not fully digesting your food and can indicate low stomach acid or a food intolerance.

ms. runny
Varying in color and generally unformed, she shows you pieces of foods you recently ate in their semi-whole, visibly identifiable form. She's what you'll see if you have eaten a food to which your body is reacting strongly and the "everybody out!" mechanism has been initiated. After a bout of diarrhea (which is multiple instances of loose stool over the course of a day or multiple days), it is important to reinoculate your gut with probiotic content.

ms. rocky
Generally dark in color and formed into small balls or pellet shapes, she's what you'll see if you are experiencing a gut flora imbalance, dehydration, stress, or if you're not eating enough soluble fiber. If she's in your toilet, your number one priority is to get rid of her! Probiotic foods (or supplements if you can't tolerate the foods), some starchy vegetables, proper hydration, and meditative breathing will all help to get her moving on out.

ms. muscles
Generally medium to dark brown in color and a shape that's a bit thicker and tougher to pass, she's what you'll see if you are eating a lot of processed forms of protein shakes, bars, or even processed meats. If you see her, swap your processed forms of protein for whole forms like grass-fed steak, pasture-raised eggs, and wild-caught fish.

ms. swim team
Generally light, greenish, or even white in color, she's what you'll see if you have eaten refined, processed, or manmade fats or refined seed oils, more natural fat than you can digest, or if your gallbladder isn't able to properly release bile in response to the fat you've eaten. Avoid bad fats, and consider having your gallbladder checked.

ms. toxic
Dark in color, strong in odor, and generally sinking to the bottom of the bowl, she's what you'll see if you have eaten too many processed or refined foods, you're eating a lot of non-organic foods, or you're experiencing a general toxicity overload from your environment, personal care products, diet, (artificial sweeteners), lifestyle habits (smoking), and use of plastics. Opt for organic, fresh, whole foods and plenty of water and seek out ways to lower toxin load in other areas of your lifestyle.

Illustration adapted from
"How to Eat, Move & Be Healthy," by Paul Chek

is your gut leaky?

- [ ] Eat whole foods and avoid modern, processed, and refined foods.
- [x] **Eat to maintain proper digestive function.**
- [ ] Eat to maintain proper blood sugar regulation.
- [ ] Follow a plan that will help you reach your own personal health goals.

IT'S IN THE GUT

When I say "gut" in this section, understand that it means your small intestine—which you already read about just a few pages back, right?

What happens in your small intestine doesn't always *stay* in your small intestine.

It is the root of your health, and much of what goes on in the rest of your body begins with what happens in this organ, otherwise known as your gut.

So, how does your gut become "leaky"? Clinically known as increased intestinal permeability, leaky gut is a condition in which the cells that line your small intestine begin to lose their integrity. Remember that the foods you eat don't actually get into the cells of your body until they have been broken down and allowed to pass through the small intestinal lining. For a myriad of reasons led strongly by the consumption of food rich in anti-nutrients day in and day out, this process stops working properly. The normal tight junctions between the cells loosen, causing the entire defense system to become compromised.

what are anti-nutrients?

They are primarily plant-based defense mechanisms that are concentrated around the reproductive force in a seed or grain. Consider this: every living thing has a defense mechanism. Plants can't run away when they're under attack, so to ensure that they continue to thrive and grow, they have internal defenses to fight against predators. To the plant, and more specifically the seed or grain of a plant (its reproductive force), your digestive system is just such a predator. These defense mechanisms in the plant fight against your digestion, blocking your ability to fully break the food down into harmless amino acids that are easily absorbed into your cells. In other words, anti-nutrients are elements within a food that either prevent or disrupt the proper digestion and absorption of the nutrients contained in that food.

the foods richest in anti-nutrients are:

- Whole grains, whole grain products, grain-like seeds and legumes that include, but is not limited to, wheat, barley, rye, oats, spelt, brown rice, corn, quinoa, lentils, red beans, black beans, pinto beans, and navy beans.
- Refined grains and refined grain products, including white rice, flour, bread, cereal, crackers, cookies, or pasta.

It's amazing, isn't it, that our culture's diet is centered around these anti-nutrient foods? If I told you I had an omelet for breakfast, a slice of quiche for lunch, and an egg soufflé for dinner, you might say, "Isn't that a lot of eggs?" Yet, if I had eaten cereal for breakfast, a sandwich for lunch, and pasta for dinner, it probably wouldn't occur to you to ask, "Isn't that a lot of grains?"

Still, if you don't think ahead about what you will eat, most of the foods you will find at the store, restaurant—pretty much everywhere—are partially grain-based. Even though our eating habits didn't center around grains for most of human history (our ancestors ate whole foods, not foods from factories), we're so accustomed to grain-based foods today—both refined and so-called "whole" grains—that we seldom question if we're overdoing it. We have been incorrectly taught that it's easy to digest grains. Not so!

why are anti-nutrients such a problem?

The truth is that we lack the digestive capacity to break down those gnarly anti-nutrients in grains. Some believe that over thousands of years of human evolution, our bodies have simply not adapted the digestive enzymes necessary to process grains. Plus, the methods of preparing grains and legumes that were used by traditional cultures are a thing of the past in the industrialized world.

It may also be that our modern upbringing has not supported the complete and healthy development of our digestive systems so that we might be able to tolerate these foods when eaten as a *small* part of our diet. So many of our modern habits contribute to weakened digestive function—a lifetime of eating refined foods, grain products, processed/pasteurized dairy products, and sugar, as well as round after round of antibiotics, stress, NSAID painkillers, and alcohol.

While your system is fully equipped to handle animal proteins that don't carry these anti-nutrients, eating large quantities of digestion-resistant foods day after day can wreak havoc. Large quantities, in this case, can mean even just one slice of bread, one cracker, or a small serving of pasta. *Any portion of grain products can cause problems in your body.* Each time you eat one of these small portions, you consume hundreds or even *thousands* of tiny anti-nutrient-bearing Trojan Horses.

Even just a few decades ago, people realized that there were ways to make grains and legumes more digestible and that simply picking them from plants and grinding them did not make them suitable for consumption. Soaking, sprouting, and fermenting them essentially "tricks" grains and legumes (as well as seeds and nuts, for that matter) into thinking that they've been planted, allowing them to release some of their anti-nutrients and make their *actual* nutrients (vitamins and minerals) available and accessible. While the outer portion of grains and legumes forms a barrier when planted, the nutrients

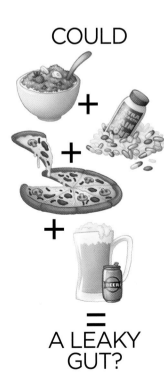

COULD

+

+

+

=

A LEAKY GUT?

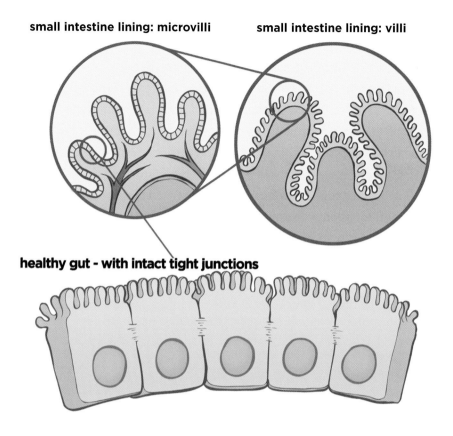

small intestine lining: microvilli   small intestine lining: villi

healthy gut - with intact tight junctions

inside are there to fuel the seed on its mission to grow into a plant.

Nevertheless, even if most people were willing to soak, sprout, and ferment their grains before eating them, these processes only help us digest grains and legumes slightly better. The reality is that meat, vegetables, and naturally occurring fats are all more nutrient-dense and less irritating to the gut than sprouted grains.

digestion run amuck

You have read about what should happen to food particles in your small intestine in the description to your digestion process, but let's discuss in more detail what happens when digestion goes awry.

When digestion is working properly, proteins are broken down into single amino acids or very short chains of amino acids before passing through the lining of your small intestine into your bloodstream. These amino acids are then available for uptake into the rest of your body for use in bodily functions and rebuilding tissues. This normal series of events does not trigger an immune system alarm.

When you consume foods that your body is not able to properly digest and assimilate—either because your body isn't functioning properly or because the foods themselves initiate the damage—food particles that are too large "slip" intact through the weakened and compromised lining of the small intestine and are seen by your body as invaders.

When these "invaders" enter your body, they interact with the immune layer on the other side of the brush border lining of your small intestine, which is known as gut associated lymphoid tissue (GALT). It is at this immune layer that inflammatory molecules called cytokines respond to these intact food particle proteins (amino acid chains) and tell your white blood cells to launch an attack. The by-products of the action of your white blood cells are called oxidants. (I'm sure you've heard about the importance of antioxidants to your health. This is why. They are needed to combat these oxidants that are created in part when you eat foods that your body interprets as harmful.) This is the same type of response that happens in your immune system when any other allergen or invader like a bacteria or virus enters your body. In an effort to fix the problem, your body reads this scenario as disease and reacts with an inflammatory response.

As you can see, your small intestine is an active part of your immune system, not just your digestive system. It's a barrier and a gatekeeper. As Alessio Fasano, M.D., gastroenterologist and leading researcher in the field of Celiac Disease,

leaky gut - with *impaired* tight junctions

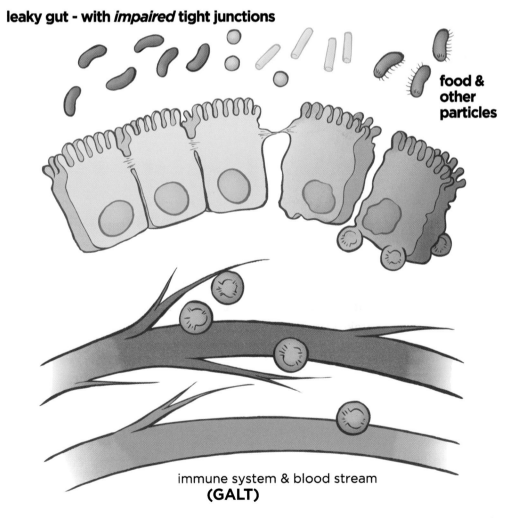

food & other particles

immune system & blood stream
(GALT)

autoimmunity, and intestinal permeability, put it: "Increased permeability ... can cause inflammation in a district distant from where the breach in intestinal barrier occurs."* This is where systemic inflammation comes into the picture.

what is systemic inflammation?

I have mentioned inflammation several times, but let's get clear on what it means inside your body. Inflammation is the biological response of your vascular tissues to infection, damaged cells, or other irritants. These irritants signal your white blood cells to launch an immune response to fix the problem. As your white blood cells do their work, they release free radicals, which are what lead to damage inside your body, and inflammation results.

The inflammatory process in and of itself is not harmful. In fact, inflammation is necessary for survival, especially when it does its job of healing cuts and helping you recover from injuries. The problem occurs when, rather than being left to handle acute issues, your immune system is overworked by chronic irritation. Then, the inflammation becomes chronic as well.

Acute inflammation, by contrast, is the type of healing process that occurs when your body has a skin lesion like a cut, scrape, burn, or bruise, or when you have a trauma like a golf ball hitting you in the head. It may also be a response to soreness after a tough workout or a minor sinus infection or cold. Our bodies are well-equipped to deal with this type of inflammation, and it's the type of damage that the immune system can remain armed to handle intermittently.

When undigested food particles get into your bloodstream on a regular basis, however, the attention of your immune system is drawn to your digestive process, leaving minimal immune response available to handle other problems as they arise. Since anywhere from 60-80% of your immune system is located in your gut as GALT, if your system is constantly bombarded with foods you don't tolerate or digest well, your ability to fight infections, allergies, cancer, diabetes, heart disease, and more will be impaired. This means that when a cold is going around the office or the pollen count skyrockets, your body may only have the ability to use about 20-40% of your potential immune response to fight it off. The rest of your immune capabilities are busy responding to the irritation from food particles in your digestive system.

That leads us to chronic inflammation in the body's systems (systemic inflammation), which is like being in a constant state of low-grade infection. Your immune system never gets downtime between healing one problem and gearing up to solve another one. With no period of recovery after its period of work, your immune system is on alert 24/7. Obviously, this takes a toll on your body, diminishing its ability to heal life-threatening issues.

Remember, inflammation is the body's response to a *perceived* problem. When your body thinks there's a *constant* problem, it lives in a *constant* state of

*source: Fasano, Alessio, M.D. "Zonulin and Its Regulation of Intestinal Barrier Function: The Biological Door to Inflammation, Autoimmunity, and Cancer." Physiol Rev., January 1, 2011 vol. 91 no. 1 151-175.

- Acne
- Allergies
- Alopecia
- Alzheimer's Disease
- Amenorrhea
- Anemia
- Anxiety
- Arthritis and Rheumatoid Arthritis
- Asthma
- Atherosclerosis
- Attention Deficit Disorder (ADD)
- Autoimmunity
- Bloating
- Bone Diseases
- Calcium Deficiency
- Cancer
- Canker Sores
- Celiac Disease
- Chronic Fatigue Syndrome
- Crohn's Disease
- Dermatitis
- Depression
- Diverticulitis
- Dyslexia
- Eczema
- Edema
- Endometriosis
- Epilepsy
- Fatigue, Lethargy
- Fibromyalgia
- Fibrosis
- Gallbladder Disease
- Gastric Ulcers
- Heart Disease
- Hepatitis
- Irritable Bowel Syndrome and Inflammatory Bowel Disease
- Infertility
- Joint Pain and Disease
- Kidney Disease
- Lactose Intolerance
- Liver Disease
- Lupus
- Migraines
- Mood Disorders
- Multiple Sclerosis
- Nephritis
- Pancreatitis
- Parkinson's Disease
- PCOS, Hormonal Imbalances
- Pre-and post-natal difficulties including difficulty with breast-feeding, infertility, miscarriages, and various obstetrical disorders
- Psoriasis
- Thyroid Disorders
- Diabetes (type 1 & 2)
- Ulcerative Colitis
- Vitamin or Mineral Deficiencies
- Vitiligo
- Weight Gain
- Weight Loss

inflammation. This chronic, constant inflammatory state underlies all chronic disease and suppressed immunity. Essentially, it's at the root of just about every disease imaginable.

Know this: Food particles that pass through your gut lining without being broken down completely are seen as invaders, and your body responds in the same way as it does toward a virus or bacterial infection.

mirror, mirror, in your cells

The resulting immune response may eventually cause any of the myriad chronic inflammatory conditions on the list, or, alternatively, it may cascade into something even more serious known as molecular mimicry. All of our cells are made up of amino acids—the same amino acids that we eat. In the case of a leaky gut, some of the undigested food particles that pass into your bloodstream contain amino acid chains that match (or mimic) body tissue proteins (self-cells), and the resulting immune attack is launched indiscriminately. **This means that your body attacks the invading food-based amino acid, as well as the amino acid chains of the self-cells. The cells under attack can be part of any body tissues—whether organs, hormones, or joint tissue. This is what is called an autoimmune condition—one in which the body begins to attack itself.**

figuring out your food intolerances

How do you know if your body can't tolerate a particular food? Most overt food allergies result in identifiable, immediate forms of discomfort to the eater. Someone with a tree-nut or shellfish allergy knows immediately if they've eaten something they shouldn't. They often experience an itchy feeling in the mouth or a closed-up throat as a result. Those who suffer with lactose intolerance can tell you how it feels shortly after they eat the offending dairy product—gas,

ARE YOU INFLAMED?
Inflammation may rear its ugly head in a myriad of ways. To work on healing your digestive process as well as a leaky gut, check out the guides on pages 74 and 88.

MOLECULAR MIMICRY EXAMPLE:

AMINO ACIDS IN A GLUTEN PROTEIN	AMINO ACIDS IN A BODY (SELF) CELL

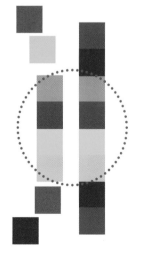

bloating, or digestive discomfort. Those are all very obvious signs.

When it comes to grains, many—perhaps even most—people experience some kind of discomfort, whether acute or chronic, but not always the expected digestive discomfort. While some people have blatant allergies to protein constituents in grains (people with Celiac disease are very seriously allergic to gluten proteins, for example), inflammatory problems are usually caused by some level of *intolerance* to grains and legumes. If someone experiences symptoms after eating, they likely blame a food *other* than the grains, or they attribute the problem to something other than food. This is what makes grain intolerance so problematic. Many of the symptoms are not easily connected to diet. Delayed onset reactions, including the chronic inflammatory conditions listed, are more often the end result of grain intolerance.

The timeframe within which you can experience food allergy or intolerance symptoms is up to 72 hours after eating a meal. This means that even a food you ate *three days ago* can cause seemingly unrelated symptoms *today*. Take your pick from the array of conditions on the list that go beyond digestive distress, not to mention that you may have a symptom that isn't on the list at all. Luckily, there's a method for determining the culprits of your symptoms.

When you identify a possible food intolerance reaction, your body is, in effect, under attack. So, until you stop eating the offending food(s) for at least two weeks (preferably three or four), you may not be able to identify the direct line between cause and effect. You must allow your body to recover from the attack, after which you can gradually reintroduce the potentially offending foods to determine your intolerances. It takes roughly two to three weeks for the entire lining of your small intestine to heal after you have stopped eating offending foods. After that, if you're intolerant to the food, you will have an identifiable response to it when you eat it again. This is what is called an "elimination-provocation diet," which is explained in more detail on page 88. It works because your immune system has had a chance to rest and calm down.

Since you didn't perceive such a severe intolerance when you were eating that food more frequently, is it possible that you'd be able to avoid food intolerances if you just ate a little of that food every day? Unfortunately, it isn't that simple. This is where the chronic, negative effects of a grain or other food intolerance really wreak havoc. It's the effects that you *don't* feel immediately that are often far worse than the ones you *do* feel. This is the difference between an *acute* inflammatory response and a *chronic* inflammatory response. In the acute response, you feel the effects right away. Your body communicates, "This isn't good; don't eat it again!" The chronic response, however, leaves your body's systems overwhelmed with inflammation and stress due to an ongoing onslaught of the food. You don't have to be aware of the problem for it to become systemic and dangerous!

"ALLERGIC" TO EVERYTHING?
If you've had a food allergy test done and the results showed allergies to 50 foods, chances are, you're not actually allergic or even intolerant to all of those foods—you probably have a leaky gut! Once you heal your gut, far fewer of those foods will be likely to cause any irritation.

Know this: If your health is not optimal, eliminate gut-irritating, anti-nutrient rich foods—grains, including gluten-containing forms; legumes; processed dairy; and other refined foods—from your diet and you'll likely experience a dramatic improvement in your health. Oh, wait, that sounds an awful lot like a Paleo diet!

guide to anti-nutrients

There are different kinds of anti-nutrients, and they affect your body in different ways. It's worth understanding a bit about how anti-nutrients work.

Phytate. Also known as phytic acid, phytate is an indigestible, mineral-binding compound that is located in the hulls of grains, legumes, nuts, and seeds. While ruminant animals like cows, sheep, and goats have adequate enzymes in their digestive systems to break down phytates, non-ruminants, like humans, do not. Phytates bind to minerals within foods, including calcium, magnesium, iron, and zinc, and this process prevents their absorption in our bodies. This means that we're unable to actually use the minerals we eat when they're blocked by the phytates we also eat in those foods.

Just how important are these minerals that are blocked by phytates? Minerals have a role in every cellular function in your body. They are responsible for proper formation and regeneration of structural tissues to prevent you from easily sustaining injuries such as fractures, broken bones, torn ligaments, and osteoporosis. Minerals also serve as anti-oxidants to help you better fight cancer, and they protect against heart disease by mediating the appropriate constriction and relaxation of blood vessels. Proper mineral reserves are also necessary to regulate hormones for fertility and stress management, among other things. There is no end to the types of body systems and tissues that require minerals for proper function. We simply need them for everything!

Magnesium alone is required to complete over 300 enzymatic processes in your body. Most of us don't obtain enough magnesium from our diets, so nutritionists frequently suggest that their clients take magnesium supplements.

Mineral deficiencies can result in a myriad of symptoms that include, but are not limited to, suppressed immunity, fatigue, insomnia, irritability, heart palpitations, muscle cramps, restless leg syndrome, muscle spasms, asthma, migraines, constipation, and hormonal imbalances like premenstrual syndrome (PMS), polycystic ovarian syndrome (PCOS), and infertility in both men and women.

We already know that soils today are depleted in mineral content, so the vegetables and fruits we eat are far less mineral-rich than those our ancestors ate. The high-stress, high-sugar, modern lifestyle also tends to deplete our systems of minerals, which means we need even more perhaps than our ancestors when we go through life events like growth spurts, puberty, pregnancy, infection, intense exercise, illness, high stress, trauma, or surgery. All of these factors create a greater need for minerals and other nutrients. Therefore, we have to make sure we not only get sufficient amounts in our diets, but that we're also able to use the minerals and other nutrients we ingest. What's the point of eating a nutrient-rich food if the nutrients are going to be inaccessible inside you?

Grains and legumes are not the only plants that contain phytates, however. Nuts and seeds contain them, too. For most nuts and seeds, their hard outer shell is the first "barrier to entry" to accessing the reproductive force of the plant. For this reason, they're well tolerated by most people in small quantities once the shell has been removed, but only when combined with a balanced, mineral-rich Paleo diet. Phytates are the main reason why large quantities of nuts and seeds are not recommended. (You will notice that nuts and seeds are eliminated entirely in some of the meal plans in the book. This is to offer the best possible chance of healing for people with specific health conditions.)

Know this: You can absorb more of the minerals you take in (from foods like leafy green vegetables and bone broth), including calcium, magnesium, iron, and zinc to name a few, simply by removing grains from your diet and not overdoing it with nuts and seeds. Remember that phytates keep minerals and other nutrients out of reach of your body's systems.

Lectins. These are sugar-binding proteins that are resistant to digestive enzymes and stomach acid. They are richly present in the seeds of plants, becoming less concentrated as plants grow. They can stick to the cells in the lining of the small intestine, impairing digestive function by altering the texture of the cell walls.

We need the cells that line our small intestine to remain intact and ready to absorb nutrients. If they become sticky from overconsumption of lectin-rich foods, like grains and legumes, digestion becomes quite difficult. Grains and legumes are actually the *seeds* of plants, and when you eat a grain product, you're eating hundreds, if not thousands, of the seeds of a plant. That's a lot of concentrated lectins!

Saponins. Bitter-tasting, soap-like molecules with the ability to puncture or create pores in cell membranes (walls); saponins are often used as carriers for vaccines due to their ability to infiltrate cells. Saponins are the main anti-

eggs contain anti-nutrients, too.

As the reproductive force of the chicken (or other animal laying them), eggs contain built-in defense mechanisms that help them to resist predation beyond simply their thin, easily cracked shells. When mama-bird gets up and walks away from guarding her nest, these anti-nutrients protect the eggs from within their shell and help to warn other animals against their consumption. While most humans are well adapted to eating eggs without issue, some people are sensitive to them for this reason.

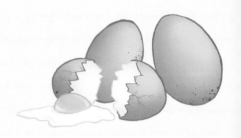

nutrient in quinoa (pronounced keen-wa). They have the ability to stimulate an immune response from within your cells and can up-regulate antibody production. When you create more antibodies, your body gets revved up and ready to launch at the first sign of an offending undigested food particle in your blood stream. This is what causes digestive distress after eating certain foods or even leads to the more behind-the-scenes chronic inflammation. Remember, you don't want to eat foods that cause an immune response of any kind.

zon-u-what?

One last—but certainly no less important—mechanism by which the lining of your small intestine may become "leaky" is through the action of a molecule called zonulin. Simply put, according to Dr. Alessio Fasano, zonulin increases leaky gut by loosening that tight junction between the cells that was mentioned at the beginning of the chapter. This process is a factor in the development of inflammation, autoimmune diseases, and cancer.

Sound dismal? Don't sweat it! Fasano says that the condition caused by zonulin and other anti-nutrients can usually be reversed through *changing your diet and lifestyle*. The glass is actually half full because you can take an active role in improving your gut barrier function, which, in turn, will improve your immunity and your ability to resist chronic diseases.

beyond food: leaky gut contributors aplenty

While dietary factors are not necessarily the *least* harmful, they are the easiest to *control* through everyday choices. Take a look at the "leaky gut contributors" on the chart on page 88. The factors listed become increasingly difficult to consciously control as you move from the bottom to the top of the list, but you *can* take steps to work on all of them, starting first with your diet and lifestyle changes.

Managing stress is one of the best ways to start to improve leaky gut. This helps to reduce cortisol, your body's fight or flight hormone. Cortisol output places extreme demands on your body. In fact, my clients have consistently reported better digestive function on days of lower stress like during weekends or vacations. Incidentally, we could probably significantly reduce the need for several classes of medications like antacids and NSAIDs by reducing physical and emotional stress. Meditation, yoga, golf, walking, listening to relaxing music, and even fun activities with friends and family can reduce stress.

If you have an autoimmune condition, you may always have a leaky gut to some degree. This doesn't mean you should throw in the towel, however, and just eat foods that you know contribute to the problem. If you have a known autoimmune condition, all the more reason to keep your diet and lifestyle "ducks" in a row. This gives your gut the best possible chance of properly digesting and assimilating nutrients from food.

Most people who change their diet report alleviation of symptoms of one or more of the chronic inflammatory conditions listed on page 74 within anywhere from two weeks to six months. Even if you cannot control all factors that have caused your leaky gut condition, you may very well be able to take control of your health in ways you never thought possible and cross a few chronic conditions off your list.

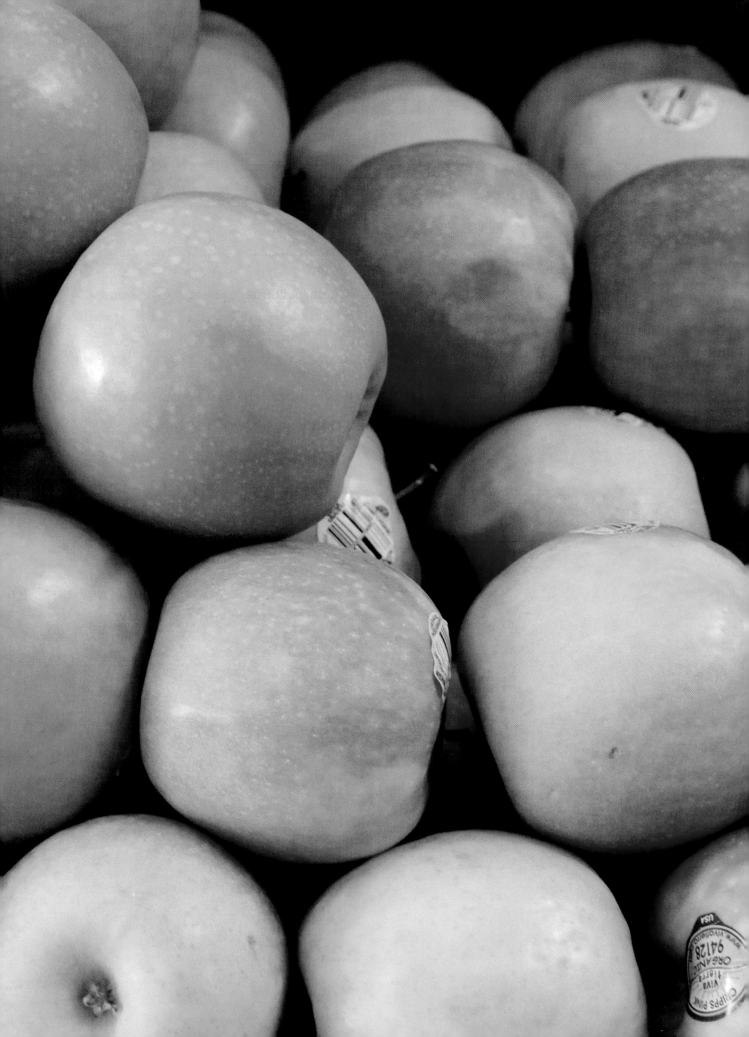

guide to: healing a leaky gut

Leaky gut (also known as intestinal permeability) is when your digestive system isn't functioning properly. Rather than only allowing fully broken-down proteins in the form of single amino acids to pass into your bloodstream, it allows larger, partially undigested proteins to pass through. This is normal in infants, as their systems are not yet fully developed, but in adults, it leads to a myriad of health concerns and uncomfortable symptoms.

signs & symptoms

gi distress:
· Constipation
· Diarrhea
· Pain
· Bloating
· Gas

nutrient malabsorption
· Undesired weight loss or weight loss resistance
· Fatty acid deficiency or vitamin and mineral deficiency

compromised immunity
· Frequent colds, flu, intense seasonal allergies, or inflammatory responses

how your gut gets leaky CONTRIBUTING FACTORS

CATEGORIES ON THE BOTTOM REPRESENT FACTORS WE MAY BE ABLE TO BETTER CONTROL VIA DAILY DIET AND LIFESTYLE CHOICES THAN THOSE ON THE TOP.

neurological
· AGEs (advanced glycation end products)
· Intestinal inflammation
· Autoimmunity

hormonal
· Thyroid imbalances
· Sex hormone imbalances
· Cortisol (chronic stress)

stress
· Decreased stomach acid
· Catecholemines
· Cortisol (chronic or acute)

infections
· H. Pylori
· Bacterial overgrowth
· Yeast overgrowth
· Intestinal virus
· Parasitic infections

medications
· NSAIDs
· Corticosteroids
· Antibiotics
· Antacids
· Xenobiotics
· Chemotherapy & radiation

diet
· Alcohol
· Grains (especially gluten)
· Dairy (especially casein)
· Legumes
· Anti-nutrients
· Processed foods
· Sugar
· Fast foods
· Trans and damaged fats

small intestine lining: microvilli   small intestine lining: villi

healthy gut - with intact tight junctions

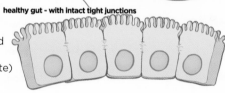

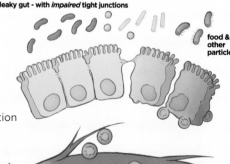
leaky gut - with *impaired* tight junctions

food & other particles

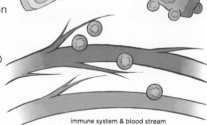
immune system & blood stream

what to do about HEALING IT

THE 4R PROTOCOL

remove
Common dietary irritants, such as processed and refined foods, alcohol, grains, legumes, dairy, refined seed oils, and sugar. If you have already removed those foods, remove nuts, seeds, coffee, and eggs as a next step.

Anti-inflammatory medications, specifically NSAIDs. Work on preventing the need for NSAIDs via diet and lifestyle.

repair
EAT adequate omega-3 fatty acids to balance out the naturally high omega-6 diet that most of us eat.

EAT adequate amounts of soluble fiber in starchy vegetables or fruits like sweet potatoes, butternut squash, and plantains.

DRINK herbal teas like peppermint and licorice root to aid in repairing the mucosal lining of your digestive system.

DRINK adequate amounts of water to prevent constipation and dehydration.

SUPPLEMENT the amino acid L-glutamine in water between meals to help with gut lining repair (5-8g per day).

SUPPLEMENT omega-3 and fat-soluble vitamin-rich fermented cod liver oil/butter oil blend (1/2-1 tsp per day) - Green Pasture brand.

SUPPLEMENT quercitin, a powerful antioxidant to help with inflammation and DGL (deglycerized licorice) to promote the repair of the mucosal lining of the gut.

reinoculate
EAT probiotic foods like raw sauerkraut or other fermented vegetables.

SUPPLEMENT with probiotics in pill or powder form if desired.

reintroduce
EAT one of the eliminated foods at each of your meals on day 31 after the elimination and note any changes to your mood, energy, mental clarity, digestive function, and your skin. Repeat the reintroduction of one eliminated food every three days to discover which are causing problems and which are not.

NOTE: the reintroduction of gluten-containing grains is not recommended.

guide to: gluten

What is it? Gluten is a protein found in wheat, rye oats, and barley. Gluten is the composite of a prolamin and a glutelin, which exist, conjoined with starch, in the endosperm of various grass-related grains. Gliadin, a water-soluble, and glutenin, a water-insoluble, (the prolamin and glutelin from wheat) compose about 80% of the protein contained in wheat seed. Being insoluble in water, they can be purified by washing away the associated starch. Worldwide, gluten is a source of protein, both in foods prepared directly from sources containing it, and as an additive to foods otherwise low in protein.

sources of gluten OR ITEMS THAT MAY CONTAIN HIDDEN GLUTEN

- Ales
- Barley
- Barley malt/extract
- Beer & lagers
- Bran
- Breading
- Broth
- Brown rice syrup
- Bulgur
- Candy coating
- Communion "wafers"
- Couscous
- Croutons
- Durum
- Einkorn
- Emmer
- Farina
- Farro
- Gloss & balms
- Graham flour
- Herbal blends
- Imitation
- Imitation seafood
- Kamut
- Lipstick
- Luncheon meats
- Malt
- Makeup
- Marinades
- Matzo flour/meal
- Meat/sausages
- Medications
- Orzo
- Panko
- Pasta
- Play dough
- Roux
- Rye
- Sauces
- Seitan
- Self-basting poultry
- Semolina
- Soup base
- Soy sauce
- Spelt
- Spice blends
- Stuffing
- Supplements
- Thickeners
- Triticale
- Udon
- Vinegar (malt only)
- Vital wheat gluten
- Vitamins
- Wafers
- Wheat
- Wheat bran
- Wheat germ
- Wheat starch

gluten-free* (BUT STILL NOT RECOMMENDED)

*Nearly all processed foods and grains carry some risk of cross-contamination. For the safest approach to a gluten-free diet, eat only whole, unprocessed foods.

- Amaranth
- Arrowroot
- Buckwheat
- Corn
- Flax
- Millet
- Montina™
- Nut flour
- Bean flour
- Potato flour
- Potato starch
- Quinoa
- Rice
- Rice bran
- Sago
- Seed flour
- Sorghum
- Soy (soya)
- Tapioca
- Teff

most common sources of HIDDEN GLUTEN

Alcohol:
Beer, malt beverages, grain alcohols

Cosmetics:
Check ingredients on makeup, shampoo, and other personal care items

Dressings:
Thickened with flour or other additives

Fried foods:
Cross contamination with breaded items in fryers

Vinegar: Malt varieties

Medications, vitamins, and supplements:
ask the pharmacist and read the labels closely

Processed / packaged foods:
Additives often contain gluten

Sauces, soups, and stews: Thickened with flour

Soy, Teriyaki, and Hoisin sauces:
Fermented with wheat

signs of gluten EXPOSURE

- Abdominal bloating
- Fatigue
- Skin problems or rashes
- Diarrhea or constipation
- Irritable, moody
- Change in energy levels
- Unexpected weight loss, mouth ulcers, depression, and even Crohn's disease are all more severe gluten allergy symptoms that you may experience.

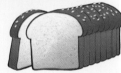

- Consult with your nutritionist or physician if you experience symptoms of a gluten exposure that result in prolonged discomfort.

gluten-free BOOZE**

- Brandy
- Bourbon
- Cognac
- Gin
- Grappa
- Rum
- Sake
- Scotch
- Sherry
- Tequila
- Vermouth
- Vodka
- Whiskey
- Wine
- Champagne
- Mead
- Hard cider
- Gluten-free beers

i am allergic TO GLUTEN

I have a severe allergy and have to follow a STRICT gluten-free diet.

I may become very ill if I eat food containing flours or grains of wheat, rye, barley, or oats.

Does this food contain flour or grains of wheat, barley rye, or oats? If you or the chef/kitchen staff are uncertain about what the food contains, please tell me.

I CAN eat food containing rice, maize, potatoes, vegetables, fruit, eggs, cheese, milk, meat, and fish as long as they are NOT cooked with wheat flour, batter, breadcrumbs, or sauce containing any of those ingredients.

Thank you for your help!

For more gluten-guides, visit: www.celiactravel.com

for more information ON GLUTEN

These sites are not necessarily "Paleo" but will give ample information for those who need to be 100% strictly gluten-free

- celiac.com
- celiac.org
- celiaccentral.org
- celiaclife.com
- celiactravel.com
- celiacsolution.com
- elanaspantry.com
- glutenfreegirl.com
- surefoodsliving.com

**According to celiac.com, all distilled alcohols are gluten-free but for someone with overt Celiac Disease, avoiding alcohols made from wheat, barley, and rye is still recommended.

The Why—Food & Your Body

a few words on stress management

Managing stress to avoid leaky gut (and the myriad other psychological and physical harmful effects of chronic stress) may require changes to your lifestyle. In my life, I certainly had to do more than just change my diet.

When I decided to pursue nutrition coaching as a full-time career, it wasn't without great reflection. I was living in a nice, top floor apartment in San Francisco with parking, laundry, a view, and a dishwasher. It was an enviable lifestyle in many ways, but keeping that fancy roof with all the trimmings over my head meant I had to work at a job that didn't feed my soul. I dreaded waking up every single morning.

Are you in a similar situation, constantly complaining about your job? Your body? Your significant other? Your friends? Your life? On an everyday basis, would you consider yourself happy? Do you live for the weekends? Are there days you dread waking up?

These questions get to the heart of the choices you make every day, and they help you to identify whether you're living a life of your own choosing. Brian Tracy, one of my favorite motivational speakers, says in his series, *The Psychology of Achievement:* "We feel good about ourselves to the exact degree to which we feel we are in control of our own lives."

Do you feel you're driving your life, or do you feel everyone or everything in your life is driving you? If you feel that having a family and the responsibility to provide financially for their needs prevents you from making a career or life change, look closely at your expenses. Do you need that bigger, fancier car? Do you need that bigger house or extra garage? It may even be as simple as asking if you need that daily latte, which can easily add up to $1,000-a-year daily habit.

When we feel out of control in our lives, we experience great stress. In *The Paleo Solution*, Robb Wolf puts it well: "Stress is an inescapable and significant factor in people's lives, and a stunning amount of ... stress is self-induced. People might benefit from considering how they want to spend their time and resources.... If you are attached to a bunch of crap that requires you to work ungodly hours to pay for it, you are missing something.... If you have weight or health issues, work yourself to death, have a closet full of clothes you never wear, and a house full of crap you never use, then maybe you need to do some thinking about how you approach your life."

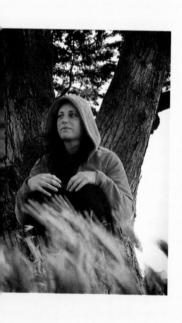

If stress is a problem in your life, it's time to make some new choices about how to drive it. Take steps to learn stress management techniques. You now know better than ever just how important it is to not just your psychological health, but also to your physical health.

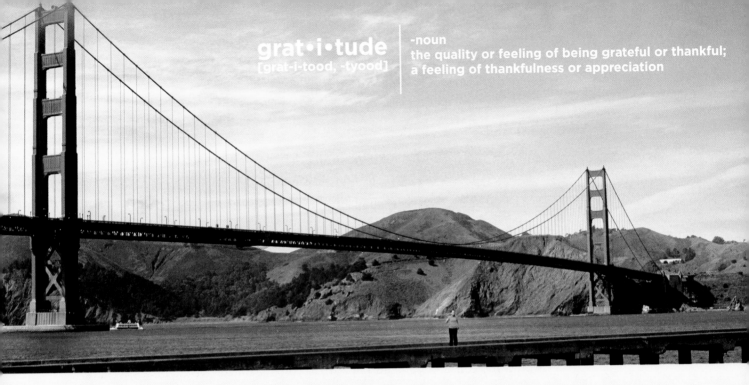

grat•i•tude
[grat-i-tood, -tyood]

-noun
the quality or feeling of being grateful or thankful;
a feeling of thankfulness or appreciation

practice an attitude of gratitude

On health educator Charles Poliquin's website (www. charlespoliquin.com), weight loss coach Jonny Bowden published a post entitled, "The Nine Habits of Highly Healthy People." One of those habits was creating a "gratitude list." He wrote: "By making a list of things you're grateful for, you focus the brain on positive energy. Gratitude is incompatible with anger and stress. Practice using your under-utilized 'right brain' and spread some love. Focusing on what you're grateful for—even for five minutes a day—has the added benefit of being one of the best stress-reduction techniques on the planet."

Some people think such a list is "hippy dippy Pollyanna nonsense," but if you are in a constant state of stress that is negatively impacting your health, it's worth a try, isn't it? After all, most of us spend our time focusing on the negatives and never stop to think about all the positives in our lives.

Bowden suggests that we create these lists daily if we can, but at the very least, it's a good idea to stop and make such a list when it crosses your mind or when you are in a particularly stressful state of mind. Simply pause, and remember what's most important to you.

You can share your list with your friends or loved ones or keep it to yourself. It doesn't matter if no one ever sees it but you. That said, I find that telling people in your life that you are grateful for their presence always yields positive results. How much would it lower your stress level if someone told you today that they appreciate you? (I thought so!) It might even help in your quest toward healing a leaky gut.

You can download a blank Gratitude List PDF from the book resources page on my website: www.balancedbites.com

The Why—Food & Your Body

blood sugar regulation: getting your carbohydrate intake right

There is a great deal of confusion about carbohydrates in the world of health and nutrition these days. Which are good, and which are bad? How many carbohydrates should you eat and how often?

Eat whole foods and avoid modern, processed, and refined foods.

Eat to maintain proper digestive function.

✓ **Eat to maintain proper blood sugar regulation.**

Follow a plan that will help you reach your own personal health goals.

Let's get one thing straight first: All carbohydrates are seen as sugar in your body, but that doesn't mean that all carbs are bad. Any food you eat that isn't a protein or a fat is a carbohydrate. There are only three different kinds of foods: proteins, fats, and carbohydrates (or some combination of the three).

good carbs, bad carbs

There are indeed "*good* carbs" and "*bad* carbs." It isn't what you think, though. I'm not going to talk about complex carbs versus simple carbs. If so, I'd be the same as most other nutritionists who suggest you eat copious amounts of whole grains. We've been there and done that, and it certainly hasn't made us healthier.

Bad carbs are those which: (1) are void of nutrients for their proper metabolism; (2) may cause digestive distress; and (3) are refined and man-made/factory-made.

Good carbs are those which: (1) contain easily digestible, bio-available nutrients that make it possible to metabolize them at a cellular level; and (2) are available from nature as whole foods.

When I say "void of nutrients," what do I mean? Well, you've heard about "empty calories." To understand this concept, you need to get a picture of how carbohydrates are processed in your body.

When you eat any kind of carbohydrate, your body expends energy in the form of micronutrients (vitamins and minerals) in order to metabolize the sugar within the food. Before the energy and nutrition from the food you eat can nourish your cells, it must be broken down into its various constituents. Your cells can't make use of a doughnut or a strawberry! In order to power *you*, your cells need macronutrients (proteins, carbs, and fats) and micronutrients (vitamins and minerals) to first power *them*.

Without both macro and micronutrients, your energy levels would

MACRO & MICRO

Protein, fat, and carbohydrates are macronutrients. They each carry calories with them to provide your body with energy. Vitamins and minerals are micronutrients. They do not carry calories, but they are required cofactors to the proper metabolism and assimilation of the fuel that macronutrients provide.

plummet. To metabolize carbohydrates and turn them into cellular energy, you need B vitamins (especially B5) and the minerals of phosphorous, magnesium, iron, copper, manganese, zinc, and chromium.

Cellular energy is your gasoline. Collectively, your cells come together to drive the engine that keeps you moving throughout the day. This is why a diet rich in bad carbs makes you tired. When you eat carbohydrates in refined forms, the food carries calories from the *macronutrients*, but lacks the *micronutrient* cofactors that help you put those calories to use at the cellular level. This is where the issue of good versus bad carbs makes a difference in your body.

Just four teaspoons of table sugar (a bad carb) delivers a total of sixty calories in carbohydrate form. That's it. It doesn't give you anything else— no nutrients at all. One small sweet potato (a good carb), on the other hand, contains about sixty calories in carbohydrate form but also gives you B vitamins, phosphorous, magnesium, iron, copper, manganese, zinc, and chromium. These are the *exact* micronutrients your body needs to metabolize carbohydrates. *This* is the difference between a whole, unrefined, nutrient-dense food and a refined, nutrient-poor food. (Incidentally, the sweet potato also gives you vitamin E, beta-carotene, vitamin C, calcium, potassium, zinc, and selenium.)

When you eat whole, nutrient-dense foods like sweet potatoes or other vegetables, fruits, roots, and tubers, you give your body everything it needs right in one "package" to effectively turn those calories into energy. In other words, eating whole, nutrient-dense foods allows you to make nutritional deposits into your body's "energy bank account." Nutrient-poor foods like sugar ask your body for a withdrawal without making a deposit.

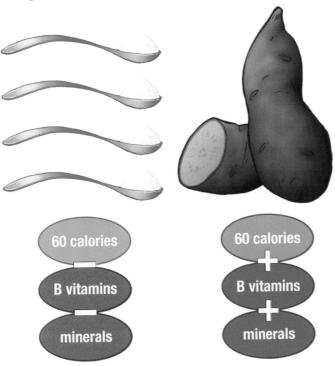

are you carb loading for your desk job?

Carbohydrates are a fast-acting fuel source and are broken down in your body into glucose (sugar) whether they begin as Pop-Tarts or fresh pineapple. If you become active shortly after eating, the glucose is then used quickly. If not, the glucose is stored in your body as one of two things: glycogen (jargon for "stored glucose") in your liver and muscles, or as fat. *Yes, fat.*

Your body can only store glycogen in two places: your liver and your muscles. When you eat carbohydrates, your body "checks" to see how much is already stored in those two places before deciding how to handle what you've just eaten. If you have been active and have used up some of your stores in your liver and muscles, your body will replenish it with the new food.

While your body has only limited places to store carbohydrates, it has *unlimited* storage sites for fat. So, what happens when you eat more carbohydrates than your body can store in your liver and muscles, and you don't use it right away through activity? The glycogen tanks aren't emptied, and your liver converts the extra carbs into one of two types of fat: triglycerides (circulating blood fat) or adipose (body fat).

Carbohydrate storage that takes place after you exercise is the exception to this rule. Your muscles have first dibs on the carbs you eat in your post-workout meal (any meal eaten between thirty minutes and two hours *after* exercise, but remember to go into rest-and-digest mode *before* eating). This allows your muscles to be replenished and restored for your next workout and is just one of the many benefits of exercise—getting carbohydrates right into your muscles rather than as fat on your bum, belly, or wherever else you don't want it.

Fat on your bum may be undesirable, but fat can *also* be stored closely around your organs. This is called visceral fat, and it's more dangerous than

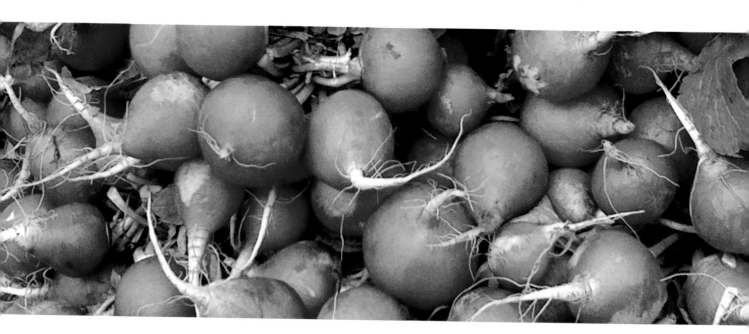

that extra junk in your trunk because it has the capacity to impede organ function due to its close proximity.

Your genes have some say in how *your* body handles the selection of where to store extra carbs as fat. You may know people, for example, who can seem to eat lots of carbs and never work out. Yet, they don't have much muscle tone. Their bodies are likely converting more of their excess carbohydrate intake into triglycerides and visceral fat than to visible body fat that makes their clothes tighter. They seem lucky because their clothing size remains the same, but they're actually in more trouble because they are probably walking around with more the visceral fat (around their organs) or high triglycerides. Unfortunately, this lack of visible cue leaves people in the dark as to their inner state of health. So, someone who isn't visibly overweight isn't necessarily healthy if they're eating more carbs than they are able to burn. While genetics are involved, you can certainly improve your health by refusing to add to the visceral fat in your body via what you eat.

carbs and exercise

Carbs can be somewhat useful in fueling moderately active lifestyles such as construction work, physical education, personal training, or other work that requires you stand on your feet all day. Carbs are mostly useful, however, in fueling higher intensity exercise that lasts for longer periods of time. High-intensity exercise like sprinting or a CrossFit style workout that lasts more than five minutes relies on carbohydrates to fuel your body, but this doesn't mean you need to "carb-load" for a five-minute or even thirty-minute workout. Regular, moderate carb intake will provide you with sufficient fuel for these activities. If you regularly perform sixty minutes of high-intensity exercise, you may need to eat more carbs on those days.

Know this: You should eat carbohydrates according to your average activity and stress levels to avoid storing extra body fat, keep triglyceride levels in a healthy place, and to prevent visceral fat development around your organs.

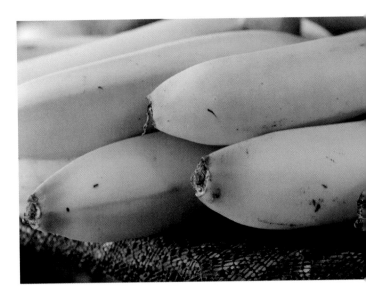

SUFFICIENT CARBOHYDRATE INTAKE (FROM GOOD CARBS!)	GENERAL LIFESTYLE FACTORS: ACTIVITY & STRESS LEVELS
very low carb*: **0-30g/day**	An inactive person or insulin-resistant person seeking to make drastic changes to their sugar metabolism; someone interested in a ketogenic diet approach (see page 176); **not recommended or necessary for most people seeking general, optimal health.**
low carb: **30-75g/day**	Not very active or participating in intense cardiovascular activity that lasts *fewer* than twenty minutes; also suitable for most weight lifting and strength-training individuals; someone interested in a ketogenic diet approach (up to ~50g of carbs) (see page 176); **this is a healthy range for many people.**
moderate carb: **75-150g/day**	Moderately active or completing intense cardiovascular activity that lasts between twenty and sixty minutes per day; a generally active job or lifestyle; a moderately stressful lifestyle; **this is a healthy range for many people.**
higher carb: **150g+/day** **(up to around 300g)**	Intense cardiovascular activity that lasts more than sixty minutes per day; a very active job with consistent movement; a very stressful lifestyle that is mentally and physically demanding; **this is a healthy range for people who are very active or have very stressful lives.**

* A prolonged very low carb approach is not recommended for most people, as we may miss out on some of the beneficial micronutrients available in carbohydrate-rich foods. While nose-to-tail animal food consumption including all organ meats would circumvent this issue, most people are not eating animals in this fashion today. Good carbs are also important for proper digestive function, as carbohydrates aid in balancing healthy gut flora (bacterial balance).

carb here often?

If you don't need to eat lots of carbs to fuel your daily life, what *do* you need to eat? That's easy—fat.

Fat serves as a perfect, long-lasting fuel source for your body, but here's the catch: Your body can't efficiently burn fat for fuel (from your food *or* from your fanny) if you are constantly eating a steady stream of carbohydrates.

In order to become what is called "fat-adapted," meaning your body knows how to effectively use fat for fuel, you have to stop giving it sugar (carbs) all day, every day. Sorry to be the bearer of bad news, but that's just how it works. Actually, this should be great news because it means you don't have to eat every couple of hours to "fuel your metabolism." Quite the contrary! When you stop feeding yourself so many carbs and stop fearing natural, healthy fats (see page 44 because this may not mean what you think), your body relearns how to make it through the day. It burns not only the fat you eat, but the extra food you have stored as body fat—the same fat you've been trying to burn off by cranking away on the elliptical machine for years.

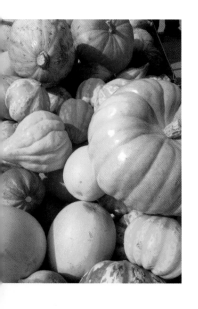

I know what you're thinking: "But how does that work? I thought I was supposed to eat lots of healthy whole grains and plenty of fruit to keep myself in shape?" Well, the answer is all about hormones and how they respond to the food you eat.

insulin is like your mom: it wants to constantly put stuff away

As I mentioned in the digestion section, insulin is a storage hormone, and your pancreas releases it primarily in response to dietary carbohydrates. It is insulin's job to take nutrients from your bloodstream (where they land after you digest your food) and deliver them into your cells for energy. So, just like your mom picks up the stuff lying around the house and puts it in its rightful place, insulin finds nutrients in your bloodstream and tries to put them in their rightful place—your cells.

Insulin does its job over a period of one to two hours after you eat a meal, so it "cleans up the mess" pretty quickly. Bad carbs make a bigger mess that sends your mom (insulin) into overdrive, putting it all away quickly.

Since high blood sugar is toxic, your body needs to respond to any amount of carbohydrate you eat by secreting insulin. This is necessary to bring your blood sugar levels back to normal, and normal is about four grams, which is equivalent to just one teaspoon of sugar. Even a little bit of sugar in your bloodstream causes insulin to respond. Within an hour or two, if insulin has been able to do its proper job, your blood sugar levels should return to this normal level.

Without insulin, you cannot get the nutrients from your food into your cells. This is why I mentioned the "wasting" phenomenon that people with Type 1 Diabetes experience. They would literally waste away without insulin injections because they do not have enough of the hormone to get nutrients to their cells.

So if insulin does such a great job as mom, what's the problem? When your hormones are out of balance, insulin can run the show entirely and constantly put stuff away without allowing your body to use enough of the stored nutrients. In other words, it's too much of a good thing.

too much of a good thing ...

Here's what happens: Over time, if your blood sugar levels remain consistently too high after meals, you can become what is called "insulin-resistant." Just like you stop noticing a messy room after a while, your body begins to lose its ability to *sense* the insulin that your pancreas has released. The insulin in your bloodstream becomes like your nagging mother. It sends signals to "pick up your room," but your body ignores those signals just like a teenager who tunes out his/her mom. Your body's receptor sites for insulin are limited, so your cells can no longer "hear" the message that there is sugar in your bloodstream. As a result, the sugar can't get into the cells and be converted into energy.

Does this mean that eating more than four grams of carbohydrates at a time is toxic? Of course not! Your body's insulin response to the carbohydrates you eat depends largely on the types and amounts of carbs you eat, as well as the frequency with which you eat them. When you eat a lot of carbohydrates, your body needs to release a lot of insulin to bring your blood sugar back down to non-toxic levels. When you eat a lot of carbohydrates *frequently*, you release a lot of insulin on a consistent basis. All of these are normal responses, but it puts you in "storage" mode all the time. Here it is in a nutshell:

> High blood sugar = high insulin response.
> High insulin = storage mode.
> Storage mode = not burning fat for fuel.

Know this: You can't have your bread and burn fat, too! In order to access and release stored body fat for energy, you need to be in "releasing" mode, not "storage" mode.

glucagon is like a teenager: it wants to play with stuff

You can better understand "releasing" mode by learning about the hormone glucagon, which is also produced by your pancreas. Unlike insulin, glucagon is like a teenager who wants to use his/her stuff rather than put it away.

Insulin and glucagon are counter-regulatory hormones. While insulin's job is to keep putting nutrients away, glucagon's job is to pull nutrients from their storage sites in your body when they're needed for fuel. When glucagon is the dominant hormone in your bloodstream, it can signal both glucose and fat to move from storage into your blood for use as fuel. When insulin is dominant, it's impossible for glucagon's actions to work. In other words, the dominant hormone dictates whether nutrients are stored or released for use. This is the difference between storage mode and release mode.

Glucagon dominance is what you want because it allows you to burn stored nutrients for fuel rather than store them away. How do you create glucagon dominance? You habitually eat a diet and live a lifestyle that promotes a strong glucagon response.

Glucagon promoter #1: Dense sources of protein. A dense source of protein is one that generally comes from an animal source and is not buried in insulin-demanding carbohydrates. Steak, for example, contains a large amount of protein and no carbohydrate at all. While protein does elicit *some* insulin response, the glucagon response is much stronger and allows glucagon to be dominant. By contrast, trying to get a glucagon response from beans doesn't work because insulin responds to the dense carbohydrates in the beans, overpowering glucagon's efforts. This is why many people who seek protein from strictly vegetarian sources have trouble losing body fat: They never release glucagon while eating carb-dense protein sources.

Glucagon promoter #2: Exercise. When you exercise, your body looks for available fuel sources to power your muscles. The very first, most easily accessible fuel comes directly from your bloodstream. You can't perform work for very long on the four grams of sugar circulating in your bloodstream, especially if it has been a while since you've eaten and insulin has cleared those nutrients away. Glucagon then goes to work to raise your blood sugar levels and power you through. Glucagon also works with cortisol, your fight-or-flight hormone, to signal to your body, "Hey! Work's happening here! Let's deliver some fuel to where it's needed!" This process goes smoothly and comfortably when your body is accustomed to burning fat for energy.

So does this mean that you should have a pre-workout snack? What if you're used to eating a lot of carbohydrates, especially in small meals every few hours like so many nutritionists and TV doctors have told you to do? Well, that's when insulin becomes the dominant hormone in your bloodstream all the time, and glucagon can't do its job properly. Let's say you're hungry an hour before you plan to exercise, and you know that within another hour, you'll be starving. That's how fast the process happens when you're burning sugar (carbs) as your primary fuel source. So in response to this hunger, you have a snack, right? Then you go to the gym, hoping to burn off body fat during your workout, but that doesn't happen. The nutrients from that recent snack are still up for grabs in your body because they haven't been pulled from your bloodstream into storage. The sugar that's in your bloodstream from your snack will be used *before* anything that is stored away. In other words: Eating extra food *too close* to a workout means you're burning off that food, *not* stored body fat. Rather than forcing your body to access what is stored, you've given it new fuel to use.

The problem is that your body burns fat as a *secondary* mechanism for energy, preferring carbs/sugar/glucose *if they're around* since they're easier and quicker to use. If glucose isn't around, your body will burn fat for energy. Therefore, if your body is well adapted to burning fat for fuel, which is what happens when you stop eating too many carbs, you won't feel the need for that pre-workout snack.

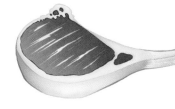

The Why—Food & Your Body

If losing body fat is your goal, becoming fat-adapted by eating more fats and proteins than carbohydrates will serve you well. Extra food before and after a workout is generally not a good idea for you. Remember: That extra food is what gets burned during your workout, not stored body fat. Extra food before and after a workout is a good idea only if you want to maintain your weight and muscle mass, not if you want to lose any weight.

How do you know if you're primarily burning sugar or fat for fuel? Can you make it through a workout without a snack right beforehand if it has been a couple of hours since you've eaten? Don't get me wrong; I'm not suggesting you challenge yourself to avoid eating if you're starving before a workout or feeling lightheaded, especially if you have passed out during a workout before. However, it is important to realize that you're probably burning sugar for fuel, and your body is not releasing enough glucagon to allow you to access stored nutrients. You are a sugar-burner who will only feel balanced if you add more sugar to the tank … unless and until you become fat-adapted. To get out of this cycle, reduce your overall carb intake (using the chart on page 96 as a guide) and allow your body to realize that it can and should use the fat you eat and the fat in your body's reserves. Glucagon will send signals to help your body do just that, but it can't do that job if insulin is always at work.

Glucagon promoter #3: Hunger. When you get hungry, your blood sugar levels drop. It is then glucagon's job to find stored sugar and bring it into your bloodstream to keep that blood sugar level at the healthy four grams. I already told you that high blood sugar is toxic, but so is low blood sugar. It's all about balance! Why is it that after twelve hours without food, you haven't passed out from hypoglycemia (which is blood sugar below four grams)? Glucagon senses the drop in blood sugar and brings sugar into your bloodstream to prevent you from passing out. Pretty cool, huh?

Eating well-balanced meals of nutrient-dense foods, including "good carbs," allows your body to easily move from a state of higher blood sugar to balanced, even blood sugar without a negative impact. Imbalanced blood sugar, for any reason, creates a stress response in your body. Eating too many bad carbs on a regular basis sends your body into a constant state of battle, fighting to keep the sugar in your bloodstream normal, which triggers the release of the stress hormone, cortisol.

blood sugar and cortisol

Cortisol, the fight-or-flight hormone, comes into play with regard to blood sugar regulation, too. When your body is stressed from constant blood sugar imbalance, you produce chronically high levels of cortisol.

Your emotional stressors are probably already causing an excess of cortisol production. Like our ancestors, we are wired to handle fairly acute stressors, followed by periods of rest or recovery. Unfortunately, the lifestyles we lead today tend to put demands on our bodies to produce marathon-like levels of stress hormones, placing us at a constant systemic stress level of 4 or 5 out of 10. We can handle a level of 7, 8, 9 or even 10, but only if it is followed by a period of very low levels of stress. Few of us get that rest period.

Add the physical stress of your body's response to carb overload, and you have even more chronically elevated cortisol, which can also create a state of chronic inflammation and disease. Furthermore, since your hormonal (endocrine) system is interdependent, and all of your stress hormones "talk" to your sex hormones and every other hormone in your body, this condition can lead to other endocrine problems. These problems include inhibited adrenal or thyroid function, low testosterone, and even infertility.

Dysglycemia is one of the biggest contributors to over-production of cortisol. Since you may not always be able to control your emotional stress levels, it makes sense to reduce your cortisol levels by controlling blood sugar through better diet and lifestyle choices.

Cortisol is released from your two triangular-shaped adrenal glands, which sit right on top of your kidneys. It works with insulin and blood sugar in a loop or circular fashion, meaning if one is high, it pushes the other one high. This, in turn, pushes the other one high yet again. As a result, high blood sugar causes high insulin release, which causes high cortisol release. Since high cortisol release tells your body it's time to "fight" or "flee," your body senses danger, and the entire loop starts over again. Your body is simply trying to prepare your muscles for fighting or fleeing by supplying them with sugar.

So what if you're stressed out all the time but want to keep your insulin levels in check? Lowering your carb intake will take you far, but it won't get you the entire way. Your hormones need to play nicely together to create this equation: fat burning = moderate insulin release + higher glucagon release + healthy cortisol release.

DYSGLYCEMIA

Dysglycemia is a constant state of high or low blood sugar. It contributes to countless hormonal and systemic issues, as well as many chronic inflammatory conditions.

when sugar takes its toll

Both *high* and *low* blood sugar can have profound effects on your ability to think clearly and maintain a positive mood. When your blood sugar levels are high, you feel foggy-headed or sleepy. People often refer to this as a "food coma." How do you feel after a lunch of a few slices of pizza, a bowl of pasta, or even rice and beans? Typically, you feel tired, full, and not quite sharp. You may sit at your desk wishing you could take a nap rather than work on the report that's due.

You know that post-Thanksgiving dinner sleepy feeling that people attribute to the tryptophan in the turkey? It is probably not due to the beneficial amino acid at all, but rather to the piles of mashed potatoes, pecans, and pumpkin pie that people eat before sitting on the couch to watch football. Too many carbohydrates can easily lead to this feeling of brain fog and fatigue. Now, if you had just come inside from *playing* football for a couple of hours before dinner, your response to that amount of carbohydrates would be totally different since your activity level had demanded that your body be replenished with more carbs.

The insulin demand of a high carbohydrate meal often results in such a strong response (this is especially true of the response from refined foods) that it can drop your blood sugar back to normal pretty quickly (if your pancreas is working as it should) and finish its job by leaving you with *low* blood sugar.

When blood sugar levels are too *low*, you feel irritable and ready to snap if anyone gets between you and your next meal or snack. When extreme hunger sets in, you're hardly able to think clearly, are you? Chances are, you can only think about one thing: food. This is how your brain feels the effects of a low blood sugar state.

blood sugar and your immune system

The stress that bad carbs put on your body, whether as a result of imbalanced blood sugar levels or consistent "energy bank account" withdrawals, can affect more than just your endocrine system. Those constant withdrawals by foods that take nutrients but don't give any back can eventually leave you broke—just like if you kept withdrawing all of your money from the bank without making any deposits. If you have no money in the bank, there is nothing to withdraw from your account, is there? Your body is similar. You need to deposit nutrients before trying to withdraw them.

Eating refined foods depletes vitamins and minerals and leads to low energy. You feel the lack of energy, but that energetic depletion is also happening at a cellular level. Not only are your cells unable to make energy for you, but they also can't do their job of repair and maintenance. This leaves your immune system vulnerable.

Know this: Much like the inflammation in your gut can lead to any chronic inflammatory condition, a state of depleted nutrient status can also lead to any condition because it has weakened your immunity.

source: Laura Knoff, NC

get off the blood sugar rollercoaster

Amusement park rides are fun but not for your metabolism. And your rollercoaster ride can start with breakfast. This is because breakfast really *is* the most important meal of the day for people with blood sugar imbalances. But what do most people eat for breakfast? A big helping of sugar, of course.

When you sit down to breakfast, do you eat a bowl of high fiber, whole grain cereal with skim or low-fat milk? Perhaps it's a bowl of steel-cut or old-fashioned oats with a banana, walnuts, brown sugar, or raisins. Maybe it's a whole wheat bagel with peanut butter and an apple or a cup of non-fat yogurt with granola and berries on top. All of these breakfasts are commonly viewed as "ideal" in today's health-oriented populations. By the "conventional wisdom" (CW) of nutrition, these foods support heart health and even fat loss, but this couldn't be further from the truth.

Starting your day this way is one of the reasons you feel the need to eat five or six times a day. You've heard this direction from countless sources, but do you *enjoy* eating that way? Every single client I've coached who was following this type of meal plan has reported to me that they:

Don't enjoy having to eat so often.
Feel stressed about choosing what to eat several times a day.

To better illustrate how it works, let's compare two common breakfasts and how they act within the body.

Both of these meals probably look pretty familiar to you. If you're a veteran of the Paleo lifestyle, one probably looks like a common morning in your past, while the other looks like a more recent morning.

Meal #1 is what we'd consider a "healthy breakfast" if we're following CW, which assures us that eating a low-fat meal rich in whole grains will provide lasting energy and nutrition to power us through the morning. Since CW also tells us that saturated fat and cholesterol are unhealthy, we're left with few

MEAL #1	MEAL #2
» 1 cup of cooked oats + 2 Tbsp of raisins + 2 tsp of brown sugar » 12 ounces of orange juice » 16 ounces of coffee + 2 ounces of skim milk + 2 teaspoons of sugar	» 3 whole eggs » 1 cup of cooked broccoli » 1/4 avocado » 2 large slices of tomato » 16 ounces of coffee + 1 ounce of half and half*

Calories: 473
Total Fat: 4g
   Saturated Fat: 1g
Cholesterol: 1mg
Total Carbohydrates: 102g
   Dietary Fiber: 5g
   Sugars: 33g
Protein: 12g
Vitamin A: 13%
Vitamin C: 266%
Calcium: 17%
Iron: 16%
	Calories: 468
	Total Fat: 32g
	   Saturated Fat: 10g
	Cholesterol: 655mg
	Total Carbohydrates: 22g
	   Dietary Fiber: 8g
	   Sugars: 7g
	Protein: 26g
	Vitamin A: 80%
	Vitamin C: 186%
	Calcium: 24%
	Iron: 20%

Meal calculations are made using nutritiondata.com

*Note: heavy cream was not available in the database at the time of calculation or it would have been used.

WHAT ABOUT FRUIT?

Fruit is a real, whole, natural food, and if you aren't concerned with dropping much body fat, avoiding it isn't a big concern. However, if you want to lose significant amounts of body fat, I recommend avoiding it. Eating too much of anything sweet, even fruit, can cause higher blood sugar levels than you want.

options for breakfast. If we're not eating eggs, what else *is* there for breakfast besides grains and fruit? Perhaps processed dairy like non-fat or low-fat yogurt? (For an egg-free breakfast plan, refer to page 131.)

meal #1 in your body

If you've made yourself Meal #1, congratulations—you've just created a lovely bowl of sugar, topped with sugar, and finished off with sugar, with a glass of sugar and some coffee with sugar and sugar added. Was that what you intended to do this morning? Sit down to a gigantic breakfast of sugar?

How do you feel after that breakfast? Pretty good, right? Sugar tastes good and I'll bet you feel amped up and powered for the morning ... until about an hour later, maybe two or three hours at the most. Then, what happens? If you're like many of my clients, you'll say, "I'm hungry again." And all from your purportedly healthy low-fat, high-carb oatmeal breakfast.

How's that working for you? It certainly hasn't worked for the thousands of people I've counseled over the years. For many, they're more than just hungry; they're shaky and even irrational, desperate to find something to eat.

When you crash from eating that oatmeal breakfast, you probably reach for whatever is around, which is usually more carbs, such as a granola bar, crackers, or nonfat yogurt to get you through until lunch. Then, noon hits, and the lunch truck rolls around. You munch on your whole wheat and turkey sandwich with chips and an iced tea. That's healthy, right?

Then, at about 3:00 p.m., you need an afternoon pick-me-up. Maybe you reach for a skim milk latte and a pastry from Starbucks. Come on, who doesn't love their Starbucks fix? Plus, it's an excuse to get out of the office.

The end of the work day arrives, and you're feeling pretty hungry again, unsure how to make it either through your 6:00 workout or the ride home in traffic before you can get to a plate of pasta for dinner. So you grab a handful of nuts on your way out of the office (finally, some fat!).

Your entire day has been a rollercoaster ride, climbing up and down the steepest of hills, and rushing back down. The flat parts of the ride are when your body can relax and burn fat for energy. When you eat your oatmeal (or other high carb, low-fat) breakfast, however, your blood sugar levels climb way up high until you head down the other side of that steep hill about an hour later when the crash of low blood sugar comes. Not as much fun as a real rollercoaster ride, is it? To your body, each part of the ride is a negative stressor.

If you continue to eat similar meals, which are high in carbs and low in fat, you'll take that rollercoaster car right back up another hill. When it comes to blood sugar regulation, that flat part of the ride before and after the hills is where your body wants to stay. Luckily, getting off the rollercoaster is easy.

Simply put, you need fat and protein to feel full for a long period of time. This feeling of fullness isn't about filling your stomach, though! Don't be fooled by the silly notion that "bulk and fiber" are what fills you from a meal. It is the nutrients that make you feel satisfied, and it is protein and fat that pack the most powerful nutrient-rich punch. The nutrients, in turn, allow your body to have a healthy hormonal response to your food. Ultimately, it is this hormonal response that determines how full you will feel in an hour, two hours, three hours, and even longer after a meal.

meal #2 in your body

Let's take a look at how your morning goes if you eat Meal #2, the real food Paleo meal. You eat this breakfast of eggs, veggies, and coffee at about 7:00 a.m., and two hours later, you feel fine. Three hours pass, and you're still fine. Four hours approach, and you may start to notice some hunger.

Noon rolls around, and you have a container of leftovers from last night's dinner ready to go. This includes some roasted chicken (recipe on page 256), perhaps over some leafy greens with carrots, avocado, and homemade dressing made with extra-virgin olive oil and lemon juice. Easy!

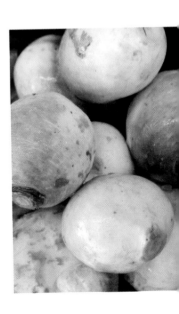

The end of your workday comes, and you head to the gym or drive home, feeling like you could eat but won't pass out if you don't. Whether you work out or simply drive home, you never feel shaky or disoriented from low blood sugar.

This is the difference between fueling your body primarily with sugar or carbs as opposed to fueling it primarily with proteins and fats. Remember, this doesn't mean you should never eat carbs! It simply means that you want to eat good carbs in an appropriate amount for your lifestyle. When you are fat-adapted, your body can access stored body fat for energy when you haven't eaten. If you never allow your body the break from burning carbohydrates as a primary fuel source, it never has the opportunity to burn fat for fuel.

The goal of most people on low-fat diets is to burn stored body fat. But these diets never give your body a chance to *learn* how to use fat as energy. Your system simply becomes accustomed to fueling on carbs. When you get hungry, which happens quickly since carbs are swiftly cleared from your bloodstream, your body is not in a hormonal state to allow stored body fat to be accessed as energy. This is a fantastic way to live and eat only if you want to keep Big Food companies in business by buying their cereal, granola bars, breads, crackers, cookies, and pastas.

So how can you plan a breakfast that will keep you satiated until lunchtime? Plan your meal around protein first, and make sure you also add good fat, followed by carbs:

- Protein: Serve yourself a breakfast consisting of *at least* 20g of protein for women, 30g for men.
- Fat: Make sure there is adequate, naturally occurring or added fat in the meal—roughly 30-50g.
- Carbs: Any carbohydrate you add to the meal should be considered in terms of your activity levels during the day. Eat roughly 10-20g of carbs in your meal if you are less active and 30-60g if you are more active.

Then, balance the rest of your meals according to your activity level. You can use the same ratios as for breakfast, shifting them slightly depending on when you exercise. Perhaps you exercise in the evening, so your breakfast and lunch have fewer carbs, while your post-workout dinner may contain a higher amount of carbs to replenish what was depleted during exercise. Again, the meal plans to come will help you make smart choices based on the information you learn in this chapter.

simplifying sweeteners

Speaking of sugar, what about the different types of sweeteners? Eating a sweetener like raw honey, molasses, or maple syrup (and I mean 100% pure maple syrup) is not the same as eating a whole, sweet food when it comes to micronutrient content. These sweeteners carry *some* micronutrients, but they are still refined to a degree. Therefore, I don't recommend eating them regularly, but they are certainly better sweetener choices than refined table sugar or artificial sweeteners.

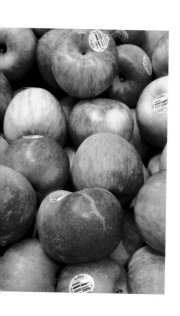

Practical Paleo

Let's compare some sweetener choices:

- A whole medjool date contains approximately 60 calories of carbohydrate, as well as small amounts of B vitamins, phosphorous, magnesium, iron, copper, manganese, and zinc.
- One tablespoon of molasses contains approximately 60 calories of carbohydrate, as well as trace amounts of B vitamins (especially B6), phosphorous, magnesium, iron, copper, manganese, zinc, and chromium.
- One tablespoon of 100% pure maple syrup contains approximately 50 calories of carbohydrate, as well as trace amounts of phosphorous, magnesium, iron, copper, manganese, and zinc.

While these less refined sweeteners are not ideal on a frequent basis, the point is that there *is* a difference between these and refined white sugar or agave nectar, for example, which is also a more refined sweetener. What about artificial and non-caloric sweeteners? I'm sure you realize by now that these are far from whole, real foods. If there are no calories, there are also no nutrients. It might seem as though an artificial sweetener doesn't require nutrients for metabolism, but that isn't the case. Your body must still do something with the substance you have ingested, even if it doesn't actually gain nutritional value from it. Again, this is one of those situations where you are withdrawing from your bank without making a deposit.

Some synthetic sweeteners initiate an insulin response in your bloodstream in a similar way to refined sugar. This is because your body is physiologically wired to release insulin in response to any sweet taste. When insulin is released despite the fact that the sweet food has provided no nutrients to support the insulin release, you are in a state of energy deficit.

The biggest issue with these artificial sweeteners, however, is that they are actually toxic. Yes, you read that correctly—they're *toxins*. Your body knows the difference between nutrients and toxins, and toxins are processed by your liver and stored away in your fat cells to keep them away from your bloodstream where they can cause damage. Most people use non-caloric sweeteners to lower overall caloric intake in an effort to lose body fat, but what they do is actually fill their fat cells with toxins. This is one reason why detoxifying from sugar and carbohydrate addiction can be painful. The release of stored toxins from fat cells often leads to headache and fatigue.

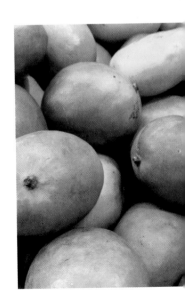

watch out for hidden sugar

Sugar is hidden in nearly all packaged, bottled, and processed foods. This is an important lesson: Turn every package of food around and read the ingredients. Even if it's a food you've bought many times before, the ingredients can change at any time. So read them again.

Even many of the seemingly "clean" dried fruits contain added sugar, which serves as a preservative or flavor enhancer. Does it make sense to you that fruit would need added sugar? It doesn't. Fruit is naturally sweet, so never buy any type of fruit or juice with sugar or any other sweeteners on the ingredient list.

When you avoid consuming added sugar, you do yourself the additional favor of eliminating many packaged, factory-made, non-whole foods from your diet. You also eliminate many other harmful added ingredients, including synthetic chemicals.

Know this: Do not trust anything written on the front of the package. Please! Remember: The word "natural" on a food label essentially means nothing. *According to the FDA food-labeling regulations, anything that originated from nature at one time can be called "natural" on a food label, no matter what has been done to it since it was in its natural state.*

Here is what the FDA has to say about it: "From a food science perspective, it is difficult to define a food product that is 'natural' because the food has probably been processed and is no longer the product of the earth. That said, the FDA has not developed a definition for use of the term "natural" or its derivatives. However, the agency has not objected to the use of the term if the food does not contain added color, artificial flavors, or synthetic substances."*

What about your breakfast cereal that says it contains 100% of the required vitamins and minerals? The truth is that your cereal has been fortified with those vitamins and minerals, and fortified foods have been refined and stripped of their nutrients from nature. This is why the nutrients have to be added back into the product. What's wrong with that? The nutrients that are added are synthetic forms, and your body is smart enough to recognize the difference.

Let's compare your cereal to the sweet potato mentioned earlier in the chapter. In that one little vegetable, you get all of the exact nutrients you need to metabolize carbohydrates. They're all present right in the "package" of the whole food sweet potato, and those nutrients are not synthetic. What's so powerful about whole food nutrition is that the nutrients work synergistically in your body in the appropriate balance for their proper use.

When we try to outsmart Mother Nature and add synthetic nutrients to foods in a factory, we make serious missteps. Manufacturers typically add the

HOW SWEET IT IS
Check out the Guide to: Sweeteners on page 111 for more information.

source: http://www. fda.gov/AboutFDA/ Transparency/Basics/ ucm214868.htm?utm_ campaign=Google2&utm_ source=fdaSearch&utm_ medium=website&utm_ term=natural%20 food%20label&utm_ content=2

latest, most popularly hyped nutrient to foods that wouldn't even contain that micronutrient naturally. The most recent trend is adding omega-3 fatty acids, known for their beneficial anti-inflammatory properties, to items like yogurt and bread. *Reality check: Omega-3s naturally occur in foods like fatty cold water fish and some nuts like walnuts and pecans, not in yogurt and bread!* When nutrients are added to foods in synthetic forms and without their other nutrient co-factors (the complementary nutrients that are needed for proper absorption and utilization in your body), you simply cannot use them appropriately.

blood sugar regulation and your overall health

Maintaining even blood sugar levels by only eating good carbs in the appropriate amount for your activity level is the key to not only satiety, but also mental clarity, positive moods, fat loss, hormonal balance, and managing inflammation. Whether your goal is fat loss or health, regulating your blood sugar is absolutely necessary.

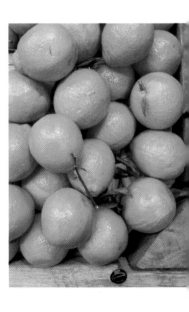

guide to: dense sources of paleo carbs

Removing grains, legumes, and refined foods from your diet doesn't mean that carbohydrates need to all disappear! Check out this list of dense sources of carbohydrates while eating a Paleo diet. While fruits and nuts are all fairly high in carbohydrates, this list is a guide to starchy vegetables to eat. Remember, these are some of your "good carbs!"

there *are* carbs beyond bread EAT UP

ITEM NAME	CARBS PER 100G	FIBER PER 100G	CARBS PER 1 CUP	OTHER NOTABLE NUTRIENTS
Cassava (raw)	38g	2g	78g	Vit C, Thiamin, Folate, Potassium, Manganese
Taro root	35g	5g	46g, sliced	B6, Vitamin E, Potassium, Manganese
Plantain	31g	2g	62g, mashed	Vitamin A (beta carotene), Vitamin C, B6, Magnesium, Potassium
Yam	27g	4g	37g, cubed	Vit C, Vitamin B6, Manganese, Potassium
White potato	22g	1g	27g, peeled	Trace Vitamin C
Sweet potato	21g	3g	58g, mashed	Vit A (beta carotene), Vit C, B6, Potassium, Manganese, Magnesium, Iron, Vitamin E
Parsnips	17g	4g	27g, sliced	Vitamin C, Manganese
Lotus root	16g	3g	19g, sliced	Vitamin C, B6, Potassium, Copper, Manganese
Winter squash	15g	4g	30g, cubed	Vitamin C, Thiamin, B6
Onion	10g	1g	21g, chopped	Vitamin C, Potassium
Beets	10g	2g	17g, sliced	Folate, Manganese
Carrots	10g	3g	13g, chopped	Vitamin A (beta carotene), Vitamin K1
Butternut squash	10g	-	22g	Vitamin A (beta carotene), Vitamin C
Rutabaga	9g	2g	21g, mashed	Vitamin C, Potassium, Manganese,
Jicama (raw)	9g	5g	12g, sliced	Vitamin C
Kohlrabi	7g	1g	11g, sliced	Vit C, B6, Potassium, Copper, Manganese
Spaghetti squash	6g	1g	9g	Trace
Turnips	5g	2g	12g, mashed	Vitamin C, Potassium, Calcium, B6, Folate, Manganese
Pumpkin	5g	1g	12g, mashed	Vitamin C, Vitamin E, Potassium

source: nutritiondata.com

110　Practical Paleo

guide to: sweeteners

How many of these sweeteners do you use or find in your favorite packaged foods? Perhaps it's time for a change! Artificial sweeteners are never recommended, while the limited use of selected, more naturally derived options can be okay for treats and special occasions. Sweeteners should not be considered "food" or nourishment.

natural USE SPARINGLY

PREFERRED CHOICES ARE IN BOLD. USE ORGANIC FORMS WHENEVER POSSIBLE

- Brown sugar
- **Dates (whole)**
- Date sugar
- Date syrup
- Cane sugar
- Raw sugar
- Turbinado

- Cane juice
- Cane juice crystals
- Coconut nectar
- Coconut sugar/crystals
- **Fruit juice (real, fresh)**
- **Fruit juice concentrate**
- **Honey (raw)**

- **Maple syrup (grade b)**
- **Molasses**
- Palm sugar
- **Stevia (green leaf or extract)**

natural BUT NOT RECOMMENDED

- Agave
- Agave nectar
- Barley malt
- Beet sugar
- Brown rice syrup
- Buttered syrup
- Caramel
- Carob syrup
- Corn syrup
- Corn syrup solids
- Demerara sugar
- Dextran
- Dextrose
- Diastatic malt

- Diastase
- Ethyl maltol
- Fructose
- Glucose / glucose solids
- Golden sugar
- Golden syrup
- Grape sugar
- High fructose corn syrup
- Invert sugar
- Lactose
- Levulose
- Light brown sugar
- Maltitol
- Malt syrup

- Maltodextrin
- Maltose
- Mannitol
- Muscovado
- Refiner's syrup
- Sorbitol
- Sorghum syrup
- Sucrose
- Treacle
- Yellow sugar
- Xylitol (or other sugar alcohols, typically they end in "-ose")

artificial NEVER CONSUME

- Acesulfame K (Sweet One)
- Aspartame (Equal, Nutra-Sweet)
- Saccharin (Sweet'N Low)
- Stevia: white/bleached (Truvia, Sun Crystals)
- Sucralose (Splenda)
- Tagatose

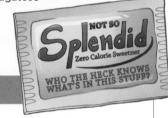

sugar is sugar BUT NOT REALLY

IT DOES MAKE A DIFFERENCE WHICH SWEETENERS YOU SELECT, CONTRARY TO POPULAR BELIEF AND THE MAINSTREAM MEDIA. WHILE ALL CALORIC SWEETENERS HAVE THE SAME NUMBER OF CALORIES (16 PER TEASPOON), EVALUATING THEIR PLACE IN YOUR DIET MAY BE DONE BY CONSIDERING A FEW FACTORS.

HOW IT'S MADE
The more highly refined a sweetener is, the worse it is for your body. For example, high fructose corn syrup (HFCS) and artificial sweeteners are all very modern, factory-made products. Honey, maple syrup, green leaf stevia (dried leaves made into powder), and molasses are all much less processed and have been made for hundreds of years. In the case of honey, almost no processing is necessary. As a result, I vote for raw, organic, local honey as the ideal natural sweetener.

WHERE IT'S USED
This is a reality check. When you read the ingredients in packaged, processed foods, it becomes obvious how most of them use highly-refined, low-quality sweeteners. Food manufacturers often even hide sugar in foods that you didn't think were sweets! Many foods that have been made low or non-fat have added sweeteners or artificial sweeteners—avoid these products!

HOW YOUR BODY PROCESSES IT
Here's where the HFCS commercials really get things wrong: your body actually does not metabolize all sugar the same way.

Interestingly enough, sweeteners like HFCS and agave nectar were viewed as better options for diabetics for quite some time since the high fructose content of both requires processing by the liver before the sugar hits your blood stream. This yielded a seemingly favorable result on blood sugar levels after consuming said sweeteners. However, it's now understood that isolated fructose metabolism is a complicated issue and that taxing the liver excessively with such sweeteners can be quite harmful to our health.

Fructose is the primary sugar in all fruit. When eating whole fruit, the micronutrients and fiber content of the fruit actually support proper metabolism and assimilation of the fruit sugar. Whole foods for the win!

The Why—Food & Your Body

frequently asked questions

Still curious about a few things? You're not alone! Here are some of the most popular questions I'm asked.

q: should I be counting calories? if not, why not?

For *general health* goals, I do not recommend counting calories. Here are the reasons:

1. When you eat a Paleo diet, calorie restriction means nutrition restriction. This is because counting calories limits intake of whole, nutrient-dense foods, thereby limiting the vitamins and minerals you need for your cells to function well.

2. Most people feel satisfied when they eat real, whole foods in reasonable portions. (See pages 128-129 for basic portion size recommendations). The hormone signals that respond to dense sources of protein, naturally-occurring fats, and vegetables will be balanced, and your body will have an even blood sugar response, which will promote long-term satiety. Translation: You aren't likely to overeat whole foods.

3. Counting calories adds stress to your life. You have to weigh and measure all of your food, log it into some kind of calculator, and worry over the minutia of what you've eaten. Adding stress to your life is not a good idea. You're already stressed enough, aren't you?

That said, calories do count at some point. For those who are struggling with fat loss, want to gain weight, or need to maintain athletic performance, counting calories can be a useful tool. The awareness that comes from logging your food intake can, of course, be a tremendous eye-opener. Often, people believe they are eating too much when they're actually not eating enough to sustain their metabolism. This means that their daily activities require more calories than they realize to keep their bodies well fueled. Eating too few or too many calories can be problematic. A numerical assessment of your overall intake is a good starting point to understand whether eating more or less will be beneficial.

For example, for most women, a minimum of 1200 calories is the baseline of necessity for simply waking up and being alive for a day. For men, the number is likely around 1600 calories. Our bodies use calories to perform basic life functions like breathing and thinking. If you restrict calories below these numbers, you will fail to supply adequate nutrients to your body for these functions, so trying to exercise on top of that nutrient deficiency can cause your body to hold onto fat as a protective mechanism versus using it for fuel.

Therefore, people who want to lose body fat often actually need to eat more. If you under-eat, you don't give your body the chance to complete metabolic processes. It's like asking your car to run without enough gas in the tank. Even if you need to reduce overall caloric intake for body fat loss, your weight loss will plateau.

If you have a metabolic issue that prevents you from feeling hunger signals, keeping track of calories can help you to make appropriate adjustments and make sure you're eating enough. If you are indeed eating too much, it's easy to figure out what you're adding that isn't necessary to feel satisfied. It may be a few extra ounces of protein or an extra tablespoon of coconut oil or nut butter. Just 2-3 extra ounces of protein at each meal can add up to an extra entire serving over the course of the day.

q: do I really need to stop eating bread, pasta, and cereal forever?

It can take some time to create new habits, and it can be difficult at first. But at the very least, it's worth eliminating these foods from your diet 100% for at least one month so that you can closely examine how you feel when you reintroduce them. You will then know just how much they affect your overall health. Review page 88 for The 4-R Protocol.

You are likely to feel significantly different after eliminating these foods. It can be pretty profound! It may make you never want to touch them again.

The main idea, of course, is to eliminate processed foods, but remember that gluten has specific properties that are detrimental to your health beyond what you feel on the surface. Gluten protein has the ability to activate the enzyme zonulin, which contributes to leaky gut. Review that chapter for more information. This is why many long-time Paleo eaters will splurge on some grains from time to time, but tend to keep the splurges to gluten-free options.

When people strive to change their diet and eliminate grain products, they sometimes forget to follow these steps, which will make it easier:

- Consider all of your options for food throughout the day ahead of time. Preparation is key!
- Pre-plan or pack a meal when you realize there might not be anything appropriate for you to eat during the course of your day.
- Review menu choices before going to a restaurant, and ask questions of the wait staff about how meals are prepared.

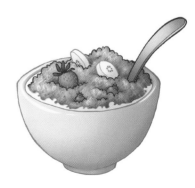

If wiping out all of your favorite foods from Day 1 feels suffocating, make use of the recipes in this book for items like squash noodles (page 308), coconut flour muffins (pages 244-247), and pumpkin pancakes (page 242), as well various other resources that have recipes for grain-free breads, pizzas, etc. These can help you make the transition away from grains and factory-made packaged foods.

q: where will I get carbs if I don't eat grains?

There are plenty of carbohydrate sources aside from refined foods and grain products. Refer to the chart dedicated to Paleo sources of dense carbs on page 110. You can easily cook sweet potatoes, for example, in the oven, or you can cook a whole, large butternut squash at once to last for several servings. Check out recipes on pages 342, 358, and 362 for a few of my favorite dense-carb go-to dishes.

q: how is vitamin K2 different from vitamin K? don't leafy greens contain vitamin K?

Yes, leafy greens contain Vitamin K (phylloquinone), which is largely responsible for supporting body functions like the clotting of blood. This is why people who take blood-thinning medications are cautioned against eating too many leafy greens. Vitamin K2 (menaquinone) is still being heavily researched for its role in human health, but information has been uncovered regarding its importance in directing the placement and proper integration of calcium throughout the body. If you want to optimize your bone and heart health, make sure you get enough Vitamin K2 from foods or concentrated food supplements. (I recommend Green Pasture brand fermented cod liver oil/butter oil blend.) K2 is found primarily in animal foods, particularly those that many people in the modern world do not include in their diets, such as hard and soft cheeses from *grass-fed* milk, egg yolks, butter from *grass-fed* cows, and liver. Dairy products from animals that are not grass-fed are *not* sources of Vitamin K2.

q: are coconut milk, almond milk, and soy milk healthy to drink?

If you aren't eating cereal, you probably won't need milk except perhaps for coffee or an occasional recipe. In that case, I recommend organic, full-fat coconut milk without added texturizers (guar gum, xanthan gum) if you can find it. If you can't find a brand that meets all three of these criteria, choose a full-fat, organic coconut milk. Thai Kitchen, Natural Value, and Whole Foods brands fall into this category. Be aware, however, that guar and xanthan gums are derived from legumes, so while most people feel fine after consuming these small amounts of legume derived ingredients, others react with digestive distress. If you find that you're using coconut milk daily, resulting in signs of inflammation, try making your own coconut milk. If that works, it was likely the additives that irritated your system. If that doesn't work, you may have an intolerance (gasp!) to coconut. Stop using the coconut milk, and see how you feel without it after two weeks.

If you know you don't tolerate coconut milk, or if you don't like it, you can also make your own fresh almond milk (or use any other nut you like). A simple web search will yield many recipes for homemade coconut milk, as well as a variety of nut milk.

As for soy milk, I recommend that everyone avoid it. Most soy milks are loaded with additives, as are most pre-packaged almond milks, which is why I recommend making your own. The first problem with soy milk, of course, is that it isn't a whole food. It's in the refined and processed category. Soy also carries compounds called trypsin-inhibitors, which can interfere with your ability to properly digest proteins. Additionally, soy has been shown to disrupt normal endocrine function and to promote estrogen-like activity. Today's environment is already loaded with many other xenoestrogens (compounds that mimic natural estrogen hormones), including BPA in plastics and cans, BHA and BHT (food preservatives), parabens found in lotions and skin care items, insecticides, fungicides, and herbicides used to treat non-organic foods. (For more on soy, check out *The Whole Soy Story* by Kaayla T. Daniel, Ph.D., CCN.)

q: what are FODMAPs? who should avoid them?

FODMAPs is an acronym that stands for fermentable-oligo-di-monosaccharides-and-polyols. These are types of carbohydrates in different foods that can be difficult for some people to digest, resulting in symptoms varying from gas and bloating to IBS-like responses of diarrhea, constipation, or a combination/alternation of the two. Unlike other types of food intolerances that are a result of incomplete digestion within the small intestine, FODMAP foods become irritating to people for different reasons:

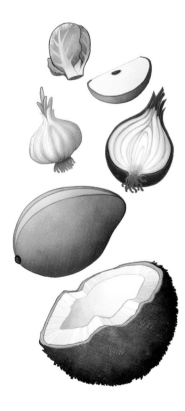

- Overgrowth of the wrong *type* of bacteria in the system (dysbiosis).
- Overgrowth of bacteria in the wrong *part* of the digestive system, usually the small intestine where bacteria don't normally live. (This condition is known as small intestinal bacterial overgrowth or SIBO.)
- Low stomach acid production/secretion, which also contributes to the previous two bacterial issues.
- A gut pathogen/infection often obtained via travel abroad.

Within the complete list of Paleo foods, FODMAP foods have been identified with an asterisk (*). If you find that you react to these foods, I recommend working with a naturopath, chiropractor, or other practitioner who submits stool tests to labs for analysis in order to determine the root cause of the intolerance.

q: what are nightshades? who should avoid them?

Nightshades are a family of plants that contain specific alkaloid compounds that can be irritating to those suffering from joint pain and inflammation. Tomatoes, white potatoes, peppers (all kinds, bell and hot), and eggplants are the most commonly consumed nightshades. Black pepper and sweet potatoes are *not* nightshades, however. Note that if a packaged food contains "spices" without listing which are included, paprika is probably one of them. These items should be avoided since paprika is derived from peppers.

Some other, less frequently consumed nightshades include tomatillos, tobacco, goji berries, cape gooseberries (not normal gooseberries), ground cherries (not regular bing or rainier cherries), garden huckleberries (not blueberries), and ashwagandha (an herb).

If you suffer from joint pain, joint inflammation, arthritis, cracking, or any other joint-related issues, eliminate nightshades from your diet for at least thirty days. See the meal plan on pages 130-137 for nightshade-free options. Also, note within the recipes in this book when nightshades may be replaced with other foods or eliminated from a recipe entirely.

q: i am currently a vegetarian (or vegan), but I want to make the switch to paleo. how should I get started?

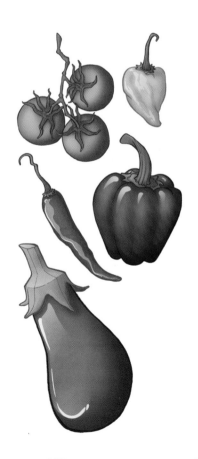

I strongly recommend that you introduce animal foods into your diet very slowly. This is especially true if you have been a vegan. If you have been eating dairy products as a vegetarian, you can introduce meat into your diet a bit faster. When you do not eat animal products, stomach acid production is usually reduced because there is less demand for it. That doesn't mean your body can't or won't bounce back to making an adequate amount, but it's best to give your body some time to adjust to digesting these foods.

Here's what you should do over the course of one month:

- Week 1: make bone broth (recipe on page 234), and sip it with meals or whenever you like for a week. You may use chicken bones at first, but work up to beef bones after a couple of days.
- Week 2: put small bits of meat into the broth that you make, chewing them well as you drink it. You can also add other vegetables to the broth to make

it a more complete soup. Eat this soup several times during the week.

- Week 3: make one of the slow-cooker recipes in this book (page 278, 282, or 284), and enjoy it several times in a week.
- Week 4: make any of the meat recipes in this book and see how you feel. If you don't feel your body was ready for a full meal or for any of the sequential steps here, just stay at the previous step for a longer period of time. You may also want to review the digestion section of this book for helpful tips for increasing stomach acid.

q: won't my cholesterol be too high if I eat lots of eggs?

According to Uffe Ravnskov, a leading researcher and expert on cholesterol, the direct effect of a lower dietary cholesterol intake on serum (blood) cholesterol measures about one half of 1%. Yes, you read that correctly.* That's it!

Cholesterol is a precursor molecule to all of our hormones. We need it, and it isn't healthy to have a cholesterol level that is too low. Our bodies make as much as we need to function properly and keep oxidative damage from taking over.

High cholesterol also doesn't run in your family unless there is a genetic predisposition for the rare condition called Familial Hypercholesterolemia (FH), which is the inability to process lipoprotein molecules properly so that levels remain extremely high in the blood. Most people with a family history of high cholesterol have a family history of poor diet and lifestyle, not an actual genetic disorder.

Typically, your cholesterol numbers will improve by medical standards on a Paleo diet as a result of the reduced stress and lowered inflammation in your system that results from removing sugar, grains, legumes, processed dairy products, and refined foods.

source: Ravnskov, Uffe. "High cholesterol may protect against infections and atherosclerosis." QJM: An International Journal of Medicine. Volume 96, Issue 12, Pp. 927-934

High levels of cholesterol is generally a sign that something else is wrong, and the body is responding with protective factors. Does high cholesterol mean you are less healthy or more prone to heart disease or death? I don't think so. In one report*, Ravnskov even shows that cholesterol can protect us against heart disease. In short, the alarm about cholesterol is unfounded. Enjoy your eggs, yolks included.

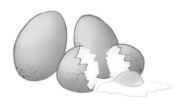

q: i'm confused about cooking fats, can you explain these a bit more?

Saturated fats are more *stable* than unsaturated fats. Ever wonder why your high quality olive oils are sold in dark green glass? It's to keep light from damaging the oil. Ever wonder why coconut oil doesn't smell rancid from sitting on the counter without a lid like vegetable oil? Air oxidizes those oils and makes them rancid.

It's safe to assume that most naturally occurring saturated fats are safe to cook with, while most unsaturated fats (called oils because they are liquid at ambient room temperature) are unsafe to cook with and are most ideal for cold uses (if appropriate for consumption at all).

Remember that manmade trans fats are never healthy to eat. These include Crisco, Earth Balance, Smart Balance, Benecol, Margarine, Country Crock, I Can't Believe It's Not Butter, and the new one claiming to be a coconut product but which actually contains soybean oil.

Seed oils are extremely high in monounsaturated fatty acids (MUFAs) and polyunsaturated fatty acids (PUFAs) at varying ratios, all of which are prone to oxidation, PUFAs most significantly. You wouldn't cook with fish oil, would you? Why would you want to cook with other oils that are very high in PUFAs? Even beyond PUFAs, MUFAs are pretty easy to damage with heat, air, etc. as well (olive oil is very high in MUFAs).

Refer to the Guide to Cooking Fats for the rankings of many popular grocery store fats and oils.

Know this: Many refined seed oils are marketed as having a high smoke point, therefore making them "ideal" choices for cooking. A higher smoke point is valid *only* if the fat or oil is fairly stable.

The process by which canola and other seed oils are made involves an expeller or screw press, high heat, and a wash with the chemical solvent (hexane). This produces a gray, foul-smelling oil that isn't smooth. It then has to be chemically bleached, deodorized, and dyed yellow before it becomes the oil you see in the bottle. That hardly sounds like a whole food, does it?

Cold-pressed fruit oils such as olive, palm, and coconut are not processed in this manner. Their processing stops after, as their name indicates, a cold-pressing application has been applied and oil has been extracted in that first step.

q: what can I eat for breakfast?

Real food! What other animal on the planet eats "breakfast foods"? You can eat anything for breakfast as long as you stick to the Paleo way of eating. You may just need an extra ten minutes to cook some meat or eggs. See page 130-137, however, for a meal plan made without any eggs at all.

q: do I need to stop drinking alcohol?

Avoid alcohol entirely if you want to see the best possible results in the shortest possible time. This may mean that you abstain for 30 to 60 days, or it may mean you need to abstain for 3-6 months. For general health, 1-2 drinks per week of gluten-free alcoholic beverages should not be problematic (see page 89). If you are dealing with a specific health condition, however, eliminating alcohol is highly recommended.

q: do I need to stop drinking coffee?

It's a healthy goal to decrease your caffeine consumption to two cups (total of 16 ounces) or fewer per day. Then, don't drink it after 12:00 p.m. if you want to get a good night's sleep. Note that one cup of regular coffee contains roughly 150mg of caffeine, and one shot of espresso contains about 50-75mg of caffeine. If you are propping yourself up on multiple cups of coffee or other caffeinated drinks (energy drinks, sodas, etc.) throughout the day, this is a sign that your system is "running on fumes."

First, try to get better and more sleep if at all possible. If you're simply staying up late and not sleeping or riding a blood sugar rollercoaster, address your diet and lifestyle habits. Focus on sleep first, and caffeine intake should be easier to limit thereafter.

If you feel you have a healthy relationship with caffeine, and you can enjoy just one cup in the morning, go ahead and drink it. Just don't lie to yourself about it. Be honest and assess your use and/or abuse of caffeine.

q: what should I drink if I'm tired of plain water?

Freshly cut and squeezed lemon, lime, or orange wedges are great ways to give your water a kick. You can also try a "spa water" approach by adding cucumber slices with fresh mint leaves, as well as other fruits or berries (just a couple of slices or pieces are plenty) to make it more interesting. Bubbly mineral water is also a good choice, either plain or with some citrus or other whole food flavors added. You can sip on warm broth as well when the weather is cooler. (See page 234 for a recipe.)

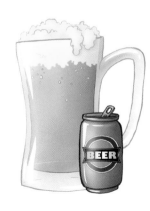

q: if I can't afford to buy everything grass-fed, wild-caught, organic, and perfectly sourced, will I still reap the health benefits of this way of eating?

The short answer is *yes!* Check out my tips for eating Paleo on a budget on page 48, but recognize that many of the health benefits you'll experience come from simply the elimination of modern, refined foods. Once you've gotten those foods out of your diet, you can work little by little to improve the quality of the foods you eat as your budget allows.

q: what's the best way to gain muscle mass but not body fat?

First of all, get adequate sleep! If you aren't sleeping well, you're at a disadvantage hormonally, and body composition is all about hormone balance. More sleep will mean better growth hormone release (which is beneficial to muscle growth, as well as fat burning). Next, make sure you are absorbing the nutrients from what you eat. Adding calories to your intake is pointless if your digestion is shot, so work on improving your digestion. If you have a leaky gut, review the steps in that chapter to heal this condition first. Don't eat foods that irritate your system. By now, you know which ones, or you know how to find out which ones bother you.

In a nutshell:

1. Ensure you are sleeping well and abundantly. More sleep = more growth hormone release.
2. Heal leaky gut.
3. Eat more protein (food, not powder), and chew your food well. Read more about protein powder on page 121 and more about why chewing matters on page 59.
4. Reduce your stress.
5. Lift heavy things. I'm not a strength coach, so turn to a well-trained expert for help there.
6. If you tolerate dairy products, add some raw, grass-fed dairy in the form of whole milk, cream, and/or kefir to your food intake.
7. Go for calorie density first and appetite drivers thereafter: In other words, eat fats like coconut milk, dried coconut, avocado, and macadamia/walnuts, or add extra-virgin olive oil on salads. Eating a few more starchy and carb-rich foods may help to increase your appetite. You can also drink smoothies. Make one with full-fat coconut milk and some fruit or even sweet potato and cinnamon.

If you are doing everything right and not adding muscle mass, get your hormone levels tested. Then, work with a practitioner to balance your levels.

q: what about protein powders?

They aren't food. Okay, I'll bend just a little: if you're looking to gain muscle mass, or you're a hard-charging athlete who needs extra fuel beyond real meals to maintain your current level of muscle mass and performance, liquid food-protein powders can be useful. First, refer to my answer to the last question if you want to add muscle mass. If your sleep and digestion are a problem, protein shakes are not a solution.

If you're on a mass-gain mission and are chowing down as much food as you can but still need to get some more calories and protein in your system, some powdered food might be okay for you. The best types of protein powder are either purely egg white or non-denatured whey protein from a grass-fed source. When you mix it into your shakes, add it at the very end and pulse it just a few times in the blender so that you don't then denature the protein. That said, these are isolated nutrients and should be viewed as supplementation sources, *not* food replacements. If you are capable of eating food, you should eat food.

For most people, powdered nutrition is not essential, and I find that it should be reserved for those with diminished capacity to chew and swallow like the elderly or someone suffering from dysphagia (inability to swallow).

q: what's the best approach to losing body fat?

Reducing body fat overall is about achieving a hormonal balance. Therefore, reducing systemic inflammation by getting your digestive function and blood sugar regulation in check are the first steps. Additionally, adequate sleep is critical, as cortisol levels are regulated during restful sleep. Cortisol is going to drive your hormonal boat either in a favorable or unfavorable direction, so keep it in check.

If you are getting great sleep, your digestion is good, and your blood sugar is well balanced throughout the day, the next steps are:

1. Monitor your carbohydrate intake relative to your activity level. This doesn't mean that everyone needs to be on a low or zero carb diet to lose body fat. It does mean, however, that if you are a very sedentary person, your carbohydrate intake should be limited to roughly 50g per day or fewer for at least 1 to 3 months to see how your body responds. If you are active daily, you may be able to take in about 50-75g of carbohydrates per day, and more if you are *very* active daily (such as in a standing/walking or manual labor-intensive job.) Reducing carbohydrate intake relative to your activity

levels will allow your body to make better use of your own stored body fat as a fuel source in between meals.

2. If you are hungry, eat more protein, which will help you to feel satiated.

3. Reduce your stress levels, as stress can undo everything you do right nutritionally. Don't let your hard work of eating well be for nothing!

q: i'm doing everything "right," but I'm not losing weight. why?

If you've been following a Paleo diet strictly for at least three months without weight loss (if you needed to lose weight), there may be other factors at play. For many people, changes in diet and lifestyle go a long way toward rebalancing their body's systems. If you're not seeing the progress you'd like to see, your problems may be a result of hormonal imbalances, heavy metal or environmental toxicity, stress, over-training, or lack of sleep. Bear in mind, too, that some people simply require longer periods of time (up to a year) of sustained intake of healthy foods before they see noticeable change. As daunting as that may sound, think about how long you have spent making poor food choices. When you think in those terms, a year isn't so long for your body to readjust. Changing your diet is not a magic bullet solution, though it can certainly work amazingly well in a very short period of time for a lot of people.

q: should I take supplements for general health?

It's easy to get caught up in a lot of hype about supplements, but your priority for at least the first three months should be to adjust your diet and lifestyle. For this reason, you'll notice that the "Squeaky Clean Paleo 30-Day Meal Plan" does not include any supplements. Once you've made significant diet and lifestyle changes, I recommend getting your Vitamin D levels tested by a doctor, holistic nutritionist, or naturopath. This is one of the most common deficiencies we see today, and Vitamin D performs a large number of functions in the body. Beyond that, proper vitamin and mineral intake can be achieved largely from a well-balanced Paleo diet if you're digesting and absorbing food properly. If you sense that you're deficient in something, find a practitioner who can help you determine if your digestion is working properly and if you need to make any adjustments regarding your diet and supplementation. There are a wide array of diagnostic tests that can be done, one of which is called an Organic Acids Panel from a lab called Meta-Metrix (only available via practitioners), that may help you discover underlying micronutrient imbalances or impairment in your body's metabolic processes.

q: should I take supplements if I have a medical condition?

The 30-Day Meal Plans in this book include supportive nutrients found in foods, as well as supplements to consider. I have not included dosages or prescriptive quantities since these vary based on each person's individual needs. The plans provide a great jumping-off point for you to create an approach that will work for you, including making smart choices regarding supplementation. I recommend working with a holistic or paleo/ancestral-health oriented practitioner if you feel that you need more assistance after about a month on a plan you have created for yourself. Ultimately, supplements should be taken just as the name suggests, on a supplemental basis in *addition* to food, not *replacing* it.

q: should I take a fish oil supplement?

I don't generally recommend isolated fish oil supplementation for a few reasons. Fish oil or any other isolated omega-3 fatty acid supplement is geared toward balancing the ratio of n3:n6 (n=omega) in your body. If you're eating a Standard American Diet, that ratio is likely 1:10 to 1:20. From an ancestral and general health perspective, this ratio should be under 1:4, if possible.

Instead of supplementation, I recommend that you eat fish (a whole food) to get omega-3. Nutrients in food are much more bio-available than supplements.

It's also difficult to know and trust the source of your isolated omega-3 supplements. Additionally, omega-3 is a polyunsaturated fatty acid (PUFA), and PUFAs are highly susceptible to damage (oxidation from heat, light, and air) if not handled carefully and appropriately. I don't trust that the delicate polyunsaturated fats in most omega-3 supplements were not damaged in the processing and extraction of the oil. Consuming damaged isolated omega-3 supplements is likely far worse than consuming none at all, so I don't recommend them.

When it comes to omega-3/omega-6 fatty acid balance, I always recommend reducing omega-6 intake drastically (as you will do when you eliminate vegetable oils, grains, and legumes) before adding any supplementation of omega-3 fatty acids like fish oil. If you're concerned about systemic inflammation, you may even want to watch your food-based intake of omega-6-rich items other than oils. Nuts high in omega-6 fatty acids include almonds, pecans, pine nuts, pistachios, and hazelnuts.

DAMAGED PUFA?
You're doing well to avoid oxidized (damaged) omega-6 fatty acids on a regular basis by not cooking with or consuming refined seed oils. What if the omega-3 supplement you are taking has been oxidized? Unless you're sure that it's safe, I recommend finding another way to increase your omega-3 intake: by eating it in whole foods.

q: i see fermented cod liver oil in a lot of the meal plans, how is it different from fish oil?

This concentrated superfood is made by a traditional, cold fermentation process versus a heat-process applied to most isolated omega-3 supplements. Furthermore, the primary benefit of fermented cod liver oil is the concentrated presence of naturally occurring fat-soluble vitamins: A, D, E and K2 that are scarce in modern diets. There are some small amounts of omega-3 fatty acids in fermented cod liver oil (FCLO), however, the cold processing, fermentation, and concentrated food-form of this supplement make it a much safer and more health-promoting option than isolated PUFA available in traditional fish oil supplements on the market. Those taking FCLO report improvements in a wide variety of inflammatory conditions and symptoms. The only brand I currently recommend for FCLO is Green Pasture (www.greenpasture.org). *Note: most people find that the cinnamon flavored gel is most palatable.*

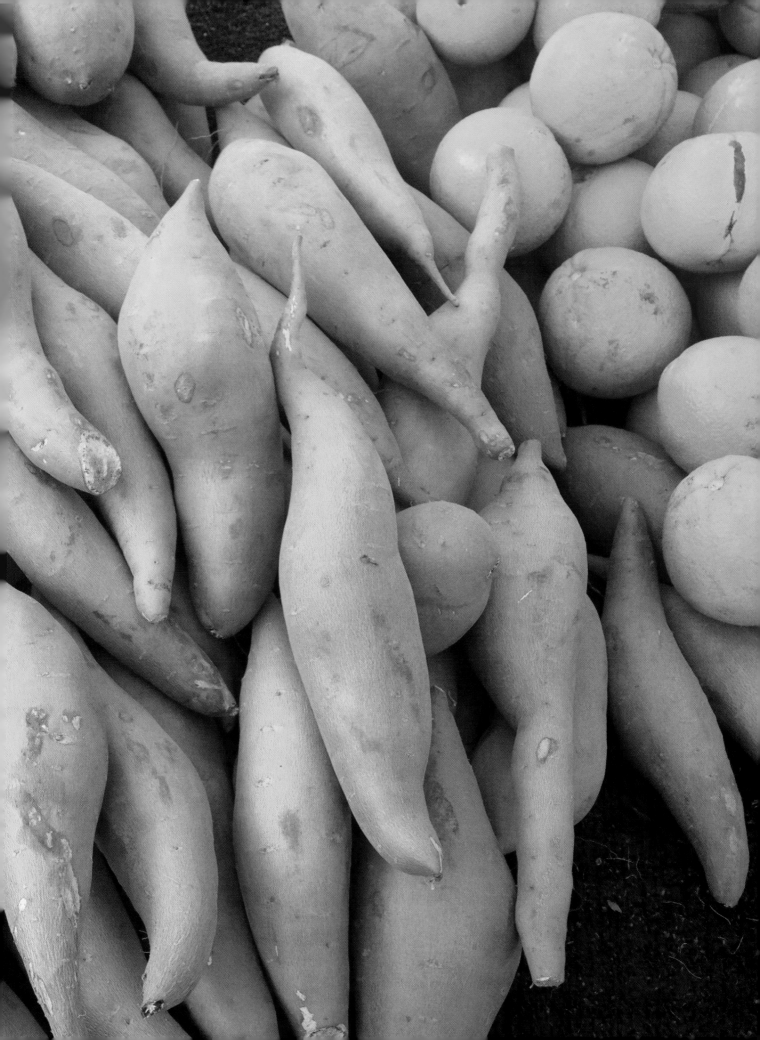

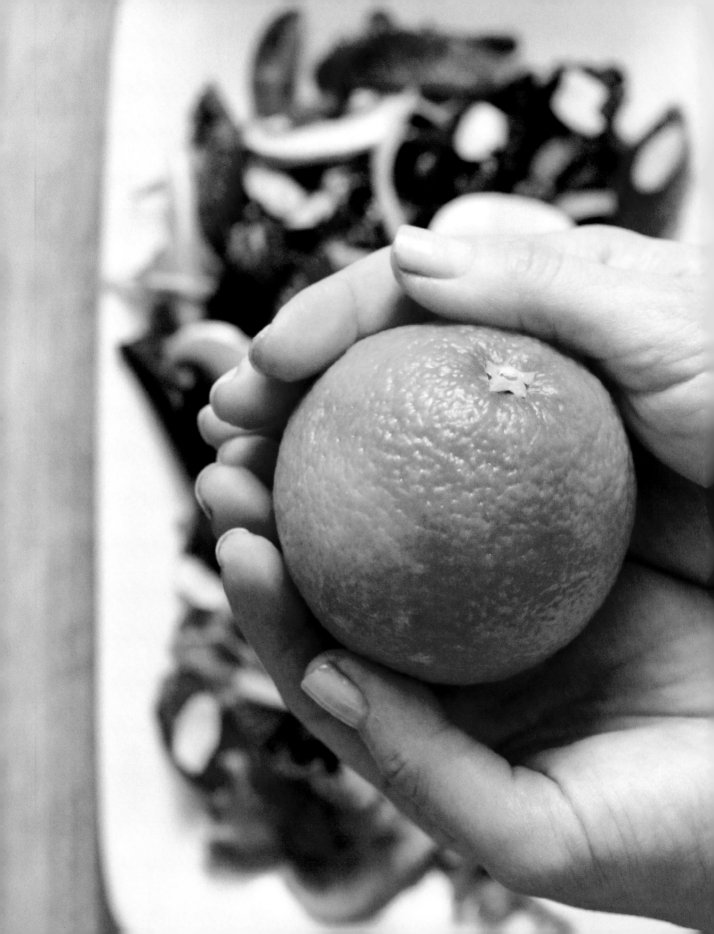

PART 2:
MEAL PLANS

navigating meal plans

☐ Eat whole foods and avoid modern, processed, and refined foods.

☐ Eat to maintain proper digestive function.

☐ Eat to maintain proper blood sugar regulation.

☑ **Follow a plan that will help you reach your own personal health goals.**

Each of the 30-Day Meal Plans focus on a specific condition, set of related conditions, or goals. They were created from a basic Paleo template using primarily recipes in this book. Although you don't have to follow the recipe guides exactly each day, it is important to note that the plans were tailored to move you in the right direction. While everyone can benefit from real, whole foods, it is impossible to make a set of meal plans that work as-is for every person. For example, nuts may appear in the meal plan you are following in a couple of places, and if you are allergic to nuts, simply work around those recommendations. While there is a lot of science behind the food recommendations I offer, creating a healthier person is not about which green, leafy vegetable you should eat today, and which starchy one you should eat tomorrow. These plans are to help you navigate, but most likely they do not factor in every one of your individual needs.

Read the [+] add and [-] avoid list at the beginning of the meal plan you want to follow before diving into it. The meal plans correspond to the recipes, and some of the recipes might need to be slightly altered, depending on which meal plan you are following. The over-arching add/avoid list should serve as a compass for navigating the meal plan and any other interesting recipes you find in this book, other books, or on the web.

Read the entire meal plan before you get started. If you see that a meal or parts of a meal repeat, you can save yourself a lot of cooking time by preparing extra so that you have the appropriate amount of leftovers.

Colored icons under the day number indicates the main protein sources used in the meals for that day. Many of the recipes can be made with interchangeable protein sources. For example, ground turkey can sometimes be used in place of beef, and in some cases chicken can be used instead of pork. If you would like to avoid certain types of protein for taste, personal, or religious reasons, these colored icons will help you plan ahead. Note that when bacon or sausage are served with eggs, eggs are noted as the main protein source since bacon and sausage are much higher in fat and not very dense sources of protein, relatively speaking.

Snacks have not been planned, as the meals should be plenty of food to satisfy your appetite. If you find you need more food, additional small servings of the foods in your meal plan are recommended.

You may choose to conduct further research on the lifestyle and supplement recommendations included with each plan in order to tailor them to your specific needs. The resources included to the left will provide a wealth of additional information on all of the conditions for which the meal plans have been created.

ADDITIONAL RESOURCES

"Life Extension: Disease Prevention and Treatment." Life Extension Media.

"Alternative Medicine: The Definitive Guide," Larry Trivieri Jr. and John W. Anderson, Editors.

"Encyclopedia of Nutritional Supplements: The Essential Guide for Improving Your Health Naturally," by Michael Murray.

portion size guidelines

FOOD TYPE	GENERAL PORTION SIZE GUIDELINES
PROTEINS	**For women: 3-8 ounces for meals, 2-4 ounces for snacks. For men: 8-12 ounces for meals, 3-6 ounces for snacks.** The higher end of the range is recommended for more active or larger individuals, and the lower end for more sedentary or smaller individuals.
NON-STARCHY VEGGIES	**Eat non-starchy veggies to satiety, do not limit them.** If they are drowning in fats or oils, you may need to monitor your intake for certain goals (as outlined in the meal plans). If a vegetable is marked with an asterisk (*), it may be interchanged with any other non-starchy vegetable that suits your needs and preferences.
STARCHY VEGGIES	**Approximately 1/2 to 1 cup in meals for women Approximately 1 to 1 1/2 cups or more for men.** Portions may vary based on your activity level and overall size/calorie needs. See the Guide to Dense Carbs for a list of starchy veggies. If these vegetables are marked with an double asterisk (**), it may be interchanged with any other starchy vegetable that suits your needs and preferences.
FRUITS	**For larger pieces of fruit, 1/2 of a piece is one serving. Around 1/2 to 1 cup of berries is a good serving size.** Again, these portion sizes may be modified and increased or decreased per the recommendations in your specific plan. Enjoy any in season fruit you like. Any fruit included in a meal plan is interchangeable, so choose whichever you enjoy. See the Guide to: Food Quality on page 31 for more information.
FATS/OILS	**1 to 2 tablespoons of a fat or oil is a serving for women. 2 to 4 tablespoons of a fat or oil is a serving for men.** A good portion of oil for a salad is around 2 tablespoons, while 1 tablespoon may be adequate for melting over steamed vegetables. This also varies by size and activity level; being a larger and/or more active person will warrant additional fat intake and, coincidentally, adding fat to meals is one of the easiest ways to add good calories and satiety if you do need more to eat.

30-DAY MEAL PLANS

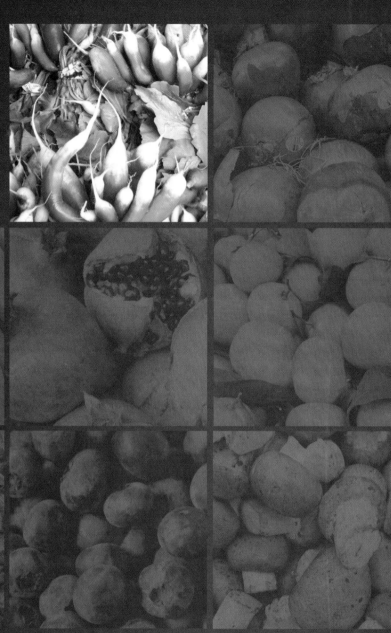

AUTOIMMUNE CONDITIONS

While the root causes and resulting symptoms may vary slightly, autoimmune conditions share underpinnings in digestive distress and, specifically, increased intestinal permeability (leaky gut). This meal plan is similar to the one for Digestive Health, but it is designed to be a more specific protocol for those diagnosed with autoimmune conditions. After completing this plan, you may find that additional therapeutic interventions for your condition will help further put your symptoms into remission. However, you may also discover that a basic Paleo approach works well for you without further limitations or omissions.

autoimmune conditions include but are not limited to:

- Addison's Disease
- Alzheimer's Disease
- Asthma
- Celiac Disease
- Chronic Fatigue Syndrome
- Crohn's Disease
- Eczema
- Grave's Disease
- Hashimoto's Thyroiditis
- Lupus
- Multiple Sclerosis
- Parkinson's Disease
- Pernicious Anemia
- Psoriasis
- Raynaud's Disease
- Rheumatoid Arthritis
- Scleroderma
- Type 1 Diabetes
- Vitiligo

All of the above conditions, as well as any chronic inflammatory condition (see page 74), can be helped by following an autoimmune protocol for at least 30 days, and a basic Paleo diet template (following the food guides throughout this book) thereafter, with varying levels of detail based on your main concerns and symptoms. Several of the above conditions also have specific meal plans later in this section.

Disclaimer: The information in this book is not intended to be a replacement for professional medical diagnosis or treatment for a medical condition. It consists solely of nutritional and lifestyle recommendations to support a healthier body.

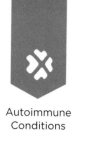

diet & lifestyle recommendations

add [+]

WELL-COOKED FOODS
Meals such as braised meats, stews, soups, and slow-cooked foods are easier to digest.

NUTRIENT-DENSE FOODS
Replenish depleted nutrient stores from eating excess refined foods over time.

SUPERFOODS
Make bone broth, and drink or cook with it regularly (recipe on page 234).

STRESS MANAGEMENT
Develop a guided meditation practice, a slow breathing practice, or begin to practice Qi Gong.

MOVEMENT
Take walks outside, or practice gentle yoga for movement without systemic stress.

Slowly begin weight training with moderate to heavy weight, not excessively demanding in terms of stress response or cortisol output.

avoid [-]

GUT-IRRITANTS
Foods with known immunological responses, including **grains, legumes, dairy (all dairy, even grass-fed for this meal plan), eggs, nuts, seeds, nightshades;** avoid large quantities of vegetables and fruits that are high in *insoluble* fiber, such as leafy greens, raspberries, and strawberries. **ALL RECIPES HAVE NOTES FOR SUBSTITUTIONS WHERE POSSIBLE. PLEASE FOLLOW THESE!**

GLUTEN
100% of the time. See the "Guide to Gluten" on page 89.

ALCOHOL, CAFFEINE, CHOCOLATE
As they can promote leaky gut.

STRESS
Make lifestyle changes to avoid stressful situations.

PAIN MEDICATIONS
Including aspirin, acetaminophen, ibuprofen, and corticosteroids as they can promote leaky gut.

HARSH CHEMICAL CLEANING OR HYGIENE PRODUCTS
Opt for gentle, natural alternatives, such as soap nuts for laundry, vinegar and water solutions for counter top cleaning, and baking soda and peroxide for cleaning and whitening surfaces, laundry, teeth, etc. Research the "No Poo" method online for hair cleansing without commercial shampoos.

HIGH INTENSITY EXERCISE
Overly intense exercise (high intensity interval training/HIIT-style workouts) and chronic cardiovascular exercise (30-60+ minutes at a steady state of intensity like jogging or biking) as it can provoke a stress-response in the body.

DISCLAIMER:
The information in this book is not intended to be a replacement for professional medical diagnosis or treatment for a medical condition. It consists solely of nutritional and lifestyle recommendations to support a healthier body.

nutritional supplements & herbs to consider

These recommendations are made as a starting point. Do your own research and determine which supplements may serve you best. It's best to get as many of your nutrients from food as possible. See the next page for specific food-based nutrients on which to focus. The items below are listed in no particular order.

» **VITAMIN A (retinol)** improves immunity when balanced with vitamin D and helps to maintain the integrity of the mucosal lining of the gut and immunity; necessary for assimilation of dietary minerals.

» **FERMENTED COD LIVER OIL/ BUTTER OIL BLEND** for fat-soluble vitamins A, D, E, and K2 as well as some omega 3 fats. I only recommend Green Pasture brand.

» **COENZYME 10 (CO-Q10, Ubiquinone)** enhances mitochondrial energy production and can help to alleviate fatigue and muscle/joint pain. It is a potent antioxidant, which statin drugs are known to deplete.

» **DIGESTIVE ENZYMES** help to break down food for absorption while your gut is healing. Look for a blend of enzymes.

» **L-GLUTAMINE** aids in the healing of the epithelial cells that line the small intestine.

» **HERBAL TEAS** that are calming to your digestive system include peppermint, ginger, kudzu, marshmallow root, and slippery elm.

» **LICORICE ROOT** is an herb that aids in repairing the mucosal lining of the gut, as well as the stomach. Look for licorice root tea, an extract of the herb, or a chewable tablet called DGL.

» **ALOE VERA JUICE** (unless it promotes loose stool).

» **MAGNESIUM** is required for more than 300 enzymatic processes in the body, and most people are deficient. It is useful in blood sugar regulation. Look for magnesium glycinate or magnesium malate forms.

» **PHOSPHATIDYLCHOLINE** enhances the integrity of the GI tract and aids in fatty acid digestion, as well as repairs the mucosal lining of the gut. This supplement is especially important when avoiding eggs.

» **PROBIOTIC SUPPLEMENTS** for better digestion. Try different brands to find one that works best for you. Start slowly with small dosages. Note that brands available via professional practitioners are often more potent than commercial brands.

» **QUERCITIN** is a potent antioxidant that promotes better immunity.

» **SELENIUM & ZINC** are antioxidants that protect against free radical damage and may need to be supplemented as it's difficult to obtain adequate amounts from food.

» **ZINC CARNOSINE** may improve gut mucosa and gut lining integrity.

YOU ARE UNIQUE

If you continue to suffer from specific symptoms, consider the food eliminations below on a continued basis or as part of an elimination-provocation test according to the 4-R protocol as outlined on page 88.

Some ways to help known issues include the following:

Joint pain, mobility issues: Eliminate nightshade vegetables, eggs, nuts, and seeds.

Skin conditions: Eliminate eggs, nuts, seeds, and all forms of dairy (even grass-fed).

supportive nutrients & foods that contain them

quick LIST

proteins

Beef
Bison
Cold water fish (salmon, herring, mackerel)
Eel
Lamb
Liver
Oysters
Shellfish

fats

Animal fats
Coconut oil
Extra-virgin olive oil
Red palm oil

vegetables

Beets
Broccoli
Brussels sprouts
Butternut squash
Cauliflower
Daikon radish
Garlic
Okra
Sweet potatoes
Swiss chard

fruits

Plantains
Bananas
Blueberries
Lemon juice

superfoods

Bone broth
Fermented cod liver oil
Fermented vegetables
Liver

spices

Basil
Cilantro
Cinnamon
Cumin
Garlic
Ginger
Oregano
Parsley
Turmeric

VITAMIN A (RETINOL)

» Liver, eel, grass-fed butter, clarified butter, or ghee (only introduce butter and ghee after the first 30-days without them)

BUTYRIC ACID

helps to decrease intestinal permeability.

» Grass-fed butter, clarified butter, or ghee (only introduce butter and ghee after the first 30-days without them)

VITAMIN C

A potent antioxidant with anti-inflammatory properties.

» Cauliflower
» Broccoli
» Daikon radish
» Lemon juice
» Garlic
» Beets
» Brussels sprouts

VITAMIN D

A potent immune system modulator that is most available from sun exposure.

» Cold water fish (salmon, herring, mackerel)
» Grass-fed butter or ghee (only introduce butter and ghee after the first 30-days without them)
» Fermented cod liver oil/butter oil blend (Green Pasture brand only)

GLYCINE

Helps to repair the gut cell lining.

» Bone broth (recipe on page 234)
» Gelatin (recipe on page 234)

OMEGA-3 FATS

An anti-inflammatory essential fatty acid that comes from limited food sources.

» Cold water fish (salmon, herring, mackerel, etc.)
» Fermented cod liver oil (Green Pasture brand only)

PROBIOTICS

Promotes healthy gut flora, which is critical to proper digestion and elimination.

» Fermented vegetables: cabbage (sauerkraut, kimchi) carrots, beets, etc.
» Kombucha (fermented tea)

SELENIUM

An antioxidant that protects against free radical damage.

» Red Swiss chard
» Turnips
» Garlic

SOLUBLE FIBER

Feeds the beneficial bacteria in your gut to promote proper motility.

» Sweet potatoes
» Butternut squash
» Plantains
» Bananas

ZINC

A potent antioxidant often deficient in people with inflammatory conditions; aids in vitamin A metabolism.

» Oysters
» Shellfish
» Lamb
» Red meat

autoimmune conditions

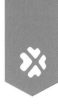

DAY	BREAKFAST	LUNCH	DINNER
1 ■ ■ ◆	Mustard Glazed Chicken Thighs (266), Sweet Potato**, Raw Sauerkraut (238)	*left-over* Mustard Glazed Chicken Thighs (266), Summer squash*	Grilled Garlic Flank Steak with Onions - no peppers (294), Baked Beets with Fennel**(362)
2 ◆ ◆ ■	*left-over* Garlic Flank Steak with Onions, Butternut Squash**	Wild Canned Salmon with Olives, Avocado, Lemon Juice, EVOO	Sage Roasted Turkey Legs (276), Sweet Potato Pancakes - make hash (298), Steamed Spinach*
3 ■ ■ ●	Chicken Thighs, *left-over* Sweet Potato Hash	*left-over* Sage Roasted Turkey Legs, Persimmon, Asparagus & Fennel Salad (380)	Lemony Lamb Dolmas (318), Cilantro Cauli-Rice (340)
4 ● ● ◆	Ground Lamb with a spice blend, Cilantro Cauli-Rice (340), Raw Sauerkraut (238)	*left-over* Lemony Lamb Dolmas, Spinach Salad with Artichokes (380)	Asian Orange Pan-Seared Scallops (304), Butternut Squash**
5 ◆ ◆ ◆	Ground beef with Curry Spice Blend (233) (omit Paprika), Butternut Squash**	Nori Salmon Handrolls (316)	Beef & Mixed Veggie Stir Fry (286), Cilantro Cauli-Rice (340)*
6 ◐ ◆ ●	Breakfast Sausage using Italian Sausage Spice Blend (233), Swiss chard*	*left-over* Beef Stir Fry with Mixed Veggies, Sweet Potato**	Lamb Lettuce Boats with Avo-Ziki Sauce (322)
7 ■ ◆ ■	Savory Baked Chicken Legs (use spices without Paprika) (264), Squash*, Raw Sauerkraut (238)	Mixed Greens with Wild Canned Salmon, Asparagus*, Lemon Juice, EVOO	Citrus & Herb Whole Roasted Chicken (256), Roasted Rosemary Roots (350)
8 ■ ■ ■	*left-over* Citrus & Herb Whole Roasted Chicken, Avocado, Apple or Blueberries	Spinach Salad with Artichokes (380), *left-over* Citrus & Herb Whole Roasted Chicken	Chinese 5-Spice Lettuce Cups (272), Sweet Potato**
9 ■ ■ ◆	Bacon-Wrapped Chicken Thighs made without Smoky Blend (262), Plantains in CO**	Indian-Spiced Turkey Burgers (268), Steamed Broccoli*	Pesto Shrimp & Squash Fettuccine (made without nuts) (308)
10 ◆ ◆ ◐	Shrimp, Avocado, Cucumbers, Apple	Simple Shrimp Ceviche without peppers (316), Mixed Greens*, EVOO	Cumin Spiced Pork Tenderloin with Root Vegetables**(328)

» *A complete shopping list for this meal plan can be found on balancedbites.com*

REMEMBER, NO:
grains	seeds
legumes	eggs
dairy	nightshades
nuts	

KEY

◆ Beef & Bison
■ Poultry
◐ Pork
● Lamb
◆ Seafood

NOTES

EVOO — Extra-virgin olive oil
CO — Coconut oil
* — or other non-starchy vegetable
** — or other starchy vegetable (refer to page 110)

If no page number is listed, simply prepare the items as noted or any way you like.
For additional protein, vegetable, and fat recommendations, refer to the QUICK LIST that is associated with your meal plan!

DAY	BREAKFAST	LUNCH	DINNER
11 ●■◆	*left-over* Cumin Spiced Pork Tenderloin and Root Vegetables	Chicken, Rainbow Red Cabbage Salad*(372) or Sautéed Cabbage	Orange Braised Beef Shanks (284), Spinach*
12 ●◆■	Breakfast Sausage using Italian Sausage Spice Blend (233), *left-over* Red Cabbage*	*left-over* Orange Braised Beef Shanks, Carrots**	Savory Baked Chicken Legs (264), Brussels Sprouts with Fennel*(350)
13 ◆■◆	Smoked Salmon, Spinach*, Raw Sauerkraut (238)	*left-over* Savory Baked Chicken Legs, *left-over* Brussels Sprouts with Fennel*	Lemon Rosemary Broiled Salmon (306), Asparagus with Lemon & Olives (338), Sweet Potato**
14 ◆■◆	*left-over* Lemon Rosemary Broiled Salmon, *left-over* Asparagus with Lemon & Olives*	Chicken Lettuce Wraps with Avocado, Salsa made from Cucumbers (296)	Red Palm & Coriander Tuna Over Daikon Noodle Salad (302), Green Salad*
15 ◆◆◆	Wild Salmon (canned) with Olives, Avocado, Lemon Juice	Spinach Salad with EVOO, *left-over* Red Palm & Coriander Tuna, Avocado, Lemon Juice	Italian-Style Stuffed Peppers (use zucchini instead of peppers) (300), Green Salad*
16 ●◆■	Breakfast Sausage using Italian Sausage Spice Blend (233), Zucchini*	*left-over* Italian-Style Stuffed Peppers (use zucchini instead of peppers), Green Salad*	Bacon-Wrapped Chicken Thighs made without Smoky Blend (262), Mixed Greens Salad*
17 ●■◆	*left-over* Breakfast Sausage, Plantains in CO***	*left-over* Bacon-Wrapped Smoky Chicken Thighs made without Smoky Blend, Green Salad*	Ground beef cooked with Garlic & Basil over Spaghetti Squash**
18 ◆◆●	Ground Beef, Bacon, *left-over* Spaghetti Squash**	Wild Salmon (canned) with Green Beans*, EVOO, Lemon	Thanksgiving Stuffing Meatballs (334), Mashed Faux-Tatoes (344)
19 ◆●◆	Wild Salmon (canned) with Olives, Avocado, Lemon Juice	*left-over* Thanksgiving Stuffing Meatballs, *left-over* Mashed Faux-Tatoes	Halibut, Lemon Roasted Romanesco*(346), Sweet potato**
20 ●◆■	Acorn Squash with Cinnamon & Coconut Butter (358), Breakfast Sausage or Bacon	*left-over* Halibut, *left-over* Lemon Roasted Romanesco	Roasted Duck with Cherry Sauce (274), Sautéed Red Cabbage with Onions and Apples*(352)

» *A complete shopping list for this meal plan can be found on balancedbites.com*

KEY
◆ Beef & Bison
■ Poultry
● Pork
● Lamb
◆ Seafood

NOTES

EVOO   Extra-virgin olive oil

CO   Coconut oil

*   or other non-starchy vegetable

**   or other starchy vegetable (refer to page 110)

If no page number is listed, simply prepare the items as noted or any way you like.

For additional protein, vegetable, and fat recommendations, refer to the QUICK LIST that is associated with your meal plan!

REMEMBER, NO:

grains	seeds
legumes	eggs
dairy	nightshades
nuts	

DAY	BREAKFAST	LUNCH	DINNER
21 ■◆●	*left-over* Roasted Duck with Cherry Sauce, Spinach*	Nori Salmon Handrolls (316)	Lamb Chops with Olive Tapenade (326), Greek Salad with Avo-Ziki (374)
22 ◆●◆	Wild Salmon (canned) with Olives, Avocado, Lemon Juice	*left-over* Lamb Chops with Olive Tapenade, *left-over* Greek Salad with Avo-Ziki	Orange Braised Beef Shanks (284), Butternut Sage Soup**(348)
23 ●◆◆	Breakfast Sausage using Italian Sausage Spice Blend (233)	*left-over* Orange Braised Beef Shanks, *left-over* Butternut Sage Soup	Hayley's Skirt Steak Tacos (292), Cucumber Salsa (296), Grilled Squash & Pineapple (342)
24 ●◆◆	Acorn Squash with Cinnamon & Coconut Butter (358), Perfectly Baked Bacon (236)	Tangy Taco Salad (296), *left-over* Cucumber Salsa	Beef burgers, Avocado, Lettuce Wraps, Red Roasted Garlic (370)
25 ◆◆◆	*left-over* Beef burgers, Avocado, Lettuce Wraps	Wild Salmon or Tuna, Green Salad*, Avocado, Olives	Asian Orange Pan-Seared Scallops (304), Baked Beets (362)
26 ■◆●	Chicken, *left-over* Beets, Orange, Orange Vinaigrette (382)	Tuna, Mixed Greens Salad with Persimmons, Asparagus & Fennel (380), Orange Vinaigrette (382)	Grandma Barbara's Stuffed Mushrooms (332), Roasted Marrow Bones (288)
27 ■●●	Mustard Glazed Chicken Thighs (266), Sweet Potato**, Raw Sauerkraut (238)	*left-over* Grandma Barbara's Stuffed Mushrooms, Mixed Greens Salad*, Balsamic Vinaigrette (378)	Spiced Lamb Meatballs with Balsamic-Fig Compote (324), Green Beans with Shallots*(358)
28 ●◆■	*left-over* Spiced Lamb Meatballs, Plantains in CO**	Wild Canned Salmon with Olives, Avocado, Lemon Juice, EVOO	Lemon & Artichoke Chicken (260), Broc-Cauli Chowder with Bacon (336)
29 ●■◆	Breakfast Sausage using Italian Sausage Spice Blend (233), Parsnips**	*left-over* Lemon & Artichoke Chicken, Kale Chips (356)	Mom's Stuffed Cabbage Rolls - leave off the Tomato Cranberry sauce (290), Green Salad*
30 ●■●	*left-over* Breakfast Sausage using Italian Sausage Spice Blend, Squash**	Turkey Meatballs, Mashed Faux-Tatoes (344)	Mediterranean Lamb Roast (320), Sautéed Spinach with Currants*(366)

» *A complete shopping list for this meal plan can be found on balancedbites.com*

KEY
◆ Beef & Bison
■ Poultry
● Pork
● Lamb
◆ Seafood

NOTES

EVOO — Extra-virgin olive oil

CO — Coconut oil

* — or other non-starchy vegetable

** — or other starchy vegetable (refer to page 110)

If no page number is listed, simply prepare the items as noted or any way you like.
For additional protein, vegetable, and fat recommendations, refer to the QUICK LIST that is associated with your meal plan!

REMEMBER, NO:

grains
legumes
dairy
nuts
seeds
eggs
nightshades

30-DAY MEAL PLANS

BLOOD SUGAR REGULATION

dysglycemia
hypoglycemia
diabetes type 1 & 2

blood sugar regulation

If you have been diagnosed with Type 1 Diabetes and have not previously used the Autoimmune Condition 30-Day Meal Plan, start with that plan with regard to food choices, and follow the lifestyle, supplement, and herbal recommendations from this plan.

blood sugar imbalances (dysglycemia)
symptoms include:

» Any blood sugar levels that are high, low, or high then low
» Energy highs and lows throughout the day, generally as a result of a high carbohydrate/refined foods diet, stress, and poor metabolic function

low blood sugar (hypoglycemia)
symptoms include:

» General fatigue
» Energy changes throughout the day
» Waking up tired/insomnia
» Inability to focus/brain fog, mental disturbances, mental confusion
» Blurred vision
» Low blood pressure
» Headaches
» Trembling
» Incoherent speech
» Weakness in legs
» Dry mouth
» Weight gain

» Mood imbalances, such as irritability, negativity, sense of gloom, crying spells, mood swings, erratic behavior, anti-social nature, depression, anxiety, hypersensitivity
» Cravings for sugar and carbohydrates
» Constant hunger
» Compulsive eating
» Loss of appetite
» Loss of sex drive
» Rapid heartbeat/fluttering in chest

DISCLAIMER:

The information in this book is not intended to be a replacement for professional medical diagnosis or treatment for a medical condition. It consists solely of nutritional and lifestyle recommendations to support a healthier body.

type 1 diabetes (hyperglycemia, autoimmune)

Type 1 Diabetes is an autoimmune condition in which the body's immune system self-attacks pancreatic beta cells and destroys them, rendering them incapable of producing insulin. A large percentage of those with Type 1 Diabetes have undiagnosed Celiac Disease and may go on to develop Hashimoto's (autoimmune thyroid condition).

symptoms include:

» Inability of pancreatic beta cells to produce insulin
» Weight loss and malabsorption with excessive thirst

» Generally diagnosed in children following infections that trigger autoimmunity
» Often correlates directly with Celiac Disease and related symptoms

type 2 diabetes (hyperglycemia)
symptoms include:

» Abdominal adiposity (belly fat)
» Weight-loss resistance despite doing "everything right"
» Fatigue, especially post-prandial (after meals)
» High blood glucose
» Poor blood markers in cholesterol (low HDL, high LDL), high triglycerides, high HbA1c (glycosylated hemoglobin), and increased C-Reactive Protein (systemic inflammation) measures

» Loss of appetite/impaired appetite signaling
» Loss of lean muscle mass
» Carbohydrate cravings
» Refer to the symptoms listed for hypoglycemia as they may be present in a Type 2 Diabetic.
» Secondary symptoms include: Metabolic syndrome, irregular periods (duration, type of flow, etc.), Polycystic Ovary Syndrome (PCOS), cardiovascular disease

Other populations who may benefit from this meal plan include those diagnosed with:

» GESTATIONAL DIABETES
» METABOLIC SYNDROME
» HORMONAL IMBALANCES (PCOS, INFERTILITY, ETC.)

You may also use this meal plan as a first step intervention before using the plans created specifically for neurological conditions, depending on how advanced they have become:

» ALZHEIMER'S DISEASE (page 176-183)
» PARKINSON'S DISEASE (page 176-183)

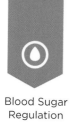

diet & lifestyle recommendations

add [+]

FAT
Many people experiencing dysglycemia patterns are unnecessarily avoiding fats and increasing carbohydrates in the diet, which contributes further to these conditions.

PROTEIN
Protein to satisfy appetite for longer periods of time (meals focused on both fat and protein will help).

NUTRIENT-DENSE FOODS
Replenish depleted nutrient stores from eating excess refined foods over time.

SUPERFOODS
As often as possible. Make and eat/drink bone broth regularly (recipe on page 234). Raw sauerkraut daily (1/4 cup), especially with breakfast (recipe on page 238).

STRESS MANAGEMENT
Develop a guided meditation practice, a slow breathing practice, or begin to practice Qi Gong.

MOVEMENT
Slowly begin weight training with moderate to heavy weight, not excessively demanding in terms of stress response or cortisol output.

Take walks outside, or practice gentle yoga for movement without systemic stress.

Ensure activity is fueled appropriately and in advance; do not exercise if you are experiencing symptoms of low blood sugar; eat a small protein/fat/carbohydrate snack 60-90 minutes before exercise to maintain blood sugar levels.

avoid [-]

GLUTEN
100% of the time. See the "Guide to Gluten" on page 89.

REFINED FOODS & SWEETENERS
Artificial sweeteners and caffeine, as they can provoke blood sugar fluctuations.

ALCOHOL, CAFFEINE, CHOCOLATE
As they can promote hypoglycemic events.

STRESS
Make lifestyle changes to avoid stressful situations.

FASTING
Fasting or going for longer than 4-5 hours without food; once blood sugar is regulated over time, you may allow more hours to pass between meals.

CHRONIC CARDIOVASCULAR EXERCISE
(meaning 30-60+ minutes at a steady state of intensity like jogging or biking), as it can lead to low blood sugar episodes, as well as provoke a stress response.

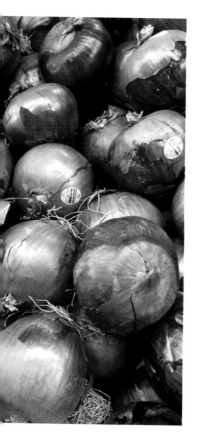

DISCLAIMER:

The information in this book is not intended to be a replacement for professional medical diagnosis or treatment for a medical condition. It consists solely of nutritional and lifestyle recommendations to support a healthier body.

nutritional supplements & herbs to consider

These recommendations are made as a starting point. Do your own research and determine which supplements may serve you best. It's best to get as many of your nutrients from food as possible. See the next page for specific food-based nutrients on which to focus. The items below are listed in no particular order.

» **FERMENTED COD LIVER OIL/ BUTTER OIL BLEND** for fat-soluble vitamins A, D, E, and K2 as well as some omega 3 fats. I only recommend Green Pasture brand.

» **VITAMIN B3 (niacin)** is supportive of blood sugar regulation and may lower cholesterol levels; the niacinamide form may be useful in healing early-onset Type 1 Diabetes.

» **VITAMIN B5 (pantothenic acid & pantethine)** may help lower cholesterol and triglycerides. Look for a B-complex for a balanced dose.

» **VITAMIN B7 (biotin)** is a coenzyme required in the metabolism of glucose, amino acids, and lipids.

» **VITAMIN C** is a potent antioxidant with anti-inflammatory properties. It helps to regenerate vitamin E and is supportive to diabetics.

» **CHROMIUM (chromium picolinate, polynicotinate, chelavite)** may improve insulin sensitivity and reduce appetite.

» **CARNITINE/L-CARNITINE** can improve insulin sensitivity and glucose storage. It optimizes fat and carbohydrate metabolism, and it may improve the utilization of fat as an energy source. Cofactors include iron, vitamin C, vitamins B3 (niacin) and B6.

» **HERBS AND TEAS:** Blood sugar-regulating and adaptogenic herbs, teas, and spices; digestive bitters; schizandra, ginseng; peppermint, ginger, cinnamon.

» **COENZYME Q10 (COQ10)** enhances mitochondrial energy production and can help to alleviate fatigue; known to be depleted by statin drugs

» **VITAMIN E** may reduce oxidative stress-induced insulin resistance.

» **L-GLUTAMINE** helps to calm sugar and carbohydrate cravings.

» **LIPOIC ACID (alpha-lipoic acid/ALA)** has antioxidant properties and may motivate greater glucose uptake from the bloodstream by promoting conversion of carbohydrates into energy.

» **MAGNESIUM** is required for more than 300 enzymatic processes in the body, and most people are deficient in it. This mineral is also useful in blood sugar regulation. Look for magnesium glycinate or magnesium malate forms.

» **N-ACETYL CYSTEINE (NAC)** may reduce the glycation processes that lead to cataract formation.

» **SELENIUM AND ZINC** are antioxidants that protect against free radical damage. Levels obtained from food may not be sufficient.

supportive nutrients
& foods that contain them

VITAMIN A (RETINOL)

» Liver, Eel
» Grass-fed butter,
  clarified butter, or ghee

VITAMIN B5

» Brewer's yeast
  (Lewis Labs brand only)

BUTYRIC ACID

Helps to decrease intestinal permeability.

» Grass-fed butter, clarified butter, or ghee

VITAMIN C

A potent antioxidant with anti-inflammatory properties.

» Cauliflower
» Broccoli
» Daikon radish
» Lemon juice
» Garlic
» Beets
» Brussels sprouts

VITAMIN D

A potent immune system modulator that
is most available from sun exposure.

» Cold water fish (salmon, herring, mackerel, etc.)
» Grass-fed butter or ghee
» Fermented cod liver oil/
  butter oil blend (Green Pasture
  brand only)

GLYCINE

Helps to repair the gut cell lining and
enhance stomach acid production.

» Bone broth
  (recipe on page 234)
» Gelatin (recipe on page 234)

OMEGA-3 FATS

An anti-inflammatory essential fatty acid
that comes from limited food sources.

» Cold water fish
  (salmon, herring, mackerel, etc.)
» Fermented cod liver oil (Green
  Pasture brand only)
» Walnuts, pecans

PROBIOTICS

Promotes healthy gut flora, which is critical to proper digestion and elimination.

» Fermented vegetables: cabbage, sauerkraut, kimchi,
  carrots
» Kombucha (fermented tea)

SELENIUM

An antioxidant that protects against free
radical damage.

» Eggs
» Red Swiss chard
» Turnips
» Garlic

SOLUBLE FIBER

Feeds the beneficial bacteria in your gut
to promote proper motility. Eat in small
amounts if your digestion needs support.

» Sweet potatoes
» Butternut squash
» Plantains

ZINC

A potent antioxidant often deficient in
people with inflammatory conditions; aids
in vitamin A metabolism.

» Oysters
» Shellfish
» Lamb
» Red meat

blood sugar regulation

DAY	BREAKFAST	LUNCH	DINNER
1 ●■◆	Swirly Crustless Quiche (240), Perfectly Baked Bacon (236), Raw Sauerkraut (238)	Mustard Glazed Chicken Thighs (266), Green Salad*, Balsamic Vinaigrette (378)	Grilled Garlic Flank Steak with Peppers & Onions (294), Baked Beets with Fennel**(362)
2 ●◆■	*left-over* Swirly Crustless Quiche, *left-over* Garlic Flank Steak with Peppers & Onions	Wild Canned Salmon with Olives, Avocado, Lemon Juice, Tomato, EVOO	Sage Roasted Turkey Legs (276), Steamed Spinach*
3 ■■●	Mustard-Glazed Chicken Thighs (266), Broccoli*	*left-over* Sage Roasted Turkey Legs, Persimmon, Asparagus & Fennel Salad (380)	Lemony Lamb Dolmas (318), Cilantro Cauli-Rice (340)
4 ●●◆	Pesto Scrambled Eggs (252), Cilantro Cauli-Rice (340), Raw Sauerkraut (238)	*left-over* Lemony Lamb Dolmas, Spinach Salad with Walnuts & Artichokes (380)	Citrus Macadamia Nut Sole (314), Kale*
5 ◆◆◆	*left-over* Citrus Macadamia Nut Sole, Spinach*	Nori Salmon Handrolls (316)	Beef & Mixed Veggie Stir Fry (286)
6 ○◆●	Pumpkin Pancakes (242), Breakfast Sausage using Italian Sausage Spice Blend (233)	*left-over* Beef Stir Fry with Mixed Veggies	Lamb Lettuce Boats with Avo-Ziki Sauce (322)
7 ●◆■	Eggs, Perfectly Baked Bacon (236), Kale*, Raw Sauerkraut (238)	Mixed Greens with Wild Canned Salmon, Asparagus*, Lemon Juice, EVOO	Citrus & Herb Whole Roasted Chicken (256), Simple Baked Kale Chips*(356)
8 ■■■	*left-over* Citrus & Herb Whole Roasted Chicken, Grain-Free Porridge (252), Berries	Spinach Salad with Walnuts & Artichokes (380), *left-over* Citrus & Herb Whole Roasted Chicken	Chinese 5-Spice Lettuce Cups (272)
9 ●■◆	Swirly Crustless Quiche (240), Steamed Broccoli*, Raw Sauerkraut (238)	Indian-Spiced Turkey Burgers (268), Steamed Broccoli*	Pesto Shrimp & Squash Fettuccine (308)
10 ●◆○	Omelet or Pesto Scrambled Eggs, *left-over* Shrimp & Avocado	Simple Shrimp Ceviche (316), Mixed Greens*, EVOO	Cumin Spiced Pork Tenderloin with Root Vegetables**(328)

» *A complete shopping list for this meal plan can be found on balancedbites.com*

KEY

◆ Beef & Bison
■ Poultry
● Eggs
○ Pork
● Lamb
◆ Seafood

NOTES

EVOO   Extra-virgin olive oil
CO   Coconut oil
*   or other non-starchy vegetable
**   or other starchy vegetable (refer to page 110)
If no page number is listed, simply prepare the items as noted or any way you like.
For additional protein, vegetable, and fat recommendations, refer to the QUICK LIST that is associated with your meal plan!

blood sugar regulation

DAY	BREAKFAST	LUNCH	DINNER
11 ●◦◆	Swirly Crustless Quiche (240) Perfectly Baked Bacon (236), *left-over* Root Vegetables*	*left-over* Cumin Spiced Pork Tenderloin, Rainbow Red Cabbage Salad*(372)	Balsamic Braised Short Ribs (278), Carrots, Spinach*
12 ●◆■	Eggs, *left-over* Rainbow Red Cabbage Salad	*left-over* Balsamic Braised Short Ribs, Green Salad*	Savory Baked Chicken Legs (264), Brussels Sprouts with Fennel*(350)
13 ●■◆	Zucchini Pancakes (248), Perfectly Baked Bacon (236), Raw Sauerkraut (238)	*left-over* Savory Baked Chicken Legs, *left-over* Brussels Sprouts with Fennel*	Lemon Rosemary Broiled Salmon (306), Asparagus with Lemon & Olives (338), Sweet Potato**
14 ◆■◆	*left-over* Lemon Rosemary Broiled Salmon, *left-over* Asparagus with Lemon & Olives*	Buffalo Chicken Lettuce Wraps (270)	Red Palm & Coriander Tuna Over Daikon Noodle Salad (302), Green Salad*
15 ●◆■	Scrambled Eggs with Olives, Steamed Spinach*, Avocado	Spinach Salad with EVOO, *left-over* Red Palm & Coriander Tuna, Avocado, Lemon Juice	Italian-Style Stuffed Peppers (300), Green Salad* with Balsamic Vinaigrette (378)
16 ◦◆■	Breakfast Sausage, Grain-Free Porridge (252),	*left-over* Italian-Style Stuffed Peppers (300), Green Salad	Bacon-Wrapped Smoky Chicken Thighs (262), Mixed Greens Salad with Beets & Blood Oranges (376)
17 ●■◆	Bacon & Egg Salad (248), Green Beans or Mixed Greens*	*left-over* Bacon-Wrapped Smoky Chicken Thighs, Green Salad	Spaghetti Squash Bolognese (280), Simple Baked Kale Chips (356)
18 ●◆◦	Pumpkin Pancakes (242), Breakfast Sausage or Bacon	*left-over* Spaghetti Squash Bolognese	Thanksgiving Stuffing Meatballs (334), Mashed Faux-Tatoes (344)
19 ●◦◆	Scrambled Eggs, Avocado, Spinach or Kale*, Raw Sauerkraut (238)	*left-over* Thanksgiving Stuffing Meatballs, *left-over* Mashed Faux-Tatoes	Citrus Macadamia Nut Sole (314), Lemon Roasted Romanesco*(346)
20 ●◆◆	Grain-Free Porridge (252), Hard Boiled Eggs	*left-over* Citrus Macadamia Nut Sole, *left-over* Lemon Roasted Romanesco	Bison & Butternut Cocoa Chili (282), Sautéed Red Cabbage with Onions and Apples*(352)

» *A complete shopping list for this meal plan can be found on balancedbites.com*

KEY

◆ Red-Meat
■ Poultry
● Eggs
◦ Pork
● Lamb
◆ Seafood

NOTES

EVOO   Extra-virgin olive oil
CO   Coconut oil
*   or other non-starchy vegetable
**   or other starchy vegetable (refer to page 110)
If no page number is listed, simply prepare the items as noted or any way you like.
For additional protein, vegetable, and fat recommendations, refer to the QUICK LIST that is associated with your meal plan!

blood sugar regulation

DAY	BREAKFAST	LUNCH	DINNER
21 ●◆●	Hard Boiled Eggs, Breakfast Sausage, Raw Sauerkraut (238)	Nori Salmon Handrolls (316)	Lamb Chops with Olive Tapenade (326), Greek Salad with Avo-Ziki (374)
22 ●●◆	Swirly Crustless Quiche (240), Breakfast Sausage	*left-over* Lamb Chops with Olive Tapenade, *left-over* Greek Salad with Avo-Ziki	Orange Braised Beef Shanks (284), Butternut Sage Soup**(348)
23 ●●◆	*left-over* Swirly Crustless Quiche (240), Perfectly Baked Bacon (236)	*left-over* Orange Braised Beef Shanks, *left-over* Butternut Sage Soup	Hayley's Skirt Steak Tacos (292), Salsa (296), Grilled Squash & Pineapple (342)
24 ○◆◆	Acorn Squash with Cinnamon & Coconut Butter (358), Breakfast Sausage or Bacon	Tangy Taco Salad (296), *left-over* Salsa	Fiery Jalapeño Burgers with Sweet Potato Pancakes (298), Red Roasted Garlic (370)
25 ●◆◆	*left-over* Sweet Potato Pancakes, Eggs, Avocado	Quick & Easy Salmon Cakes (310), Green Salad*, Avocado, Olives	Asian Orange Pan-Seared Scallops (304), Tomatillo Shrimp Cocktail (312), Zucchini*
26 ●◆○	Zucchini Pancakes (248), Perfectly Baked Bacon (236)	Tuna, Mixed Greens Salad with Persimmons, Asparagus & Fennel (380), Orange Vinaigrette (382)	Grandma Barbara's Stuffed Mushrooms (332), Roasted Marrow Bones (288), Spinach
27 ○○●	Grain-Free Porridge (252), Breakfast Sausage using Italian Sausage Spice Blend (233)	*left-over* Grandma Barbara's Stuffed Mushrooms, Mixed Greens Salad, Balsamic Vinaigrette (378)	Greek-Style Lamb Kabobs (326), Cilantro or other herb Cauli-Rice (340)
28 ●◆■	*left-over* Greek-Style Lamb Kabobs, Spinach or Cabbage*	Wild Canned Salmon with Olives, Avocado, Lemon Juice, Tomato, EVOO	Lemon & Artichoke Chicken (260), Broc-Cauli Chowder with Bacon (336)
29 ●■◆	Apple Streusel Egg Muffins (254), Bacon or Breakfast Sausage	*left-over* Lemon & Artichoke Chicken, Kale & Carrot Salad with Lemon-Tahini Dressing (376)	Mom's Stuffed Cabbage Rolls with Tomato Cranberry Sauce (290), Green Salad*
30 ●●○	*left-over* Apple Streusel Egg Muffins (254), Bacon or Breakfast Sausage	Chorizo Meatballs (330), Mixed Greens Salad* with Avocado, Lemon Juice, and EVOO	Mediterranean Lamb Roast (320), Sautéed Spinach with Pine Nuts & Currants*(366)

» *A complete shopping list for this meal plan can be found on balancedbites.com*

KEY
◆ Red-Meat
■ Poultry
● Eggs
○ Pork
● Lamb
◆ Seafood

NOTES
EVOO — Extra-virgin olive oil
CO — Coconut oil
* — or other non-starchy vegetable
** — or other starchy vegetable (refer to page 110)
If no page number is listed, simply prepare the items as noted or any way you like.
For additional protein, vegetable, and fat recommendations, refer to the QUICK LIST that is associated with your meal plan!

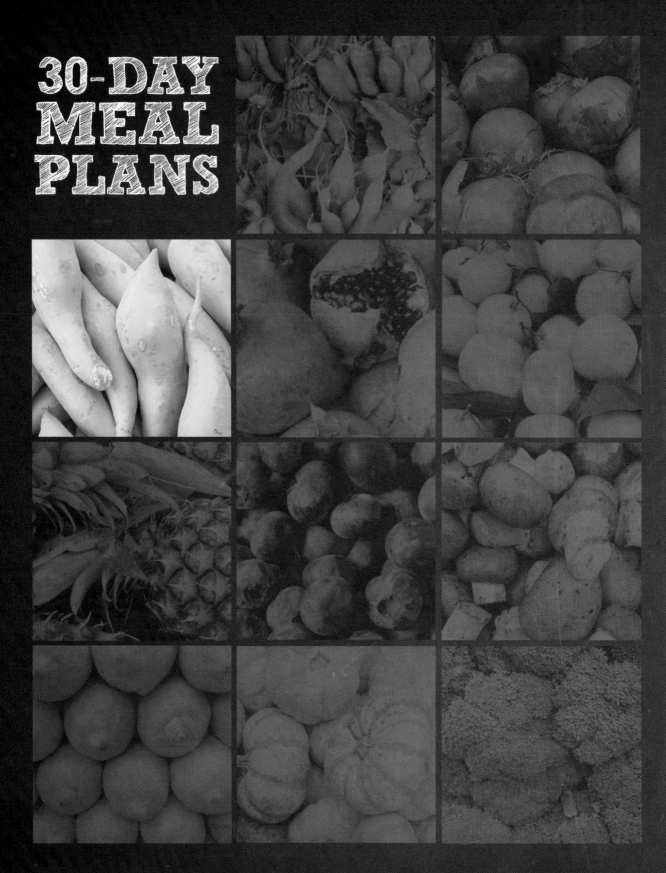

30-DAY MEAL PLANS

DIGESTIVE HEALTH

leaky gut

irritable bowel syndrome

inflammatory bowel disease

crohn's disease

colitis and ulcerative colitis

celiac disease

digestive health

If your symptoms are very severe, I recommend that you start with the Autoimmune Condition 30-Day Meal Plan with regard to food choices and use the lifestyle, supplement, and herbal recommendations from this plan.

leaky gut
symptoms include:

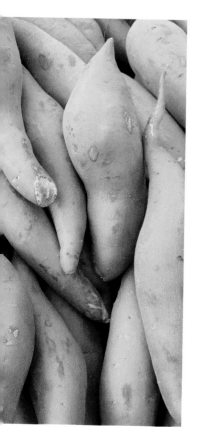

- » Undesired weight loss or weight loss resistance
- » Digestive distress
- » Food allergies or intolerances in response to a wide variety of seemingly unrelated foods; "allergic to everything" types of reactions or even food allergy tests that show an extremely high number of allergenic foods
- » Chronic inflammatory and autoimmune conditions

irritable bowel syndrome (IBS)
symptoms include:

- » Abdominal pain with change in bowel habits that may alternate between IBS-C (constipation) and IBS-D (diarrhea) and/or gas and bloating that is relieved by defecation
- » Altered elimination frequency, form, and ease of passage
- » Mucous in stools
- » Feeling that there is more stool left in the body after defecation
- » Leaky gut and/or food allergy/intolerance symptoms

inflammatory bowel disease (IBD)
symptoms include:

- » Aching all over (often occurs after an infection or trauma)
- » Similar symptoms to IBS but more severe and chronic
- » Encompasses Crohn's, Colitis, and Ulcerative Colitis

crohn's disease
symptoms include:

- » Inflammation or swelling anywhere along the GI tract, typically in the ileum and may affect all layers of the gut lining
- » Inflammatory patches can become strictures
- » Experience of extreme bouts of diarrhea (10-20x/day)
- » Pain and tenderness in the lower right of abdomen
- » Serious symptoms of malnutrition and fatigue

DISCLAIMER:
The information in this book is not intended to be a replacement for professional medical diagnosis or treatment for a medical condition. It consists solely of nutritional and lifestyle recommendations to support a healthier body.

colitis and ulcerative colitis
symptoms include:

» Similar symptoms to Crohn's, but the problem is located in the colon and/or rectum; inflammation is limited to the top layer of epithelial cells (gut lining)

» Symptoms may be intermittent with periods of remission

celiac disease (autoimmune)
symptoms include:

» A severe intolerance to gluten (found primarily in wheat, barley, rye, oats, spelt, kamut, and tritcale) and other grain proteins resulting in the autoimmune, self-cell attacking of the small intestine lining

» A latent, silent, or "non-classical celiac disease" sufferer may experience symptoms that mimic those of any of the previously listed digestive conditions or any chronic inflammatory or autoimmune condition

diet & lifestyle recommendations

add [+]

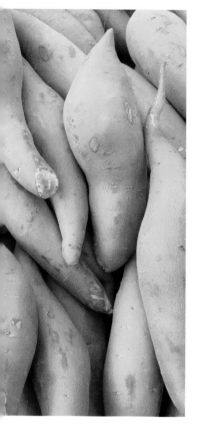

WELL-COOKED FOODS
Meals such as braised meats, stews, soups, and slow-cooked foods are easier to digest.

NUTRIENT-DENSE FOODS
Replenish depleted nutrient stores from eating excess refined foods over time.

SUPERFOODS: BONE BROTH
Make and eat/drink bone broth regularly for its gut-healing properties: minerals, glycine, gelatin, and collagen recipe on page 234).

SOLUBLE FIBER
Eat soluble fiber from starchy vegetables such as sweet potatoes, butternut squash, carrots, and cassava (to name a few) to feed the beneficial bacteria in your gut and promote proper stool motility.

STRESS MANAGEMENT
Develop a guided meditation practice, a slow breathing practice, or begin to practice Qi Gong.

MOVEMENT
Take walks outside, or practice gentle yoga for movement without systemic stress.

Slowly begin weight training with moderate to heavy weight, not excessively demanding in terms of stress response or cortisol output.

avoid [-]

GLUTEN
100% of the time. See the "Guide to Gluten" on page 89.

GUT-IRRITANTS
Foods with known immunological responses, including **grains, legumes, dairy (all dairy, even grass-fed for this meal plan), eggs (optionally - if you choose to eliminate eggs as a test, refer to the breakfast items in the Autoimmune Conditions meal plan), nuts, seeds**; avoid large quantities of foods high in *insoluble* fiber, such as leafy greens, raspberries, strawberries, nuts, seeds.

Optional: You may find that avoiding FODMAP foods helps for a period of time. FODMAPs are denoted on the Guide to Paleo Foods as well as on each recipe. The meal plan in this section includes FODMAP foods since most people tolerate them well, but remove them if you need to.

ALCOHOL, CAFFEINE, CHOCOLATE
As they can promote leaky gut.

PAIN MEDICATIONS
Including aspirin, acetaminophen, ibuprofen, naproxen, and corticosteroids.

HARSH CHEMICAL CLEANING OR HYGIENE PRODUCTS
Opt for gentle, natural alternatives, such as soap nuts for laundry, vinegar and water solutions for counter top cleaning, and baking soda and peroxide for cleaning and whitening surfaces, laundry, teeth, etc.

HIGH INTENSITY EXERCISE
Overly intense exercise (high intensity interval training/HIIT style workouts) and chronic cardiovascular exercise (30-60+ minutes at a steady state of intensity like jogging or biking) as it can provoke a stress-response in the body.

DISCLAIMER:
The information in this book is not intended to be a replacement for professional medical diagnosis or treatment for a medical condition. It consists solely of nutritional and lifestyle recommendations to support a healthier body.

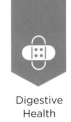

nutritional supplements & herbs to consider

These recommendations are made as a starting point. Do your own research and determine which supplements may serve you best. It's best to get as many of your nutrients from food as possible. See the next page for specific food-based nutrients on which to focus. The items below are listed in no particular order.

» **VITAMIN A (retinol)** improves immunity when balanced with vitamin D and helps to maintain immunity and the integrity of the mucosal lining of the gut; necessary for assimilation of dietary minerals.

» **FERMENTED COD LIVER OIL/BUTTER OIL BLEND** for fat-soluble vitamins A, D, E, and K2 as well as some omega 3 fats. I only recommend Green Pasture brand.

» **ARTICHOKE LEAF EXTRACT** has antioxidant properties and offers liver support; heals the chronic inflammatory state of digestive distress and aids in the digestion of fats. If you are avoiding FODMAPs, this supplement may not be ideal for you.

» **DIGESTIVE ENZYMES** help to break down food for absorption while your gut is healing. Look for a blend of enzymes.

» **L-GLUTAMINE** aids in the healing of the epithelial cells that line the small intestine.

» **HERBAL TEAS** that are calming to your digestive system are peppermint, ginger, kudzu, marshmallow root, and slippery elm.

» **LICORICE ROOT** is an herb that aids in repairing the mucosal lining of the gut, as well as the stomach. Look for licorice root tea, an extract of the herb, or a chewable tablet called DGL.

» **ALOE VERA JUICE** (unless it promotes loose stool).

» **MAGNESIUM** is required for more than 300 enzymatic processes in the body, and most people are deficient. It is useful in blood sugar regulation. Look for magnesium glycinate or magnesium malate forms.

» **OX BILE / BILE SALTS** are supportive for those without a gallbladder, as they help the body to emulsify dietary fats, especially unsaturated forms.

» **PHOSPHATIDYLCHOLINE** enhances the integrity of the GI tract and aids in fatty acid digestion, as well as repairs the mucosal lining of the gut. This supplement is especially important if you are avoiding eggs.

» **QUERCETIN** is a potent antioxidant that promotes better immunity.

» **SELENIUM & ZINC** are antioxidants that protect against free radical damage and may need to be supplemented as it's difficult to obtain adequate amounts from food.

» **ZINC CARNOSINE** may improve gut mucosa and gut lining integrity.

Digestive
Health

supportive nutrients
& foods that contain them

quick LIST

proteins

Beef
Bison
Cold water fish (salmon, herring, mackerel, etc.)
Eel
Lamb
Liver
Oysters
Shellfish

fats

Coconut oil
Extra-virgin olive oil
Grass-fed butter/ghee

vegetables

Beets
Broccoli (cooked)
Brussels sprouts
Butternut squash
Cauliflower (cooked)
Daikon radish
Okra
Spinach
Squash (all kinds)
Sweet potatoes

fruits

Bananas
Blueberries
Lemon juice
Plantains

superfoods

Bone broth
Fermented cod liver oil
Liver
Sauerkraut

spices

Basil
Cilantro
Cinnamon
Cumin
Garlic
Ginger
Oregano
Parsley
Turmeric

VITAMIN A (RETINOL)
» Liver
» Eel
» Grass-fed butter, clarified butter, or ghee

BROMELAIN
An enzyme with anti-inflammatory properties.
» Pineapple

BUTYRIC ACID
Helps to decrease intestinal permeability.
» Grass-fed butter, clarified butter, or ghee

VITAMIN C
A potent antioxidant with anti-inflammatory properties.
» Adrenal glands of pasture-raised animals
» Cauliflower, broccoli, daikon radish, lemon juice, garlic, beets, Brussels sprouts

VITAMIN D
A potent immune system modulator that is most available from sun exposure.
» Cold water fish (salmon, herring, mackerel)
» Grass-fed butter or ghee
» Fermented cod liver oil/butter oil blend (Green Pasture brand only)

GLYCINE
Helps to repair the gut cell lining and enhance stomach acid production.
» Bone broth (recipe on page 234)
» Gelatin (recipe on page 234)

OMEGA-3 FATS
An anti-inflammatory essential fatty acid that comes from limited food sources.
» Cold water fish (salmon, herring, mackerel), fermented cod liver oil (Green Pasture brand only)

PROBIOTICS
Promotes healthy gut flora, which is critical to proper digestion and elimination.
» Fermented vegetables: cabbage (sauerkraut/kimchi), carrots, beets
» Kombucha (fermented tea)

SELENIUM
An antioxidant that protects against free radical damage.
» Eggs
» Red Swiss chard
» Turnips
» Garlic

SOLUBLE FIBER
Feeds the beneficial bacteria in your gut to promote proper cell motility.
» Sweet potatoes
» Butternut squash
» Plantains
» Bananas

ZINC
A potent antioxidant often deficient in people with inflammatory conditions; aids in vitamin A metabolism.
» Oyster
» Shellfish
» Lamb
» Red meat

digestive health

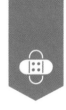

DAY	BREAKFAST	LUNCH	DINNER
1 ●■◆	Swirly Crustless Quiche (240), Perfectly Baked Bacon (236), Raw Sauerkraut (238)	Mustard Glazed Chicken Thighs (266), Butternut Squash**	Grilled Garlic Flank Steak with Peppers & Onions (294), Baked Beets with Fennel**(362)
2 ●◆■	*left-over* Swirly Crustless Quiche, *left-over* Garlic Flank Steak with Peppers & Onions	Wild Canned Salmon with Olives, Avocado, Lemon Juice, Tomato, EVOO	Sage Roasted Turkey Legs (276), Sweet Potato Pancakes (298), Steamed Spinach*
3 ■■●	*left-over* Sweet Potato Pancakes, *left-over* Mustard-Glazed Chicken Thighs (266)	*left-over* Sage Roasted Turkey Legs, Persimmon, Asparagus & Fennel Salad (380)	Lemony Lamb Dolmas (318), Cilantro Cauli-Rice (340)
4 ●●◆	Pesto Scrambled Eggs (252), *left-over* Cilantro Cauli-Rice, Raw Sauerkraut (238)	*left-over* Lemony Lamb Dolmas, Steamed Spinach*	Asian Orange Pan-Seared Scallops (304), Butternut Squash**
5 ◆◆◆	Eggs, Perfectly Baked Bacon (236), *left-over* Butternut Squash**	Nori Salmon Handrolls (316)	Beef & Mixed Veggie Stir Fry (286), Cilantro Cauli-Rice (340)*
6 ●◆●	Pumpkin Pancakes (242), Breakfast Sausage using Italian Sausage Spice Blend (233)	*left-over* Beef Stir Fry with Mixed Veggies	Lamb Lettuce Boats with Avo-Ziki Sauce (322)
7 ●◆■	Eggs, Perfectly Baked Bacon (236), Kale*, Raw Sauerkraut (238)	Mixed Greens with Wild Canned Salmon, Asparagus*, Lemon Juice, EVOO	Citrus & Herb Whole Roasted Chicken (256), Roasted Rosemary Roots (350)
8 ■■■	*left-over* Citrus & Herb Whole Roasted Chicken, Apple Streusel Egg Muffins (254)	Green Salad*, *left-over* Citrus & Herb Whole Roasted Chicken	Chinese 5-Spice Lettuce Cups (272), Sweet Potato**
9 ●■◆	Swirly Crustless Quiche (240), Steamed Broccoli*, Raw Sauerkraut (238)	Indian-Spiced Turkey Burgers (268), Steamed Broccoli*	Pesto Shrimp & Squash Fettuccine (no nuts) (308)
10 ●◆●	Omelet or Pesto Scrambled Eggs, *left-over* Shrimp & Avocado	Simple Shrimp Ceviche (316), Mixed Greens*, EVOO	Cumin Spiced Pork Tenderloin with Root Vegetables**(328)

» *A complete shopping list for this meal plan can be found on balancedbites.com*

KEY
◆ **Beef & Bison**
■ **Poultry**
● **Eggs**
● **Pork**
● **Lamb**
◆ **Seafood**

NOTES

EVOO	Extra-virgin olive oil
CO	Coconut oil
*	or other non-starchy vegetable
**	or other starchy vegetable (refer to page 110)

If no page number is listed, simply prepare the items as noted or any way you like.

For additional protein, vegetable, and fat recommendations, refer to the QUICK LIST that is associated with your meal plan!

DAY	BREAKFAST	LUNCH	DINNER
11 ● ● ● ◆	Swirly Crustless Quiche (240) Perfectly Baked Bacon (236), *left-over* Root Vegetables	*left-over* Cumin Spiced Pork Tenderloin, Rainbow Red Cabbage Salad*(372) or Sautéed Red Cabbage (352)	Balsamic Braised Short Ribs (278), Candied Carrots (340), Spinach*
12 ● ◆ ■	Eggs, *left-over* Red Cabbage	*left-over* Balsamic Braised Short Ribs, *left-over* Candied Carrots, Green Salad*	Savory Baked Chicken Legs (264), Brussels Sprouts with Fennel*(350)
13 ● ■ ◆	Zucchini Pancakes (248), Perfectly Baked Bacon (236), Raw Sauerkraut (238)	*left-over* Savory Baked Chicken Legs, *left-over* Brussels Sprouts with Fennel*	Lemon Rosemary Broiled Salmon (306), Asparagus with Lemon & Olives (338), Sweet Potato**
14 ◆ ■ ◆	*left-over* Lemon Rosemary Broiled Salmon, *left-over* Asparagus with Lemon & Olives*	Buffalo Chicken Lettuce Wraps (270)	Red Palm & Coriander Tuna Over Daikon Noodle Salad (302), Green Salad*
15 ● ◆ ◆	Scrambled Eggs with Olives, Avocado, Squash**	Spinach Salad with EVOO, *left-over* Red Palm & Coriander Tuna, Avocado, Lemon Juice	Italian-Style Stuffed Peppers (300), Green Salad* with Balsamic Vinaigrette (378)
16 ● ◆ ■	Apple Streusel Egg Muffins (254), Breakfast Sausage	*left-over* Italian-Style Stuffed Peppers (300)	Bacon-Wrapped Smoky Chicken Thighs (262), Mixed Greens Salad with Beets & Blood Oranges* (376)
17 ● ■ ■ ◆	Bacon & Egg Salad (248), Sweet Potato or Beets**	*left-over* Bacon-Wrapped Smoky Chicken Thighs, Green Beans*	Spaghetti Squash Bolognese (280)
18 ● ◆ ●	Pumpkin Pancakes (242), Breakfast Sausage or Bacon	*left-over* Spaghetti Squash Bolognese	Thanksgiving Stuffing Meatballs (334), Mashed Faux-Tatoes (344)
19 ● ● ◆	Scrambled Eggs, Avocado, Raw Sauerkraut (238)	*left-over* Thanksgiving Stuffing Meatballs, *left-over* Mashed Faux-Tatoes	Citrus Macadamia Nut Sole (314), Lemon Roasted Romanesco*(346)
20 ● ◆ ■	Acorn Squash with Cinnamon & Coconut Butter (358), Breakfast Sausage or Bacon	*left-over* Citrus Macadamia Nut Sole, *left-over* Lemon Roasted Romanesco	Roasted Duck with Cherry Sauce (274), Sautéed Red Cabbage with Onions and Apples*(352)

» A complete shopping list for this meal plan can be found on balancedbites.com

KEY
◆ Red-Meat
■ Poultry
● Eggs
● Pork
● Lamb
◆ Seafood

NOTES
EVOO   Extra-virgin olive oil
CO   Coconut oil
*   or other non-starchy vegetable
**   or other starchy vegetable (refer to page 110)
If no page number is listed, simply prepare the items as noted or any way you like.
For additional protein, vegetable, and fat recommendations, refer to the QUICK LIST that is associated with your meal plan!

digestive health

DAY	BREAKFAST	LUNCH	DINNER
21 ●◆●	Hard Boiled Eggs, Breakfast Sausage, Raw Sauerkraut (238)	Nori Salmon Handrolls (316)	Lamb Chops with Olive Tapenade (326), Greek Salad with Avo-Ziki (374)
22 ●●◆	Swirly Crustless Quiche (240), Breakfast Sausage	*left-over* Lamb Chops with Olive Tapenade, *left-over* Greek Salad with Avo-Ziki	Orange Braised Beef Shanks (284), Butternut Sage Soup**(348)
23 ●◆◆	*left-over* Swirly Crustless Quiche Perfectly Baked Bacon (236)	*left-over* Orange Braised Beef Shanks, *left-over* Butternut Sage Soup	Hayley's Skirt Steak Tacos (292), Salsa (296), Grilled Squash & Pineapple (342)
24 ○◆◆	Acorn Squash with Cinnamon & Coconut Butter (358), Breakfast Sausage or Bacon	Tangy Taco Salad (296), *left-over* Salsa	Fiery Jalapeño Burgers with Sweet Potato Pancakes (298), Red Roasted Garlic (370)
25 ●◆◆	*left-over* Sweet Potato Pancakes, Eggs, Avocado	Quick & Easy Salmon Cakes (310), Green Salad*, Avocado, Olives	Asian Orange Pan-Seared Scallops (304), Tomatillo Shrimp Cocktail (312), Zucchini*
26 ●◆○	Zucchini Pancakes (248), Perfectly Baked Bacon (236)	Tuna, Mixed Greens Salad with Persimmons, Asparagus & Fennel (380), Orange Vinaigrette (382)	Grandma Barbara's Stuffed Mushrooms (332), Roasted Marrow Bones (288)
27 ○●●	Breakfast Sausage using Italian Sausage Spice Blend (233), Butternut Squash**	*left-over* Grandma Barbara's Stuffed Mushrooms, Mixed Greens Salad, Balsamic Vinaigrette (378)	Spiced Lamb Meatballs with Balsamic-Fig Compote (324), Green Beans with Shallots*(358)
28 ●◆■	*left-over* Spiced Lamb Meatballs, Spinach or Cabbage*	Wild Canned Salmon with Olives, Avocado, Lemon Juice, Tomato, EVOO	Lemon & Artichoke Chicken (260), Broc-Cauli Chowder with Bacon (336)
29 ●■◆	Apple Streusel Egg Muffins (254), Bacon or Breakfast Sausage	*left-over* Lemon & Artichoke Chicken, Kale & Carrot Salad with Lemon-Tahini Dressing (376)	Mom's Stuffed Cabbage Rolls with Tomato Cranberry Sauce (290)
30 ●○●	*left-over* Apple Streusel Egg Muffins (254), Bacon or Breakfast Sausage	Chorizo Meatballs (330), Mashed Faux-Tatoes (344)	Mediterranean Lamb Roast (320), Sautéed Spinach with Currants*(366)

» *A complete shopping list for this meal plan can be found on balancedbites.com*

KEY
- ◆ **Beef & Bison**
- ■ **Poultry**
- ● **Eggs**
- ○ **Pork**
- ● **Lamb**
- ◆ **Seafood**

NOTES

EVOO	Extra-virgin olive oil
CO	Coconut oil
*	or other non-starchy vegetable
**	or other starchy vegetable (refer to page 110)

If no page number is listed, simply prepare the items as noted or any way you like.

For additional protein, vegetable, and fat recommendations, refer to the QUICK LIST that is associated with your meal plan!

30-DAY MEAL PLANS

THYROID HEALTH

If you have been recently diagnosed with a thyroid condition or you are new to a Paleo way of eating, I recommend that you start with the Autoimmune Condition 30-Day Meal Plan with regard to food choices and follow the lifestyle, supplement, and herbal recommendations from this plan.

Thyroid disorders can be very delicate to balance, so it's strongly recommended that you work closely with a trusted practitioner in making dietary, lifestyle, and nutritional supplement changes.

hypothyroidism (autoimmune Hashimoto's or otherwise)
symptoms include:

- Weight loss resistance
- Sudden weight gain
- Constipation
- Fatigue
- Lethargy
- Low energy
- Irregular menstrual cycles, female hormonal imbalances
- Low body temperature

hyperthyroidism
symptoms include:

- Enlarged thyroid
- Bulging eyes
- Rash on lower legs
- Rapid heartbeat
- Weight loss
- Fatigue
- Anxiety
- Diarrhea

Note: hyperthyroidism is less common than hypothyroidism.

Disclaimer: The information in this book is not intended to be a replacement for professional medical diagnosis or treatment for a medical condition. It consists solely of nutritional and lifestyle recommendations to support a healthier body.

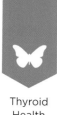

diet & lifestyle recommendations

add [+]

PROTEIN

Add protein to satisfy appetite for longer periods of time (meals focused on both fat and protein will help).

NUTRIENT-DENSE FOODS

Replenish depleted nutrient stores from eating excess refined foods over time.

SUPERFOODS

Eat superfoods often as possible. Make and eat/drink bone broth and liver regularly (recipes on page 234 and 384). Use the sauerkraut recipe on page 238 to make fermented carrots or beets and eat them daily (1/4 cup), especially with breakfast to aid in gastrointestinal motility and eliminations.

SUN EXPOSURE

Safe sun exposure daily for about ten minutes when the sun is at its peak or longer when the sun is not as strong to promote vitamin D production; do not burn.

STRESS MANAGEMENT

Manage stress to keep systemic inflammation low and avoid blood sugar imbalances. Develop a guided meditation practice, or begin to practice Qi Gong.

MOVEMENT

Take walks outside, or practice gentle yoga for movement without systemic stress.

avoid [-]

GLUTEN

100% of the time. See the "Guide to Gluten" on page 89.

EXCESS GOITROGENIC FOODS

Eat cooked goitrogenic (potentially thyroid inhibiting) foods only if possible, avoid raw and fermented goitrogenic vegetables (like cabbage) as fermentation increases their goitrogen levels. See page 29 for the list of Paleo foods with goitrogens denoted.

REFINED FOODS, SWEETENERS & CAFFEINE

These can all provoke blood sugar fluctuations and systemic stress, which inhibit thyroid function.

ALCOHOL

As it can induce hypoglycemic events which inhibit thyroid function.

STRESS

Make lifestyle changes to avoid stressful situations.

CHRONIC CARDIOVASCULAR EXERCISE

(meaning 30-60+ minutes at a steady state of intensity like jogging or biking), as it can lead to low blood sugar episodes, as well as provoke a stress response.

DISCLAIMER:

The information in this book is not intended to be a replacement for professional medical diagnosis or treatment for a medical condition. It consists solely of nutritional and lifestyle recommendations to support a healthier body.

nutritional supplements & herbs to consider

These recommendations are made as a starting point. Do your own research and determine which supplements may serve you best. It's best to get as many of your nutrients from food as possible. See the next page for specific food-based nutrients on which to focus. The items below are listed in no particular order.

» **VITAMIN A (retinol)** helps to maintain the integrity of the mucosal lining of the gut; helps to maintain immunity when balanced with vitamin D; necessary for the assimilation of dietary minerals.

» **FERMENTED COD LIVER OIL/ BUTTER OIL BLEND** for fat-soluble vitamins A, D, E, and K2 as well as some omega 3 fats. I only recommend Green Pasture brand.

» **ADAPTOGENIC HERBS** help modulate energy up or down as your body requires. Rotate amongst: Ashwagandha, Holy Basil, Rhodiola

» **VITAMIN B5 (pantothenic acid & pantethine)** is beneficial to energy production, especially in the manufacture of adrenal hormones and red blood cells.

» **VITAMIN B7 (biotin)** is a coenzyme required in the metabolism of glucose, amino acids, and lipids.

» **VITAMIN B12 (cobalamin)** supports energy metabolism and immune function, and it may help to regulate circadian rhythms by improving melatonin secretion. (In other words, it may help you sleep better.)

» **VITAMIN C** supports immune function, and it is a potent antioxidant with anti-inflammatory properties.

» **CHROMIUM (chromium picolinate, polynicotinate, chelavite)** may improve insulin sensitivity and reduce appetite.

» **VITAMIN D** is a potent immune system modulator. Proper balance with vitamin A is important, and it is most available via sun exposure.

» **VITAMIN E** is an antioxidant that benefits cellular communication and may reduce oxidative stress-induced insulin resistance.

» **IODINE** may support healing of *hyper*thyroidism or non-autoimmune thyroiditis. Supplementation for those with Hashimoto's/ autoimmune thyroiditis (the largest cause of hypothyroidism in the U.S.) may exacerbate the problem. If you have Hashimoto's or are unsure of the type of hypothyroidism you have, do not supplement with iodine foods. Consult a practitioner before supplementing with iodine.

» **MAGNESIUM** is required for more than 300 enzymatic processes in the body, and most people are deficient in it. Look for magnesium glycinate or magnesium malate forms.

» **OMEGA-3 FATS** are anti-inflammatory essential fatty acids. I only recommend Green Pasture brand fermented cod liver oil.

» **PROBIOTICS** promote healthy gut flora, which is critical to proper digestion and elimination. Use a supplement, if necessary. *Hypo*thyroidism is commonly associated with constipation.

» **SELENIUM** is an antioxidant that is important in the production of thyroid hormone. It is antagonistic to heavy metals like lead, mercury, cadmium, and aluminum. Absorption may be decreased by high zinc intake, so it must be balanced with zinc.

» **THYROID GLANDULAR** (for *hypo*thyroidism)—Work with your doctor or other practitioner to determine if this is right for you.

» **ZINC** is a potent antioxidant often deficient in people with inflammatory conditions; aids in vitamin A metabolism.

Thyroid
Health

supportive nutrients
& foods that contain them

quick LIST

proteins

Beef
Herring
Lamb
Mackerel
Oysters
Salmon
Sardines
Shellfish
Tuna

fats

Coconut oil
Grass-fed butter/ghee
Animal fats
Extra-virgin olive oil

vegetables

Beets
Carrots
Fennel
Green beans
Green bell pepper
Lettuces
Mushrooms
Parsnips
Squash
Swiss chard

fruits

Cantaloupe
Citrus
Strawberries
Tropical fruits

superfoods

Bone broth
Fermented carrots
Fermented cod liver oil
Liver

spices

Basil
Black pepper
Chili powder
Cilantro
Cinnamon
Cloves
Garlic
Thyme
Turmeric

VITAMIN A (RETINOL)
» Liver, eel, grass-fed butter, clarified butter, or ghee

VITAMIN B5
» Liver, brewer's yeast (Lewis Labs brand only)
» Mushrooms
» Trace amounts: pecans, sunflower seeds

VITAMIN B7
» Liver, brewer's yeast (Lewis Labs brand only)
» Trace amounts: Swiss chard, walnuts, pecans, almonds

VITAMIN B12
(only in animal foods)
» Liver, clams, kidney
» Oysters, sardines, trout, salmon, tuna, lamb, beef, eggs, cheeses, flounder, scallops, halibut

VITAMIN C
» Beets, bell peppers, cantaloupe, garlic, kiwi, lemons, oranges, papaya, pineapple
» (limited/cooked) Brussels sprouts, cauliflower, collard greens, broccoli, daikon radish,

CHOLINE
An important nutrient for cell membrane integrity, nerve-to-muscle communication, and optimal liver function.
» Eggs, liver, heart meat, kidney meat, fish roe (eggs), caviar, Cod
» Cauliflower (cooked)

CHROMIUM
» Liver, grass-fed cheese
» Brewer's yeast (Lewis Labs brand only)
» Trace amounts: green pepper, apple, parsnips, spinach, carrots

VITAMIN E
» Extra-virgin olive oil, pecans
» (limited/cooked) Broccoli, Brussels sprouts, spinach

IODINE
» Wild fish, seaweed, kelp, dulse

LIPOIC ACID
(ALPHA-LIPOIC ACID/ALA)
» Red meat, organ meats

MANGANESE
Beneficial for blood sugar regulation, energy metabolism, and thyroid hormone function. Intake should be balanced with that of magnesium, calcium, iron, copper, and zinc.
» Pecans, walnuts, turnip greens, rhubarb, beet greens, cloves, cinnamon, thyme, turmeric

OMEGA-3 FATS
An anti-inflammatory essential fatty acid that comes from limited food sources.
» Cold water fish (salmon, herring, mackerel, etc.), fermented cod liver oil (Green Pasture brand only)
» Walnuts, pecans

PROBIOTICS
Promote healthy gut flora, which is critical to proper digestion and elimination.
» Fermented vegetables: carrots, beets, or other non-goitogenic vegetables
» Kombucha (fermented tea)

SELENIUM
An antioxidant that protects against free radical damage.
» Eggs
» Red Swiss chard, turnips, garlic

ZINC
» Oysters, shellfish, lamb, red meat, pumpkin seeds (pepitas)

thyroid health

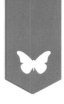

DAY	BREAKFAST	LUNCH	DINNER
1 ● ■ ◆	Swirly Crustless Quiche (240), Perfectly Baked Bacon (236), Raw Fermented Carrots - use Sauerkraut recipe (238)	Mustard Glazed Chicken Thighs (266), Green Salad*, Balsamic Vinaigrette (378)	Grilled Garlic Flank Steak with Peppers & Onions (294), Baked Beets with Fennel**(362)
2 ● ◆ ■	*left-over* Swirly Crustless Quiche, *left-over* Garlic Flank Steak with Peppers & Onions	Wild Canned Salmon with Olives, Avocado, Lemon Juice, Tomato, EVOO	Sage Roasted Turkey Legs (276), Sweet Potato Pancakes (298), Steamed Spinach*
3 ■ ■ ●	*left-over* Sweet Potato Pancakes, Mustard-Glazed Chicken Thighs (266)	*left-over* Sage Roasted Turkey Legs, Persimmon, Asparagus & Fennel Salad (380)	Lemony Lamb Dolmas (318), Cilantro Cauli-Rice (340)
4 ● ● ◆	Pesto Scrambled Eggs (252), Cilantro Cauli-Rice (340), Raw Fermented Carrots	*left-over* Lemony Lamb Dolmas, Swiss Chard, EVOO	Citrus Macadamia Nut Sole (314), Butternut Squash**
5 ◆ ◆ ◆	*left-over* Citrus Macadamia Nut Sole, Butternut Squash**	Nori Salmon Handrolls (316)	Beef & Mixed Veggie Stir Fry (286)
6 ● ◆ ●	Pumpkin Pancakes (242), Breakfast Sausage using Italian Sausage Spice Blend (233)	*left-over* Beef Stir Fry with Mixed Veggies	Lamb Lettuce Boats with Avo-Ziki Sauce (322), Parsnips**
7 ● ◆ ■	Eggs, Perfectly Baked Bacon (236), Green Beans, Raw Fermented Carrots	Mixed Greens with Wild Canned Salmon, Asparagus*, Lemon Juice, EVOO	Citrus & Herb Whole Roasted Chicken (256), Roasted Rosemary Roots** (350)
8 ■ ■ ■	Grain-Free Porridge (252), Berries, *left-over* Citrus & Herb Whole Roasted Chicken	Spinach Salad with Walnuts & Artichokes (380), *left-over* Citrus & Herb Whole Roasted Chicken	Chinese 5-Spice Lettuce Cups (272)
9 ● ■ ◆	Swirly Crustless Quiche (240), Raw Fermented Carrots	Indian-Spiced Turkey Burgers (268), Steamed Broccoli*	Pesto Shrimp & Squash Fettuccine (308)
10 ● ◆ ●	Omelet or Pesto Scrambled Eggs, *left-over* Shrimp & Avocado	Simple Shrimp Ceviche (316), Mixed Greens*, EVOO	Cumin Spiced Pork Tenderloin with Root Vegetables**(328)

» *A complete shopping list for this meal plan can be found on balancedbites.com*

KEY

◆ Red-Meat
■ Poultry
● Eggs
○ Pork
● Lamb
◆ Seafood

NOTES

EVOO	Extra-virgin olive oil
CO	Coconut oil
*	or other non-starchy vegetable
**	or other starchy vegetable (refer to page 110)

If no page number is listed, simply prepare the items as noted or any way you like.

For additional protein, vegetable, and fat recommendations, refer to the QUICK LIST that is associated with your meal plan!

DAY	BREAKFAST	LUNCH	DINNER
11 ● ○ ◆	Swirly Crustless Quiche (240) Perfectly Baked Bacon (236), *left-over* Root Vegetables	*left-over* Cumin Spiced Pork Tenderloin, Mixed Greens Salad	Balsamic Braised Short Ribs (278), Candied Carrots (340), Steamed Spinach*
12 ● ◆ ■	Eggs, Mixed Greens Salad with EVOO & Lemon, Avocado	*left-over* Balsamic Braised Short Ribs, *left-over* Candied Carrots, Green Salad*	Savory Baked Chicken Legs (264), Bell Peppers, Mushrooms*
13 ● ■ ◆	Zucchini Pancakes (248), Perfectly Baked Bacon (236), Raw Fermented Carrots	*left-over* Savory Baked Chicken Legs, *left-over* Brussels Sprouts with Fennel*	Lemon Rosemary Broiled Salmon (306), Asparagus with Lemon & Olives (338), Butternut Squash**
14 ◆ ■ ◆	*left-over* Lemon Rosemary Broiled Salmon, *left-over* Asparagus with Lemon & Olives*	Buffalo Chicken Lettuce Wraps (270)	Red Palm & Coriander Tuna Over Daikon Noodle Salad (302), Green Salad*
15 ● ◆ ◆	Scrambled Eggs with Olives, Steamed Swiss Chard*, Avocado	Spinach Salad with EVOO, *left-over* Red Palm & Coriander Tuna, Avocado, Lemon Juice	Italian-Style Stuffed Peppers (300), Green Salad* with Balsamic Vinaigrette (378)
16 ○ ◆ ■	Grain-Free Porridge (252), Breakfast Sausage	*left-over* Italian-Style Stuffed Peppers (300), Green Salad	Bacon-Wrapped Smoky Chicken Thighs (262), Mixed Greens Salad with Beets & Blood Oranges (376)
17 ● ■ ◆	Bacon & Egg Salad (248), Beets**	*left-over* Bacon-Wrapped Smoky Chicken Thighs, Green Salad*	Spaghetti Squash Bolognese (280)
18 ● ◆ ○	Pumpkin Pancakes (242), Breakfast Sausage or Bacon	*left-over* Spaghetti Squash Bolognese	Thanksgiving Stuffing Meatballs (334), Mashed Parsnips (344, replace Cauliflower with Parsnips)
19 ● ○ ◆	Scrambled Eggs, Avocado, Raw Fermented Carrots	*left-over* Thanksgiving Stuffing Meatballs, *left-over* Mashed Parsnips	Citrus Macadamia Nut Sole (314), Green Beans*
20 ● ◆ ■	Grain-Free Porridge (252), Hard Boiled Eggs	*left-over* Citrus Macadamia Nut Sole, Lemon Roasted Romanesco (346)	Roasted Duck with Cherry Sauce (274), Carrots**

» *A complete shopping list for this meal plan can be found on balancedbites.com*

KEY

◆ **Red-Meat**
■ **Poultry**
● **Eggs**
○ **Pork**
● **Lamb**
◆ **Seafood**

NOTES

EVOO   Extra-virgin olive oil
CO   Coconut oil
*   or other non-starchy vegetable
**   or other starchy vegetable (refer to page 110)
If no page number is listed, simply prepare the items as noted or any way you like.
For additional protein, vegetable, and fat recommendations, refer to the QUICK LIST that is associated with your meal plan!

thyroid health

DAY	BREAKFAST	LUNCH	DINNER
21 ●◆●	Hard Boiled Eggs, Breakfast Sausage, Raw Fermented Carrots - use Sauerkraut recipe (238)	Nori Salmon Handrolls (316)	Lamb Chops with Olive Tapenade (326), Greek Salad with Avo-Ziki (374)
22 ●●◆	Swirly Crustless Quiche (240), Breakfast Sausage	*left-over* Lamb Chops with Olive Tapenade, *left-over* Greek Salad with Avo-Ziki	Orange Braised Beef Shanks (284), Butternut Sage Soup**(348)
23 ●◆◆	*left-over* Swirly Crustless Quiche, Perfectly Baked Bacon (236)	*left-over* Orange Braised Beef Shanks, *left-over* Butternut Sage Soup	Hayley's Skirt Steak Tacos (292), Salsa (296), Grilled Squash & Pineapple (342)
24 ●◆◆	Acorn Squash with Cinnamon & Coconut Butter (358), Breakfast Sausage or Bacon	Tangy Taco Salad (296), *left-over* Salsa	Fiery Jalapeño Burgers with Sweet Potato Pancakes (298), Red Roasted Garlic (370)
25 ●◆◆	*left-over* Sweet Potato Pancakes, Eggs, Avocado	Quick & Easy Salmon Cakes (310), Green Salad*, Avocado, Olives	Asian Orange Pan-Seared Scallops (304), Tomatillo Shrimp Cocktail (312), Zucchini*
26 ●◆●	Zucchini Pancakes (248), Perfectly Baked Bacon (236), Raw Fermented Carrots	Tuna, Mixed Greens Salad with Persimmons, Asparagus & Fennel (380), Orange Vinaigrette (382)	Grandma Barbara's Stuffed Mushrooms (332), Roasted Marrow Bones (288), Spinach*
27 ●●●	Grain-Free Porridge (252), Breakfast Sausage using Italian Sausage Spice Blend (233)	*left-over* Grandma Barbara's Stuffed Mushrooms, Mixed Greens Salad, Balsamic Vinaigrette (378)	Spiced Lamb Meatballs with Balsamic-Fig Compote (324), Green Beans with Shallots*(358)
28 ●◆■	*left-over* Spiced Lamb Meatballs, Parsnips**	Wild Canned Salmon with Olives, Avocado, Lemon Juice, Tomato, EVOO	Lemon & Artichoke Chicken (260), Broc-Cauli Chowder with Bacon (336)
29 ●■◆	Apple Streusel Egg Muffins (254), Bacon or Breakfast Sausage	*left-over* Lemon & Artichoke Chicken, Kale* (cooked in CO)	Mom's Stuffed Cabbage Rolls (290) with Tomato Cranberry Sauce (388)
30 ●●●	*left-over* Apple Streusel Egg Muffins (254), Bacon or Breakfast Sausage	Chorizo Meatballs (330), Mixed Greens Salad* with Avocado, Lemon Juice, and EVOO	Mediterranean Lamb Roast (320), Steamed Swiss chard*

» *A complete shopping list for this meal plan can be found on balancedbites.com*

KEY
- ◆ Red-Meat
- ■ Poultry
- ● Eggs
- ● Pork
- ● Lamb
- ◆ Seafood

NOTES

EVOO	Extra-virgin olive oil
CO	Coconut oil
*	or other non-starchy vegetable
**	or other starchy vegetable (refer to page 110)

If no page number is listed, simply prepare the items as noted or any way you like.

For additional protein, vegetable, and fat recommendations, refer to the QUICK LIST that is associated with your meal plan!

30-DAY MEAL PLANS

MULTIPLE SCLEROSIS, FIBROMYALGIA, & CHRONIC FATIGUE

multiple sclerosis, fibromyalgia, and chronic fatigue syndrome

I recommend that you start with the Autoimmune Condition 30-Day Meal Plan with regard to food choices while following the lifestyle, supplement, and herbal recommendations from this plan.

multiple sclerosis
symptoms include:

- » Muscle wasting
- » Weakness
- » Dysphagia (difficulty or inability to swallow)
- » Jerking
- » Spastic movements
- » Loss of balance
- » Twitches
- » Tics
- » Tingling (pins & needles)
- » Sensitivity to heat and cold
- » Loss of sensation and electric shock sensations

- » Loss of muscle and speech coordination and paralysis (complete or partial)
- » Blurred or double vision
- » Eye pain
- » Blindness
- » Urinary urgency
- » Incontinence, hesitancy, or retention
- » Cognitive dysfunction such as memory problems (short or long-term)
- » Depression
- » May lead to complete incapacitation / a bed-ridden state

For more information on an approach for MS, I also recommend checking out: Dr. Terry Wahls' website - www.terrywahls.com

fibromyalgia
symptoms include:

- » Tightening and thickening of myofascia (connective tissue)
- » Aching all over (often occurs after an infection or trauma)

chronic fatigue syndrome
symptoms include:

» Unexplained fatigue that is not a result of exertion, is not resolved by bed rest, and is severe enough to reduce previously maintained daily activity levels.

For at least six months:

» Unexplained or new headaches
» Short-term memory or concentration impairment
» Muscle pain
» Pain/redness/swelling in multiple joints

» Unrestful sleep
» Post-exertion malaise lasting for more than 24-hours
» Sore throat
» Tender lymph nodes in the neck or armpits

Other populations who may benefit from this meal plan include those diagnosed with:

» SCLERODERMA
» ARTHRITIS, OSTEOARTHRITIS, OR RHEUMATOID ARTHRITIS

diet & lifestyle recommendations

add [+]

NUTRIENT-DENSE FOODS

Replenish depleted nutrient stores from eating excess refined foods over time.

SUPERFOODS

Eat superfoods often as possible. Make and eat/drink bone broth and liver regularly (recipes on page 234 and 384).

Use the sauerkraut recipe on page 238 and eat it daily (1/4 cup), especially with breakfast to aid in gastrointestinal motility & eliminations.

ORGANIC FOODS

Eat as often as possible to avoid toxins.

POSITIVE MINDSET

Focus on maintaining a positive attitude, and create a Gratitude List (see book resources on www.balancedbites.com) regularly.

STRESS MANAGEMENT

Manage stress to keep systemic inflammation low. Develop a guided meditation practice, or begin to practice Qi Gong. Practice meditation, biofeedback, Tai Chi, and/or guided imagery for deep relaxation.

MOVEMENT

Take walks outside, or practice gentle yoga for movement without systemic stress.

MASSAGE

Get gentle massages, look into the Feldenkrais method and find a practitioner.

avoid [-]

NIGHTSHADE FOODS

(if pain you experience is also in your joints) Nightshade vegetables: tomatoes, potatoes, peppers, and eggplants. See page 29 for the list of Paleo foods with nightshades denoted. Also use the substitutions and modifications in recipes that contain nightshades.

RESTAURANTS/DINING OUT

Avoid damaged and manmade fats most often used in restaurant foods.

REFINED FOODS, SWEETENERS, CAFFEINE & ALCOHOL

These can all provoke blood sugar fluctuations and systemic stress.

HARSH CHEMICAL CLEANING OR HYGIENE PRODUCTS

Opt for gentle, natural alternatives, such as soap nuts for laundry, vinegar and water solutions for counter top cleaning, and baking soda and peroxide for cleaning and whitening surfaces, laundry, teeth, etc. Research the "No Poo" method online for hair cleansing without commercial shampoos.

HEATING PADS, CHLORINATED WATER, AND FLUORIDE

DENTAL AMALGAMS

(silver fillings) Consider safe/biological-dentistry to remove existing amalgams.

HIGH INTENSITY EXERCISE

Overly intense exercise (high intensity interval training/HIIT style workouts) and chronic cardiovascular exercise (30-60+ minutes at a steady state of intensity like jogging or biking) as it can lead to low blood sugar episodes, as well as provoke a stress-response in the body.

DISCLAIMER:

The information in this book is not intended to be a replacement for professional medical diagnosis or treatment for a medical condition. It consists solely of nutritional and lifestyle recommendations to support a healthier body.

nutritional supplements & herbs to consider

These recommendations are made as a starting point. Do your own research and determine which supplements may serve you best. It's best to get as many of your nutrients from food as possible. See the next page for specific food-based nutrients on which to focus. The items below are listed in no particular order.

- » **ACETYL L-CARNITINE** may help to preserve glutathione levels in the body. Glutathione is an important neuro-protective nutrient.

- » **VITAMIN C** supports immune function, and it is a potent antioxidant with anti-inflammatory properties.

- » **COENZYME Q10 (CoQ10)** enhances mitochondrial (cellular) energy production and can help alleviate fatigue.

- » **CURCUMIN** is a potent antioxidant.

- » **VITAMIN D** is a potent immune system modulator. Proper balance with vitamin A is important, and it is most available via sun exposure.

- » **FERMENTED COD LIVER OIL/ BUTTER OIL BLEND** for fat-soluble vitamins A, D, E, and K2 as well as some omega 3 fats. I only recommend Green Pasture brand.

- » **DIGESTIVE ENZYMES** help to break down food for absorption while your gut is healing. Look for a blend of enzymes.

- » **GABA** is a calming neurotransmitter that can be helpful if you have trouble sleeping.

- » **GINKGO BILOBA** is a potent antioxidant herb.

- » **5-HTP** can help to increase dopamine and possibly alleviate pain.

- » **MAGNESIUM** is required for more than 300 enzymatic processes in the body, and most people are deficient in it. Look for magnesium glycinate or magnesium malate forms.

- » **MILK THISTLE** supports liver detox and is available in herbal tea, tincture, or capsule form.

- » **N-ACETYL CYSTEINE (NAC)** supports liver function.

- » **OMEGA-3 FATS** are anti-inflammatory essential fatty acids. I only recommend Green Pasture brand fermented cod liver oil.

- » **PROBIOTICS** promote healthy gut flora, which is critical to proper digestion and elimination. Use a supplement, if necessary.

- » **SAM-e** may help to prevent oxidative damage, maintain cognitive function, and improve mental outlook.

MS, FM,
& CFS

supportive nutrients
& foods that contain them

quick LIST

proteins

Beef
Bison
Eel
Eggs
Lamb
Mackerel
Oysters
Salmon
Shellfish

fats

Coconut oil
Extra-virgin olive oil
Grass-fed butter/ghee
Pumpkin seeds

vegetables

Beets
Broccoli
Brussels sprouts
Butternut squash
Carrots
Cauliflower
Daikon radish
Okra
Spinach
Sweet potato

fruits

Bananas
Blueberries
Lemon
Pineapple

superfoods

Bone broth
Fermented cod liver oil
Liver
Sauerkraut

spices

Basil
Cilantro
Cinnamon
Cumin
Garlic
Ginger
Oregano
Parsley
Turmeric

B VITAMINS
B Vitamins are critical to assisting neurotransmitters for improved brain health, as well as nerve and muscular activities.
» Liver, bison, brewer's yeast (Lewis Labs brand only)
» Mushrooms
» Trace amounts: Pecan, sunflower seeds, broccoli, Brussels sprouts

BROMELAIN
An enzyme with anti-inflammatory properties.
» Pineapple

VITAMIN C
A potent antioxidant with anti-inflammatory properties.
» Beets, bell peppers, cantaloupe, garlic, kiwi, lemons, oranges, papaya, pineapple
» Brussels sprouts, cauliflower, collard greens, broccoli, daikon radish, kale

VITAMIN D
A potent immune system modulator and is most available via sun exposure.
» Egg yolks, cold water fish (salmon, herring, mackerel, etc.)
» Grass-fed butter or ghee
» Fermented cod liver oil (Green Pasture brand only)

CARNITINE
Essential for fat metabolism and the transport of fatty acids into cells for normal tissue function.
» Red meat

CHOLINE
Important for cell membrane integrity, nerve-to-muscle communication, and optimal liver function.
» Eggs, liver, heart meat, kidney meat, fish roe (eggs), caviar, cod, cauliflower (cooked)

VITAMIN E
An antioxidant that benefits neurological function, smooth muscle growth, and cellular communication.
» Extra-virgin olive oil
» Pecans, spinach, broccoli, Brussels sprouts

GLUTATHIONE
An antioxidant that aids in liver detox processes.
» Asparagus, broccoli, avocado, garlic, turmeric, curcumin

MAGNESIUM
Magnesium is critical to cellular energy production in order to battle fatigue and maintain proper calcium metabolism for vascular health.
» Kale, green leafy vegetables
» Beets
» Pumpkin seeds/pepitas

OMEGA-3 FATS
An anti-inflammatory essential fatty acid that comes from limited food sources.
» Cold water fish (salmon, herring, mackerel, etc.), fermented cod liver oil (Green Pasture brand only)
» Walnuts, pecans

PROBIOTICS
Promote healthy gut flora, which is critical to proper digestion and elimination.
» Fermented vegetables: cabbage (sauerkraut) carrots, beets or other vegetables
» Kombucha (fermented tea)

ZINC
» Oysters, shellfish
» Lamb, red meat
» Pumpkin seeds (pepitas)

multiple sclerosis, fibromyalgia, chronic fatigue syndrome

DAY	BREAKFAST	LUNCH	DINNER
1 ●■◆	Swirly Crustless Quiche (240), Perfectly Baked Bacon (236), Raw Sauerkraut (238)	Mustard Glazed Chicken Thighs (266), Green Salad*, Balsamic Vinaigrette (378)	Grilled Garlic Flank Steak with Peppers & Onions (294), Baked Beets with Fennel**(362)
2 ●◆■	*left-over* Swirly Crustless Quiche, *left-over* Garlic Flank Steak with Peppers & Onions	Wild Canned Salmon with Olives, Avocado, Lemon Juice, Tomato, EVOO	Sage Roasted Turkey Legs (276), Sweet Potato Pancakes (298), Steamed Spinach*
3 ■■●	*left-over* Sweet Potato Pancakes, *left-over* Mustard-Glazed Chicken Thighs	*left-over* Sage Roasted Turkey Legs, Persimmon, Asparagus & Fennel Salad (380)	Lemony Lamb Dolmas (318), Cilantro Cauli-Rice (340)
4 ●●◆	Pesto Scrambled Eggs (252), Cilantro Cauli-Rice (340), Raw Sauerkraut (238)	*left-over* Lemony Lamb Dolmas, Spinach Salad with Walnuts & Artichokes (380)	Citrus Macadamia Nut Sole (314), Butternut Squash**
5 ◆◆◆	*left-over* Citrus Macadamia Nut Sole, Butternut Squash**	Nori Salmon Handrolls (316)	Beef & Mixed Veggie Stir Fry (286)
6 ●◆●	Pumpkin Pancakes (242), Breakfast Sausage using Italian Sausage Spice Blend (233)	*left-over* Beef Stir Fry with Mixed Veggies	Lamb Lettuce Boats with Avo-Ziki Sauce (322)
7 ●◆■	Eggs, Perfectly Baked Bacon (236), Kale*, Raw Sauerkraut (238)	Mixed Greens with Wild Canned Salmon, Asparagus*, Lemon Juice, EVOO	Citrus & Herb Whole Roasted Chicken (256), Roasted Rosemary Roots (350), Kale Chips*(356)
8 ■■■	Grain-Free Porridge (252), Berries, *left-over* Citrus & Herb Whole Roasted Chicken	Spinach Salad with Walnuts & Artichokes (380), *left-over* Citrus & Herb Whole Roasted Chicken	Chinese 5-Spice Lettuce Cups (272)
9 ●■◆	Swirly Crustless Quiche (240), Steamed Broccoli*, Raw Sauerkraut (238)	Indian-Spiced Turkey Burgers (268), Steamed Broccoli*	Pesto Shrimp & Squash Fettuccine (308)
10 ●◆●	Omelet or Pesto Scrambled Eggs, *left-over* Shrimp & Avocado	Simple Shrimp Ceviche (316), Mixed Greens*, EVOO	Cumin Spiced Pork Tenderloin with Root Vegetables**(328)

» *A complete shopping list for this meal plan can be found on balancedbites.com*

KEY

◆ **Red-Meat**
■ **Poultry**
● **Eggs**
● **Pork**
● **Lamb**
◆ **Seafood**

NOTES

EVOO	Extra-virgin olive oil
CO	Coconut oil
*	or other non-starchy vegetable
**	or other starchy vegetable (refer to page 110)

If no page number is listed, simply prepare the items as noted or any way you like.

For additional protein, vegetable, and fat recommendations, refer to the QUICK LIST that is associated with your meal plan!

multiple sclerosis, fibromyalgia, chronic fatigue syndrome

DAY	BREAKFAST	LUNCH	DINNER
11 ● ● ◆	Swirly Crustless Quiche (240) Perfectly Baked Bacon (236), *left-over* Root Vegetables	*left-over* Cumin Spiced Pork Tenderloin, Sautéed Red Cabbage (352)	Balsamic Braised Short Ribs (278), Candied Carrots (340), Spinach*
12 ● ◆ ■	Eggs, *left-over* Red Cabbage	*left-over* Balsamic Braised Short Ribs, *left-over* Candied Carrots, Green Salad*	Savory Baked Chicken Legs (264), Brussels Sprouts with Fennel*(350)
13 ● ■ ◆	Zucchini Pancakes (248), Perfectly Baked Bacon (236), Raw Sauerkraut (238)	*left-over* Savory Baked Chicken Legs, *left-over* Brussels Sprouts with Fennel*	Lemon Rosemary Broiled Salmon (306), Asparagus with Lemon & Olives (338), Sweet Potato**
14 ◆ ■ ◆	*left-over* Lemon Rosemary Broiled Salmon, *left-over* Asparagus with Lemon & Olives*	Buffalo Chicken Lettuce Wraps (270)	Red Palm & Coriander Tuna Over Daikon Noodle Salad (302), Green Salad*
15 ● ◆ ◆	Scrambled Eggs with Olives, Steamed Spinach*, Avocado	Spinach Salad with EVOO, *left-over* Red Palm & Coriander Tuna, Avocado, Lemon Juice	Italian-Style Stuffed Peppers (300), Green Salad* with Balsamic Vinaigrette (378)
16 ● ◆ ■	Grain-Free Porridge (252), Breakfast Sausage	*left-over* Italian-Style Stuffed Peppers (300), Green Salad*	Bacon-Wrapped Smoky Chicken Thighs (262), Mixed Greens Salad with Beets & Blood Oranges (376)
17 ● ■ ◆	Bacon & Egg Salad (248), Sweet Potato or Beets**	*left-over* Bacon-Wrapped Smoky Chicken Thighs, Green Salad*	Spaghetti Squash Bolognese (280), Kale Chips (356)
18 ● ◆ ●	Pumpkin Pancakes (242), Breakfast Sausage or Bacon	*left-over* Spaghetti Squash Bolognese	Thanksgiving Stuffing Meatballs (334), Mashed Faux-Tatoes (344)
19 ● ● ◆	Scrambled Eggs, Avocado, Spinach or Kale*, Raw Sauerkraut (238)	*left-over* Thanksgiving Stuffing Meatballs, *left-over* Mashed Faux-Tatoes	Citrus Macadamia Nut Sole (314), Lemon Roasted Romanesco*(346), Sweet & Savory Potatoes**(362)
20 ● ◆ ■	Grain-Free Porridge (252), Hard Boiled Eggs	*left-over* Citrus Macadamia Nut Sole, *left-over* Lemon Roasted Romanesco	Roasted Duck with Cherry Sauce (274), Sautéed Red Cabbage with Onions and Apples*(352)

» *A complete shopping list for this meal plan can be found on balancedbites.com*

KEY
◆ **Red-Meat**
■ **Poultry**
● **Eggs**
● **Pork**
● **Lamb**
◆ **Seafood**

NOTES

EVOO	Extra-virgin olive oil
CO	Coconut oil
*	or other non-starchy vegetable
**	or other starchy vegetable (refer to page 110)

If no page number is listed, simply prepare the items as noted or any way you like.

For additional protein, vegetable, and fat recommendations, refer to the QUICK LIST that is associated with your meal plan!

DAY	BREAKFAST	LUNCH	DINNER
21 ●◆●	Hard Boiled Eggs, Breakfast Sausage, Raw Sauerkraut (238)	Nori Salmon Handrolls (316)	Lamb Chops with Olive Tapenade (326), Greek Salad with Avo-Ziki (374)
22 ●●◆	Swirly Crustless Quiche (240), Breakfast Sausage	*left-over* Lamb Chops with Olive Tapenade, *left-over* Greek Salad with Avo-Ziki	Orange Braised Beef Shanks (284), Butternut Sage Soup**(348)
23 ●◆◆	*left-over* Swirly Crustless Quiche, Perfectly Baked Bacon (236)	*left-over* Orange Braised Beef Shanks, *left-over* Butternut Sage Soup**	Hayley's Skirt Steak Tacos (292), Salsa (296), Grilled Squash & Pineapple (342)
24 ●◆◆	Acorn Squash with Cinnamon & Coconut Butter (358), Breakfast Sausage or Bacon	Tangy Taco Salad (296), *left-over* Salsa	Fiery Jalapeño Burgers with Sweet Potato Pancakes (298), Red Roasted Garlic (370)
25 ●◆◆	*left-over* Sweet Potato Pancakes, Eggs, Avocado	Quick & Easy Salmon Cakes (310), Green Salad*, Avocado, Olives	Asian Orange Pan-Seared Scallops (304), Tomatillo Shrimp Cocktail (312), Zucchini*
26 ●◆●	Zucchini Pancakes (248), Perfectly Baked Bacon (236)	Tuna, Mixed Greens Salad with Persimmons, Asparagus & Fennel (380), Orange Vinaigrette (382)	Grandma Barbara's Stuffed Mushrooms (332), Roasted Marrow Bones (288), Spinach
27 ●●●	Grain-Free Porridge (252), Breakfast Sausage using Italian Sausage Spice Blend (233)	*left-over* Grandma Barbara's Stuffed Mushrooms, Mixed Greens Salad, Balsamic Vinaigrette (378)	Spiced Lamb Meatballs with Balsamic-Fig Compote (324), Green Beans with Shallots*(358)
28 ●◆■	*left-over* Spiced Lamb Meatballs, Spinach or Cabbage*	Wild Canned Salmon with Olives, Avocado, Lemon Juice, Tomato, EVOO	Lemon & Artichoke Chicken (260), Broc-Cauli Chowder with Bacon (336)
29 ●■◆	Apple Streusel Egg Muffins (254), Bacon or Breakfast Sausage	*left-over* Lemon & Artichoke Chicken, Kale & Carrot Salad with Lemon-Tahini Dressing (376)	Mom's Stuffed Cabbage Rolls with Tomato Cranberry Sauce (290), Green Salad*
30 ●●●	*left-over* Apple Streusel Egg Muffins (254), Bacon or Breakfast Sausage	Chorizo Meatballs (330), Mixed Greens Salad* with Avocado, Lemon Juice, and EVOO	Mediterranean Lamb Roast (320), Sautéed Spinach with Pine Nuts & Currants*(366)

» *A complete shopping list for this meal plan can be found on balancedbites.com*

KEY
◆ Red-Meat
■ Poultry
● Eggs
● Pork
● Lamb
◆ Seafood

NOTES
EVOO   Extra-virgin olive oil
CO   Coconut oil
*   or other non-starchy vegetable
**   or other starchy vegetable (refer to page 110)

If no page number is listed, simply prepare the items as noted or any way you like.
For additional protein, vegetable, and fat recommendations, refer to the QUICK LIST that is associated with your meal plan!

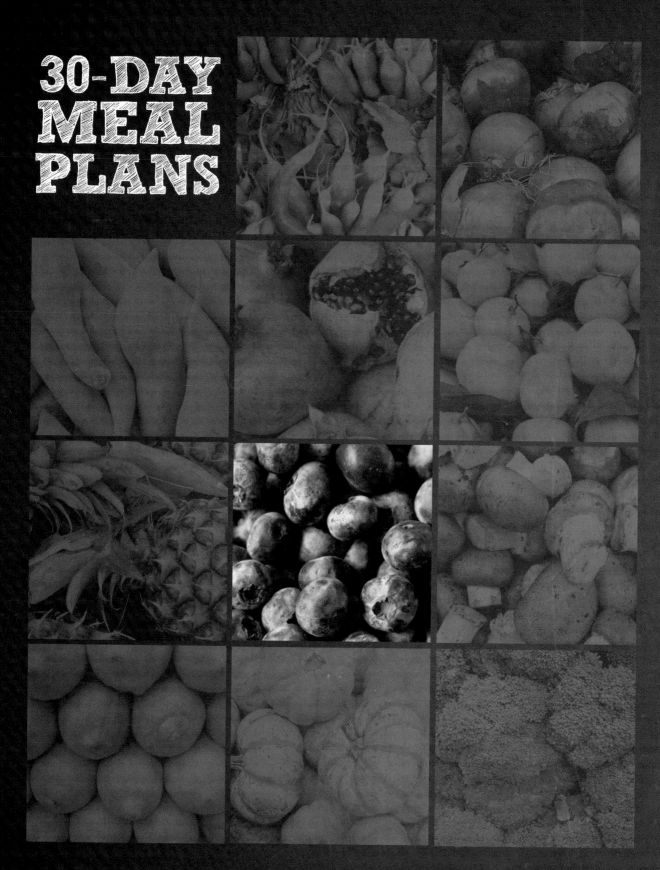

30-DAY MEAL PLANS

NEUROLOGICAL HEALTH

For an initial dietary intervention before this slightly more limited plan, you may want to try the Blood Sugar Regulation 30-Day Meal Plan first with regard to food choices and follow the lifestyle, supplement, and herbal recommendations from this plan.

parkinson's disease

symptoms include:

» Slowed movement
» Muscular rigidity and tightness
» Resting tremor that improves with movement
» Postural instability (a shuffle or tiny steps used to maintain balance)

alzheimer's disease

symptoms include:

» Memory loss, progressive short and long-term impairment that is more severe than is typically associated with age
» Repetitive questioning
» Decline in vocabulary or "word-loss"
» Forgetting of familiar names
» Difficulty with numbers, spatial relations, and time relations

Other populations who may benefit from this meal plan include those diagnosed with:

» EPILEPSY
» TYPE 2 DIABETES
» ANYONE SEEKING A KETOGENIC DIET APPROACH

Disclaimer: The information in this book is not intended to be a replacement for professional medical diagnosis or treatment for a medical condition. It consists solely of nutritional and lifestyle recommendations to support a healthier body.

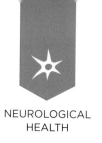

diet & lifestyle recommendations

add [+]

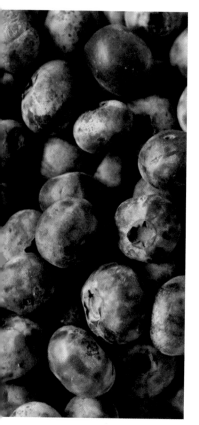

FATS

Eat more fats in order to support the brain in on ketones versus glucose as a primary source. See page 44 for the Guide to Fats & Oils. Coconut oil is especially therapeutic.

ANTIOXIDANT-RICH FOODS

Eat deeply colored foods like leafy greens, berries, and carrots.

ORGANIC

Eat as often as possible to avoid toxins.

POSITIVE MINDSET

Focus on maintaining a positive attitude, and create a Gratitude List regularly. (See the book resources on www.balancedbites. com.)

STRESS MANAGEMENT

Manage stress to keep systemic inflammation low. Develop a guided meditation practice, or begin to practice Qi Gong. Practice meditation, biofeedback, Tai Chi, and/or guided imagery for deep relaxation.

DETOX

Consider detoxification methods for heavy metals (particularly mercury).

MENTAL EXERCISES

Practice mental exercises to keep the brain active and engaged, such as reading, puzzles, games, and anything else that is mentally stimulating and enjoyable.

HYDROTHERAPY

Try hydrotherapy, a water-based pain relief physiotherapy treatment.

MASSAGE

(For Parkinson's Disease specifically) Get gentle massages, look into the Feldenkrais method and find a practitioner.

avoid [-]

GLUTEN & DAIRY

100% of the time. See the "Guide to Gluten" on page 89. Avoid dairy for potential morphine-like effect that is promoted by casein/casomorphin.
(Butter and ghee are okay.)

STARCHY CARBOHYDRATES

Maintain a total carbohydrate intake of around 50g per day. Measure and create a food journal if necessary to keep track.

RESTAURANTS/DINING OUT

Avoid damaged and manmade fats most often used in restaurant foods.

SWEETENERS, CAFFEINE

These can all provoke blood sugar fluctuations and systemic stress.

ALCOHOL, TOBACCO, NICOTINE & MSG (MONOSODIUM GLUTAMATE)

These are products that require detoxification and/or may have some neurotoxic effects.

HARSH CHEMICAL CLEANING OR HYGIENE PRODUCTS

Opt for gentle, natural alternatives, such as soap nuts for laundry, vinegar and water solutions for counter top cleaning, and baking soda and peroxide for cleaning and whitening surfaces, laundry, teeth, etc.

TYRAMINES

Contained in fermented foods if you are prone to migraines.

DENTAL AMALGAMS

(silver fillings) Consider safe/biological-dentistry to remove existing amalgams.

HIGH INTENSITY EXERCISE

High intensity training can be too taxing on the system and cause a stress-response.

DISCLAIMER:

The information in this book is not intended to be a replacement for professional medical diagnosis or treatment for a medical condition. It consists solely of nutritional and lifestyle recommendations to support a healthier body.

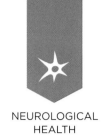

nutritional supplements & herbs to consider

These recommendations are made as a starting point. Do your own research and determine which supplements may serve you best. It's best to get as many of your nutrients from food as possible. See the next page for specific food-based nutrients on which to focus. The items below are listed in no particular order.

» **LIPOIC ACID (alpha-lipoic acid)** is an antioxidant that may improve cellular energy production and support liver function.

» **ACETYL L-CARNITINE** may help to preserve glutathione levels in the body. Glutathione is an important neuro-protective nutrient.

» **VITAMIN C** supports immune function, and it is a potent antioxidant with anti-inflammatory properties that helps to regenerate vitamin E.

» **COENZYME Q10 (CoQ10)** enhances mitochondrial (cellular) energy production and can help alleviate fatigue. It is known to be depleted by statin drugs.

» **VITAMIN D** is a potent immune system modulator. Proper balance with vitamin A is important, and it is most available via sun exposure.

» **FERMENTED COD LIVER OIL/ BUTTER OIL BLEND** for fat-soluble vitamins A, D, E, and K2 as well as some omega 3 fats. I only recommend Green Pasture brand. If migraines persist, omit this supplement.

» **GABA** is a calming neurotransmitter that can be helpful if you have trouble sleeping.

» **GINKGO BILOBA** is a potent antioxidant herb.

» **5-HTP** can help to increase dopamine and possibly alleviate pain.

» **MAGNESIUM** is required for more than 300 enzymatic processes in the body, and most people are deficient in it. Look for magnesium glycinate or magnesium malate forms.

» **MILK THISTLE** supports liver detox and is available in herbal tea, tincture, or capsule form.

» **N-ACETYL CYSTEINE (NAC)** supports liver function.

» **OMEGA-3 FATS** are anti-inflammatory essential fatty acids. I only recommend Green Pasture brand fermented cod liver oil.

» **PASSIONFLOWER** (for Parkinson's Disease) may help to reduce tremors.

» **PHOSPHATIDYLCHOLINE** enhances the integrity of the GI tract and aids in fatty acid digestion, as well as repairs the mucosal lining of the gut.

» **PHOSPHATIDYLSERINE** supports cell membrane integrity and may improve memory and cognition. It has been shown to blunt the release of cortisol in response to stress.

» **PROBIOTICS** promote healthy gut flora, which is critical to proper digestion and elimination. Use a supplement, if necessary.

» **SAM-e** may help to prevent oxidative damage, maintain cognitive function, and improve mental outlook.

» **SELENIUM** is an antioxidant that is antagonistic to heavy metals like lead, mercury, cadmium, and aluminum; it supports cancer recovery, immune function, cardiac health, inflammatory conditions, vision, and proper fetal growth. Absorption may be decreased by high zinc intake - these minerals should be balanced.

» **SUPER OXIDE DISMUTASE (SOD)** is an anti-inflammatory that prevents free radical damage.

» **DIGESTIVE ENZYMES** help to break down food for absorption while your gut is healing. Look for a blend of enzymes.

» **ZINC** is a potent antioxidant that aids in vitamin A metabolism. People with inflammatory conditions are often deficient in zinc; it should be balanced with selenium

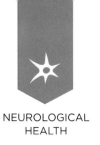

supportive nutrients & foods that contain them

B VITAMINS

B Vitamins are critical to assisting neurotransmitters for improved brain health, as well as nerve and muscular activities.

» Liver, bison, lamb, flounder, haddock, salmon, trout, tuna
» Brewer's yeast (Lewis Labs brand only)
» Mushrooms
» Hazelnuts, walnuts
» Trace amounts: pecan, sunflower seeds, broccoli, Brussels sprouts, other dark leafy greens

VITAMIN C

A potent antioxidant with anti-inflammatory properties.

» Adrenal glands, beets, bell peppers, garlic, lemons, Brussels sprouts, cauliflower, collard greens, broccoli, daikon radish, kale, mustard greens, parsley, spinach, strawberries

VITAMIN D

A potent immune system modulator and is most available via sun exposure.

» Egg yolks, cold water fish (salmon, herring, mackerel, etc.)
» Grass-fed butter or ghee
» Fermented cod liver oil (Green Pasture brand only)

CHOLINE

An important for cell membrane integrity, nerve-to-muscle communication, and optimal liver function

» Eggs, liver, heart meat, kidney meat, fish roe (eggs), caviar, cod
» Cauliflower (cooked)

VITAMIN E

An antioxidant that benefits neurological function, smooth muscle growth, and cellular communication.

» Extra-virgin olive oil
» Pecans, spinach, broccoli, Brussels sprouts

GLUTATHIONE

An antioxidant that aids in liver detox.

» Asparagus, broccoli, avocado, garlic, turmeric, curcumin

LIPOIC ACID (ALPHA-LIPOIC ACID/ALA)

» Red meat, organ meats

MAGNESIUM

Magnesium is critical to cellular energy production in order to battle fatigue and maintain proper calcium metabolism for vascular health.

» Kale, green leafy vegetables, beets, pumpkin seeds/pepitas

OMEGA-3 FATS

An anti-inflammatory essential fatty acid that comes from limited food sources.

» Cold water fish (salmon, herring, mackerel, etc.), fermented cod liver oil (Green Pasture brand only)
» Walnuts, pecans

POTASSIUM

» Avocado, spinach, Swiss chard

PROBIOTICS

Promote healthy gut flora, which is critical to proper digestion and elimination. Limit or avoid these foods if you are prone to migraines.

» Fermented vegetables: cabbage (sauerkraut) carrots, beets or other vegetables
» Kombucha (fermented tea)

SELENIUM

» Brazil nuts, red Swiss chard, turnips, garlic

ZINC

» Oysters, shellfish, lamb, red meat
» Pumpkin seeds/pepitas

neurological health

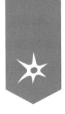

DAY	BREAKFAST	LUNCH	DINNER
1 ●■◆	Swirly Crustless Quiche (240), Perfectly Baked Bacon (236), Raw Sauerkraut (238)	Mustard Glazed Chicken Thighs (266), Green Salad*, Balsamic Vinaigrette (378)	Grilled Garlic Flank Steak with Peppers & Onions (294), Green Salad, EVOO
2 ●◆■	*left-over* Swirly Crustless Quiche, *left-over* Garlic Flank Steak with Peppers & Onions	Wild Canned Salmon with Olives, Avocado, Lemon Juice, Tomato, EVOO	Sage Roasted Turkey Legs (276), Steamed Spinach*
3 ●■●	Hard boiled eggs, Broccoli*	*left-over* Sage Roasted Turkey Legs, Mixed Greens with Asparagus & Fennel, EVOO, Lemon	Lemony Lamb Dolmas (318), Cilantro Cauli-Rice (340)
4 ●●◆	Pesto Scrambled Eggs (252), *left-over* Cilantro Cauli-Rice, Raw Sauerkraut (238)	*left-over* Lemony Lamb Dolmas, Spinach Salad with Walnuts & Artichokes (380)	Citrus Macadamia Nut Sole (314), Kale*
5 ◆◆◆	*left-over* Citrus Macadamia Nut Sole, Carrots	Nori Salmon Handrolls (316)	Beef & Mixed Veggie Stir Fry (286)
6 ○◆●	Breakfast Sausage using Italian Sausage Spice Blend (233), Cauliflower*	*left-over* Beef Stir Fry with Mixed Veggies	Lamb Lettuce Boats with Avo-Ziki Sauce (322)
7 ●◆■	Eggs, Perfectly Baked Bacon (236), Kale*, Raw Sauerkraut (238)	Mixed Greens with Wild Canned Salmon, Asparagus*, Lemon Juice, EVOO	Citrus & Herb Whole Roasted Chicken (256), Simple Baked Kale Chips*(356)
8 ■■■	Grain-Free Porridge (252), *left-over* Citrus & Herb Whole Roasted Chicken	Spinach Salad with Walnuts & Artichokes (380), *left-over* Citrus & Herb Whole Roasted Chicken	Chinese 5-Spice Lettuce Cups (272)
9 ●■◆	Swirly Crustless Quiche (240), Steamed Broccoli*, Raw Sauerkraut (238)	Indian-Spiced Turkey Burgers (268), Steamed Broccoli*	Pesto Shrimp & Squash Fettuccine (308)
10 ●◆○	Omelet or Pesto Scrambled Eggs, *left-over* Shrimp & Avocado	Simple Shrimp Ceviche (316), Mixed Greens*, EVOO	Cumin Spiced Pork Tenderloin with Root Vegetables (328)

» *A complete shopping list for this meal plan can be found on balancedbites.com*

KEY

◆ Red-Meat
■ Poultry
● Eggs
○ Pork
● Lamb
◆ Seafood

NOTES

EVOO   Extra-virgin olive oil
CO   Coconut oil
*   or other non-starchy vegetable

If no page number is listed, simply prepare the items as noted or any way you like. For additional protein, vegetable, and fat recommendations, refer to the QUICK LIST that is associated with your meal plan!

For Parkinson's Disease: If you take Levodopa, do not eat foods rich in vitamin B6 (like bananas, liver, and fish) when taking the medication. Stick to smaller protein portions before doses, and a larger portion of protein in the evening after your final dose.

DAY	BREAKFAST	LUNCH	DINNER
11 ● ● ◆	Swirly Crustless Quiche (240) Perfectly Baked Bacon (236), Raw Sauerkraut (238)	*left-over* Cumin Spiced Pork Tenderloin, Rainbow Red Cabbage Salad*(372)	Balsamic Braised Short Ribs (278), Carrots, Spinach*
12 ● ◆ ■	Eggs, *left-over* Rainbow Red Cabbage Salad	*left-over* Balsamic Braised Short Ribs, *left-over* Carrots, Green Salad*	Savory Baked Chicken Legs (264), Brussels Sprouts with Fennel*(350)
13 ● ■ ◆	Zucchini Pancakes (248), Perfectly Baked Bacon (236), Raw Sauerkraut (238)	*left-over* Savory Baked Chicken Legs, *left-over* Brussels Sprouts with Fennel*	Lemon Rosemary Broiled Salmon (306), Asparagus with Lemon & Olives (338)
14 ◆ ■ ◆	*left-over* Lemon Rosemary Broiled Salmon, *left-over* Asparagus with Lemon & Olives*	Buffalo Chicken Lettuce Wraps (270)	Red Palm & Coriander Tuna Over Daikon Noodle Salad (302), Green Salad*
15 ● ◆ ◆	Scrambled Eggs with Olives, Steamed Spinach*, Avocado	Spinach Salad with EVOO, *left-over* Red Palm & Coriander Tuna, Avocado, Lemon Juice	Italian-Style Stuffed Peppers (300), Green Salad* with Balsamic Vinaigrette (378)
16 ● ◆ ■	Grain-Free Porridge (252), Breakfast Sausage	*left-over* Italian-Style Stuffed Peppers (300), Green Salad	Bacon-Wrapped Smoky Chicken Thighs (262), Mixed Greens Salad with Beets & Blood Oranges (376)
17 ● ■ ◆	Bacon & Egg Salad (248), Broccoli*	*left-over* Bacon-Wrapped Smoky Chicken Thighs, Green Salad*	Spaghetti Squash Bolognese (280), Kale Chips*(356)
18 ● ◆ ●	Pumpkin Pancakes (242), Breakfast Sausage or Bacon	*left-over* Spaghetti Squash Bolognese	Thanksgiving Stuffing Meatballs (334), Mashed Faux-Tatoes (344)
19 ● ● ◆	Scrambled Eggs, Avocado, Spinach or Kale*, Raw Sauerkraut (238)	*left-over* Thanksgiving Stuffing Meatballs, *left-over* Mashed Faux-Tatoes	Citrus Macadamia Nut Sole (314), Lemon Roasted Romanesco*(346)
20 ● ◆ ■	Grain-Free Porridge (252), Hard Boiled Eggs	*left-over* Citrus Macadamia Nut Sole, *left-over* Lemon Roasted Romanesco	Roasted Duck with Cherry Sauce (274), Sautéed Red Cabbage with Onions and Apples*(352)

» *A complete shopping list for this meal plan can be found on balancedbites.com*

KEY
◆ Red-Meat
■ Poultry
● Eggs
● Pork
● Lamb
◆ Seafood

NOTES

EVOO   Extra-virgin olive oil

CO   Coconut oil

*   or other non-starchy vegetable

If no page number is listed, simply prepare the items as noted or any way you like.

For additional protein, vegetable, and fat recommendations, refer to the QUICK LIST that is associated with your meal plan!

For Parkinson's Disease: If you take Levodopa, do not eat foods rich in vitamin B6 (like bananas, liver, and fish) when taking the medication. Stick to smaller protein portions before doses, and a larger portion of protein in the evening after your final dose.

neurological health

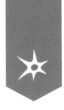

DAY	BREAKFAST	LUNCH	DINNER
21 ●◆●	Hard Boiled Eggs, Breakfast Sausage, Raw Sauerkraut (238)	Nori Salmon Handrolls (316)	Lamb Chops with Olive Tapenade (326), Greek Salad with Avo-Ziki (374)
22 ●●◆	Swirly Crustless Quiche (240), Breakfast Sausage	*left-over* Lamb Chops with Olive Tapenade, *left-over* Greek Salad with Avo-Ziki	Orange Braised Beef Shanks (284), Green Salad
23 ●◆◆	*left-over* Swirly Crustless Quiche, Perfectly Baked Bacon (236)	*left-over* Orange Braised Beef Shanks, Green Salad*	Hayley's Skirt Steak Tacos (292), Salsa (tomato or cucumber, not fruit) (296)
24 ◆◆◆	Smoked Salmon, Cucumber, Green Beans in CO*	Tangy Taco Salad (296), *left-over* Salsa	Fiery Jalapeño Burgers with Sweet Potato Pancakes (298), Red Roasted Garlic (370)
25 ●◆◆	*left-over* Sweet Potato Pancakes, Eggs, Avocado	Quick & Easy Salmon Cakes (310), Green Salad*, Avocado, Olives	Asian Orange Pan-Seared Scallops (304), Tomatillo Shrimp Cocktail (312), Zucchini*
26 ●◆○	Pesto Scrambled Eggs(252), Perfectly Baked Bacon (236)	Tuna, Mixed Greens Salad with Persimmons, Asparagus & Fennel (380), Orange Vinaigrette (382)	Grandma Barbara's Stuffed Mushrooms (332), Roasted Marrow Bones (288), Spinach
27 ○●●	Grain-Free Porridge (252), Breakfast Sausage using Italian Sausage Spice Blend (233)	*left-over* Grandma Barbara's Stuffed Mushrooms, Mixed Greens Salad, Balsamic Vinaigrette (378)	Spiced Lamb Meatballs with Balsamic-Fig Compote (324), Green Beans with Shallots*(358)
28 ●◆■	*left-over* Spiced Lamb Meatballs, Spinach or Cabbage*	Wild Canned Salmon with Olives, Avocado, Lemon Juice, Tomato, EVOO	Lemon & Artichoke Chicken (260), Broc-Cauli Chowder with Bacon (336)
29 ●■◆	Zucchini Pancakes (248), Bacon or Breakfast Sausage	*left-over* Lemon & Artichoke Chicken, Kale & Carrot Salad with Lemon-Tahini Dressing (376)	Mom's Stuffed Cabbage Rolls with Tomato Cranberry Sauce (290), Green Salad*
30 ●○●	*left-over* Zucchini Pancakes, Bacon or Breakfast Sausage	Chorizo Meatballs (330), Mixed Greens Salad* with Avocado, Lemon Juice, and EVOO	Mediterranean Lamb Roast (320), Sautéed Spinach with Pine Nuts & Currants*(366)

» *A complete shopping list for this meal plan can be found on balancedbites.com*

KEY
- ◆ Red-Meat
- ■ Poultry
- ● Eggs
- ○ Pork
- ● Lamb
- ◆ Seafood

NOTES

EVOO	Extra-virgin olive oil
CO	Coconut oil
*	or other non-starchy vegetable

For Parkinson's Disease: If you take Levodopa, do not eat foods rich in vitamin B6 (like bananas, liver, and fish) when taking the medication. Stick to smaller protein portions before doses, and a larger portion of protein in the evening after your final dose.

If no page number is listed, simply prepare the items as noted or any way you like. For additional protein, vegetable, and fat recommendations, refer to the QUICK LIST that is associated with your meal plan!

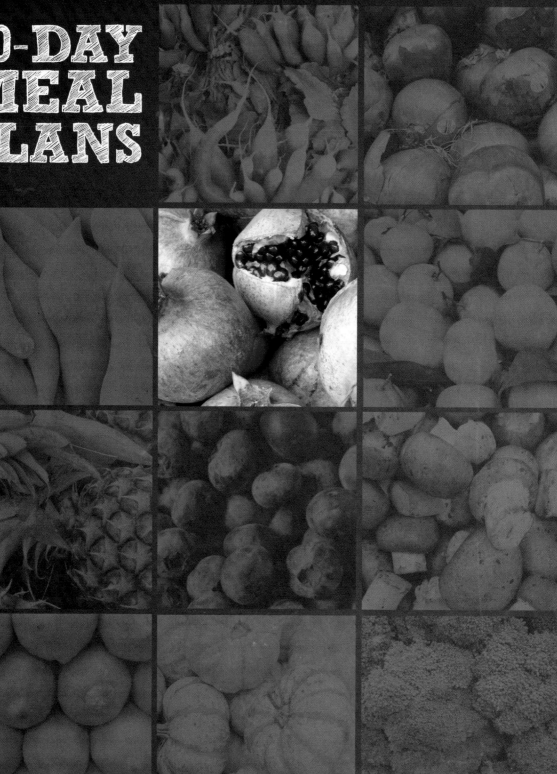

30-DAY MEAL PLANS

HEART HEALTH

For an initial dietary intervention before this slightly more specific plan, you may want to try the Squeaky Clean Paleo 30-Day Meal Plan first.

cholesterol concerns
may cause one or more of the following:

» Low blood markers for high-density lipoproteins (HDL)
» High blood markers for low-density lipoproteins (LDL)
» High triglycerides (circulating blood lipids)
» Total:HDL ratio outside of an ideal range between 3-4 (divide your total cholesterol by your HDL marker to find this number)
» High blood markers of oxidized LDL (if you have access to such tests)

blood pressure concerns
may cause one or more of the following:

» General fatigue
» Energy changes throughout the day
» Waking up tired
» Insomnia
» Inability to focus/brain fog; mental disturbances; mental confusion
» Blurred vision
» Low blood pressure
» Headaches
» Trembling
» Incoherent speech
» Weakness in legs
» Dry mouth
» Weight gain
» Mood imbalances, such as irritability, negativity, sense of gloom, crying spells, mood swings, erratic behavior, anti-social nature, depression, anxiety, hypersensitivity
» Cravings for sugar and carbohydrates
» Constant hunger
» Compulsive eating
» Loss of appetite
» Loss of sex drive
» Rapid heartbeat/fluttering in chest

Disclaimer: The information in this book is not intended to be a replacement for professional medical diagnosis or treatment for a medical condition. It consists solely of nutritional and lifestyle recommendations to support a healthier body.

diet & lifestyle recommendations

add [+]

NUTRIENT-DENSE FOODS
Replenish depleted nutrient stores from eating excess refined foods over time.

STRESS MANAGEMENT
Manage stress to keep systemic inflammation low. Develop a guided meditation practice, or begin to practice Qi Gong. Practice meditation, biofeedback, Tai Chi, and/or guided imagery for deep relaxation.

MOVEMENT
Take walks outside, or practice gentle yoga for movement without systemic stress.

Slowly begin weight training with moderate to heavy weight, not excessively demanding in terms of stress response or cortisol output.

avoid [-]

GLUTEN
100% of the time. See the "Guide to Gluten" on page 89.

RESTAURANTS/DINING OUT
Avoid damaged and manmade fats most often used in restaurant foods.

REFINED FOODS, BAD CARBS, SWEETENERS, CAFFEINE, ALCOHOL, & MSG (MONOSODIUM GLUTAMATE)
These can all provoke blood sugar fluctuations and systemic stress. Avoid packaged foods with excess sodium.

ALCOHOL, TOBACCO, NICOTINE
These are products that require detoxification and may impair liver function and promote systemic inflammation.

STRESS
Make lifestyle changes to avoid stressful situations.

CHRONIC CARDIOVASCULAR EXERCISE
(meaning 30-60+ minutes at a steady state of intensity like jogging or biking), as it can provoke a stress response.

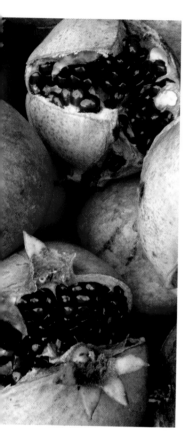

DISCLAIMER:
The information in this book is not intended to be a replacement for professional medical diagnosis or treatment for a medical condition. It consists solely of nutritional and lifestyle recommendations to support a healthier body.

nutritional supplements & herbs to consider

These recommendations are made as a starting point. Do your own research and determine which supplements may serve you best. It's best to get as many of your nutrients from food as possible. See the next page for specific food-based nutrients on which to focus. The items below are listed in no particular order.

» **VITAMIN A (retinol)** helps to maintain the integrity of the mucosal lining of the gut; helps to maintain immunity when balanced with vitamin D; necessary for the assimilation of dietary minerals.

» **FERMENTED COD LIVER OIL/ BUTTER OIL BLEND** for fat-soluble vitamins A, D, E, and K2 as well as some omega 3 fats. I only recommend Green Pasture brand.

» **VITAMIN B3 (niacin)** is supportive of blood sugar regulation and may lower cholesterol levels.

» **VITAMIN B5 (pantothenic acid & pantethine)** may lower cholesterol and triglycerides in the pantethine form, especially in diabetics.

» **VITAMIN B7 (biotin)** is a coenzyme required for the metabolism of glucose, amino acids and lipids.

» **VITAMIN B9 (folate)** supports healthy red blood cells, boosts growth, and reduces risks of birth defects. Look for a B-complex supplement for a balanced dose.

» **VITAMIN C** s is a potent antioxidant with anti-inflammatory properties that helps to regenerate vitamin E.

» **COENZYME Q10 (CoQ10)** enhances mitochondrial (cellular) energy production and can help to alleviate fatigue. It is also known to be depleted by statin drugs.

» **VITAMIN E** is an antioxidant that protects against free radical damage.

» **LIPOIC ACID (alpha-lipoic acid)** may improve cellular energy production and has antioxidant properties. It may also be helpful to cardiac patients.

» **MAGNESIUM** is required for more than 300 enzymatic processes in the body, and most people are deficient in it. Look for magnesium glycinate or magnesium malate forms.

» **OMEGA-3 FATS** are anti-inflammatory essential fatty acids. I only recommend Green Pasture brand fermented cod liver oil.

» **SELENIUM & ZINC** are antioxidants that protect against free radical damage, and it is difficult to get sufficient amounts solely from food sources.

supportive nutrients
& foods that contain them

quick LIST

proteins

Chicken
Eggs
Herring
Mackerel
Oysters
Pork
Salmon
Shellfish
Tuna

fats

Coconut oil
Extra-virgin olive oil
Grass-fed butter/ghee
Walnuts

vegetables

Asparagus
Avocado
Beets
Brussels sprouts
Broccoli
Cabbage
Cauliflower
Squash
Swiss chard
Yams

fruits

Berries
Citrus
Melon
Papaya

superfoods

Bone broth
Fermented cod liver oil
Liver
Sauerkraut

spices

Basil
Black pepper
Cardamom
Cinnamon
Cloves
Garlic
Oregano
Thyme
Turmeric

B VITAMINS

(especially B3, B6, B9)
» Liver, chicken, tuna, lamb, salmon, egg yolks, sardines, grass-fed dairy, brewer's yeast (Lewis Labs brand only)
» Trace amounts: sesame seeds, sunflower seeds, almonds, walnuts, pecans, mushrooms, romaine lettuce, cauliflower

VITAMIN C

» Adrenal glands from pasture-raised animals, beets, bell peppers, garlic, lemons, Brussels sprouts, cauliflower, collard greens, broccoli, daikon radish, kale, mustard greens, parsley, spinach, strawberries

CALCIUM

» Dark leafy greens (be sure to also eat grass-fed butter or a K2 supplement like the fermented cod liver oil/butter oil blend from Green Pasture to assimilate calcium appropriately)

CHOLESTEROL

Cholesterol helps to maintain proper cell membrane structure and is a precursor to hormones and bile. It is necessary for converting sunlight into usable vitamin D and is critical for proper brain function and hormone production and should not be feared in foods.
» Eggs (yolks), seafood/shellfish, Beef, lamb

VITAMIN D

A potent immune system modulator and is most available via sun exposure.
» Egg yolks, cold water fish (salmon, herring, mackerel, etc.)
» Grass-fed butter or ghee
» Fermented cod liver oil (Green Pasture brand only)

LIPOIC ACID
(ALPHA-LIPOIC ACID/ALA)

» Red meat, organ meats

MAGNESIUM

Magnesium is critical to cellular energy production in order to battle fatigue and maintain proper calcium metabolism for vascular health.
» Kale, green leafy vegetables, beets, pumpkin seeds/pepitas

OMEGA-3 FATS

An anti-inflammatory essential fatty acid that comes from limited food sources.
» Cold water fish (salmon, herring, mackerel, etc.), fermented cod liver oil (Green Pasture brand only)
» Walnuts, pecans

POTASSIUM

» Asparagus, avocado, spinach, Swiss chard, papaya, banana, honeydew, cantaloupe, necta ines, oranges, grapefruit, yams

PROBIOTICS

Promote healthy gut flora, which is critical to proper digestion and elimination.
» Fermented vegetables: cabbage (sauerkraut) carrots, beets or other vegetables
» Kombucha (fermented tea)

SELENIUM

» Eggs, Brazil nuts
» Red Swiss chard, turnips, garlic

SODIUM

An unrefined, mineral-rich sea salt that is unprocessed (Celtic or Real Salt brand).

ZINC

» Oysters, Shellfish, lamb, red meat
» Pumpkin seeds (pepitas)

heart health

DAY	BREAKFAST	LUNCH	DINNER
1 ●■■ ◆	Swirly Crustless Quiche (240), Perfectly Baked Bacon (236), Raw Sauerkraut (238)	Mustard Glazed Chicken Thighs (266), Green Salad*, Balsamic Vinaigrette (378)	Grilled Garlic Flank Steak with Peppers & Onions (294), Baked Beets with Fennel**(362)
2 ●◆■	*left-over* Swirly Crustless Quiche, *left-over* Garlic Flank Steak with Peppers & Onions	Wild Canned Salmon with Olives, Avocado, Lemon Juice, Tomato, EVOO	Sage Roasted Turkey Legs (276), Sweet Potato Pancakes (298), Steamed Spinach*
3 ■■●	*left-over* Sweet Potato Pancakes, *left-over* Mustard-Glazed Chicken Thighs	*left-over* Sage Roasted Turkey Legs, Persimmon, Asparagus & Fennel Salad (380)	Lemony Lamb Dolmas (318), Cilantro Cauli-Rice (340)
4 ●●◆	Pesto Scrambled Eggs (252), *left-over* Cilantro Cauli-Rice	*left-over* Lemony Lamb Dolmas, Spinach Salad with Walnuts & Artichokes (380)	Citrus Macadamia Nut Sole (314), Butternut Squash**
5 ◆◆◆	*left-over* Citrus Macadamia Nut Sole, Butternut Squash**	Nori Salmon Handrolls (316)	Beef & Mixed Veggie Stir Fry (286)
6 ○◆●	Pumpkin Pancakes (242), Breakfast Sausage using Italian Sausage Spice Blend (233)	*left-over* Beef Stir Fry with Mixed Veggies	Lamb Lettuce Boats with Avo-Ziki Sauce (322)
7 ●◆■	Eggs, Perfectly Baked Bacon (236), Raw Sauerkraut (238)	Mixed Greens with Wild Canned Salmon, Asparagus*, Lemon Juice, EVOO	Citrus & Herb Whole Roasted Chicken (256), Roasted Rosemary Roots (350), Simple Baked Kale Chips*(356)
8 ■■■	Grain-Free Porridge (252), Berries, *left-over* Citrus & Herb Whole Roasted Chicken	Spinach Salad with Walnuts & Artichokes (380), *left-over* Citrus & Herb Whole Roasted Chicken	Chicken Liver Pâté (384), Cucumber, Kale*, Berries
9 ●■◆	Swirly Crustless Quiche (240), Steamed Broccoli*, Raw Sauerkraut (238)	*left-over* Chicken Liver Pâté, Green Salad*, Melon	Pesto Shrimp & Squash Fettuccine (308)
10 ●◆○	Omelet or Pesto Scrambled Eggs, *left-over* Shrimp & Avocado	Simple Shrimp Ceviche (316), Mixed Greens*, EVOO	Cumin Spiced Pork Tenderloin with Root Vegetables**(328)

» *A complete shopping list for this meal plan can be found on balancedbites.com*

KEY

◆ Red-Meat
■ Poultry
● Eggs
○ Pork
● Lamb
◆ Seafood

NOTES

EVOO   Extra-virgin olive oil
CO   Coconut oil
*   or other non-starchy vegetable
**   or other starchy vegetable (refer to page 110)
If no page number is listed, simply prepare the items as noted or any way you like.
For additional protein, vegetable, and fat recommendations, refer to the QUICK LIST that is associated with your meal plan!

DAY	BREAKFAST	LUNCH	DINNER
11 ● ○ ◆	Swirly Crustless Quiche (240) Perfectly Baked Bacon (236), *left-over* Root Vegetables**	*left-over* Cumin Spiced Pork Tenderloin, Rainbow Red Cabbage Salad*(372)	Balsamic Braised Short Ribs (278), Candied Carrots (340), Spinach*
12 ● ◆ ■	Eggs, *left-over* Rainbow Red Cabbage Salad*	*left-over* Balsamic Braised Short Ribs, *left-over* Candied Carrots, Green Salad*	Savory Baked Chicken Legs (264), Brussels Sprouts with Fennel*(350)
13 ● ■ ◆	Zucchini Pancakes (248), Perfectly Baked Bacon (236), Raw Sauerkraut (238)	*left-over* Savory Baked Chicken Legs, *left-over* Brussels Sprouts with Fennel*	Lemon Rosemary Broiled Salmon (306), Asparagus with Lemon & Olives (338), Sweet Potato**
14 ◆ ■ ◆	*left-over* Lemon Rosemary Broiled Salmon, *left-over* Asparagus with Lemon & Olives*	Buffalo Chicken Lettuce Wraps (270)	Red Palm & Coriander Tuna Over Daikon Noodle Salad (302), Green Salad*
15 ● ◆ ◆	Scrambled Eggs with Olives, Steamed Spinach*, Avocado	Spinach Salad with EVOO, *left-over* Red Palm & Coriander Tuna, Avocado, Lemon Juice	Italian-Style Stuffed Peppers (300), Green Salad* with Balsamic Vinaigrette (378)
16 ● ◆ ■	Grain-Free Porridge (252), Breakfast Sausage	*left-over* Italian-Style Stuffed Peppers (300), Green Salad*	Chicken Liver Pâté (384), Cucumber, Mixed Greens Salad with Beets & Blood Oranges (376)
17 ● ■ ◆	Bacon & Egg Salad (248), Sweet Potato or Beets**	*left-over* Chicken Liver Pâté, Cucumber, Green Salad*	Spaghetti Squash Bolognese (280), Baked Kale Chips* (356)
18 ● ◆ ○	Pumpkin Pancakes (242), Breakfast Sausage or Bacon	*left-over* Spaghetti Squash Bolognese	Thanksgiving Stuffing Meatballs (334), Mashed Faux-Tatoes (344)
19 ● ○ ◆	Scrambled Eggs, Avocado, Spinach or Kale*, Raw Sauerkraut (238)	*left-over* Thanksgiving Stuffing Meatballs, *left-over* Mashed Faux-Tatoes	Citrus Macadamia Nut Sole (314), Lemon Roasted Romanesco*(346), Sweet & Savory Potatoes**(362)
20 ● ◆ ■	Grain-Free Porridge (252), Hard Boiled Eggs	*left-over* Citrus Macadamia Nut Sole, *left-over* Lemon Roasted Romanesco*	Roasted Duck with Cherry Sauce (274), Sautéed Red Cabbage with Onions and Apples*(352)

» *A complete shopping list for this meal plan can be found on balancedbites.com*

KEY

◆ Red-Meat
■ Poultry
● Eggs
● Pork
● Lamb
◆ Seafood

NOTES

EVOO   Extra-virgin olive oil
CO   Coconut oil
*   or other non-starchy vegetable
**   or other starchy vegetable (refer to page 110)
If no page number is listed, simply prepare the items as noted or any way you like.
For additional protein, vegetable, and fat recommendations, refer to the QUICK LIST that is associated with your meal plan!

DAY	BREAKFAST	LUNCH	DINNER
21 ●◆●	Hard Boiled Eggs, Breakfast Sausage, Raw Sauerkraut (238)	Nori Salmon Handroll (316)	Lamb Chops with Olive Tapenade (326), Greek Salad with Avo-Ziki (374)
22 ●●◆	Swirly Crustless Quiche (240), Breakfast Sausage	*left-over* Lamb Chops with Olive Tapenade, *left-over* Greek Salad with Avo-Ziki	Orange Braised Beef Shanks (284), Butternut Sage Soup**(348)
23 ●◆◆	*left-over* Swirly Crustless Quiche, Perfectly Baked Bacon (236)	*left-over* Orange Braised Beef Shanks, *left-over* Butternut Sage Soup	Hayley's Skirt Steak Tacos (292), Salsa (296), Grilled Squash & Pineapple (342)
24 ●◆◆	Acorn Squash with Cinnamon & Coconut Butter (358), Breakfast Sausage or Bacon	Tangy Taco Salad (296), *left-over* Salsa	Fiery Jalapeño Burgers with Sweet Potato Pancakes (298), Red Roasted Garlic (370)
25 ●◆◆	*left-over* Sweet Potato Pancakes, Eggs, Avocado	Quick & Easy Salmon Cakes (310), Green Salad*, Avocado, Olives	Asian Orange Pan-Seared Scallops (304), Tomatillo Shrimp Cocktail (312), Zucchini*
26 ●◆●	Zucchini Pancakes (248), Perfectly Baked Bacon (236), Raw Sauerkraut (238)	Tuna, Mixed Greens Salad with Persimmons, Asparagus & Fennel (380), Orange Vinaigrette (382)	Grandma Barbara's Stuffed Mushrooms (332), Roasted Marrow Bones (288), Spinach*
27 ●●●	Grain-Free Porridge (252), Breakfast Sausage using Italian Sausage Spice Blend (233)	*left-over* Grandma Barbara's Stuffed Mushrooms, Mixed Greens Salad*, Balsamic Vinaigrette (378)	Spiced Lamb Meatballs with Balsamic-Fig Compote (324), Green Beans with Shallots*(358)
28 ●◆■	*left-over* Spiced Lamb Meatballs, Spinach or Cabbage*	Wild Canned Salmon with Olives, Avocado, Lemon Juice, Tomato, EVOO	Lemon & Artichoke Chicken (260), Broc-Cauli Chowder with Bacon (336)
29 ●■◆	Apple Streusel Egg Muffins (254), Bacon or Breakfast Sausage	*left-over* Lemon & Artichoke Chicken, Kale & Carrot Salad with Lemon-Tahini Dressing (376)	Mom's Stuffed Cabbage Rolls with Tomato Cranberry Sauce (290), Green Salad*
30 ●●●	*left-over* Apple Streusel Egg Muffins (254), Bacon or Breakfast Sausage	Chorizo Meatballs (330), Mixed Greens Salad* with Avocado, Lemon Juice, and EVOO	Mediterranean Lamb Roast (320), Sautéed Spinach with Pine Nuts & Currants*(366)

» *A complete shopping list for this meal plan can be found on balancedbites.com*

KEY

- ◆ Red-Meat
- ■ Poultry
- ● Eggs
- ● Pork
- ● Lamb
- ◆ Seafood

NOTES

EVOO   Extra-virgin olive oil

CO   Coconut oil

*   or other non-starchy vegetable

**   or other starchy vegetable (refer to page 110)

If no page number is listed, simply prepare the items as noted or any way you like.

For additional protein, vegetable, and fat recommendations, refer to the QUICK LIST that is associated with your meal plan!

30-DAY MEAL PLANS

CANCER RECOVERY

While an anti-inflammatory diet and lifestyle are the cornerstones of supporting your body in *preventing* cancer, we can't always control every aspect of what may cause our bodies to fall ill. That said, there are many ways to give yourself the best possible chance for recovery. Many people find a new way of eating while dealing with illness to be overwhelming, but it can provide your body with what it needs to heal. Along with an intensely strong positive mental outlook, food provides the raw materials for your cells to rebuild anew.

If you are interested in a ketogenic diet approach to cancer recovery, you may also want to consider incorporating aspects of the Neurological Health "Diet & Lifestyle Recommendations" on page 178 (specifically regarding minimal carbohydrate intake from starchy vegetables and fruits).

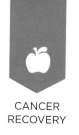

diet & lifestyle recommendations

add [+]

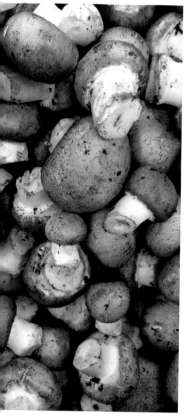

NUTRIENT-DENSE FOODS

Replenish depleted nutrient stores from eating excess refined foods over time.

SUPERFOODS

Eat superfoods often as possible. Make and eat/drink bone broth and liver regularly (recipes on page 234 and 384). Make sauerkraut (recipe on page 238) and eat it daily (1/4 cup), especially with breakfast to aid in gastrointestinal motility & eliminations.

PROTEIN

Protein helps to heal the gut lining (amino acids are the building blocks).

MEDICINAL MUSHROOMS

Such as reishi, shiitake, and maitake counter the side effects of chemotherapy and radiation (in food or extract form).

ANTIOXIDANT-RICH FOODS

Eat deeply colored foods like leafy greens, berries, and sweet potatoes.

STRESS MANAGEMENT

Manage stress to keep systemic inflammation low. Develop a guided meditation practice, or begin to practice Qi Gong. Practice meditation, biofeedback, Tai Chi, and/or guided imagery for deep relaxation.

SLEEP

Melatonin production while asleep in a dark room overnight is a potent antioxidant necessary to recharge and power your immune system.

MOVEMENT

Take walks outside, or practice gentle yoga for movement without systemic stress.

avoid [-]

GLUTEN

100% of the time. See the "Guide to Gluten" on page 89.

DAIRY

Avoid for its potential growth-promotion effects. (Butter and ghee are okay.)

RESTAURANTS/DINING OUT

Avoid damaged and man-made fats. (This applies to everyone but is especially critical for people with these conditions.)

REFINED FOODS, SWEETENERS, CAFFEINE

Cancer cells feed on sugar; they have about eight times the receptors for sugar as normal cells. Eat only nutrient-dense carbohydrates in the form of vegetables and fruits.

ALCOHOL, TOBACCO, NICOTINE & MSG (MONOSODIUM GLUTAMATE)

These are products that require detoxification and/or may have some neurotoxic effects.

PROCESSED MEATS

Processed meats with synthetic chemical preservatives added such as BHA and/or BHT. Read ingredient lists carefully for these items.

CHARRED FOODS

NON-ORGANIC FOODS & COMMERCIALLY RAISED MEATS

Avoid excess toxins.

HARSH CHEMICAL CLEANING OR HYGIENE PRODUCTS

Opt for gentle, natural alternatives, such as soap nuts for laundry, vinegar and water solutions for counter top cleaning, and baking soda and peroxide for cleaning and whitening surfaces, laundry, teeth, etc.

DISCLAIMER:

The information in this book is not intended to be a replacement for professional medical diagnosis or treatment for a medical condition. It consists solely of nutritional and lifestyle recommendations to support a healthier body.

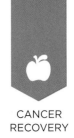
nutritional supplements & herbs to consider

These recommendations are made as a starting point. Do your own research and determine which supplements may serve you best. It's best to get as many of your nutrients from food as possible. See the next page for specific food-based nutrients on which to focus. The items below are listed in no particular order.

» **VITAMIN A (retinol)** helps to maintain the integrity of the mucosal lining of the gut and may preserve/improve vision. It is also helpful in maintaining immunity when balanced with vitamin D, and it is necessary for the assimilation of dietary minerals.

» **FERMENTED COD LIVER OIL/ BUTTER OIL BLEND** for fat-soluble vitamins A, D, E, and K2 as well as some omega 3 fats. I only recommend Green Pasture brand.

» **B VITAMINS** are critical in assisting neurotransmitters for improved brain health, as well as nerve and muscular activities. Look for a B-complex supplement with B12.

» **VITAMIN C** is a potent antioxidant.

» **CURCUMIN** is a potent antioxidant that supports immune health.

» **COENZYME Q10 (CoQ10, ubiquinone)** enhances mitochondrial (cellular) energy production, and it can help alleviate fatigue, as well as muscle/joint pain. It is also a potent antioxidant; statin drugs are known to deplete CoQ10.

» **DIINDOYLMETHANE (DIM)** may inhibit tumor formation and help to induce cancer cell apoptosis (cell death) in breast, colon, prostate, and lung cancers.

» **VITAMIN E** is an antioxidant that benefits neurological function, smooth muscle growth, and cellular communication. It may also reduce oxidative stress-induced insulin resistance.

» **EPIGALLOCATECHIN GALLATE (EGCG/green tea extract)** is a potent antioxidant flavonoid that promotes angiogenesis. It may be best to wait three weeks post-chemo to consume.

» **GLUTATHIONE** is an antioxidant that aids in liver detox processes and the regeneration of vitamins A, C, and E.

» **HERBS AND TEAS:** Green tea (for EGCG), ginger

» **L-GLUTAMINE** aids in the healing of the epithelial cells that line the small intestine.

» **LIPOIC ACID (alpha-lipoic acid/ALA)** has antioxidant properties and may motivate greater glucose uptake from the bloodstream by promoting the conversion of carbohydrates into energy.

» **MAGNESIUM** is required for more than 300 enzymatic processes in the body, and most people are deficient in it. Look for magnesium glycinate or magnesium malate forms.

» **N-ACETYL CYSTEINE (NAC)** supports liver function.

» **OMEGA-3 FATS** are anti-inflammatory essential fatty acids. I only recommend Green Pasture brand fermented cod liver oil.

» **PROTEOLYTIC ENZYMES** are anti-inflammatory and may alter cytokine (inflammatory mediator) expression.

» **SELENIUM & ZINC** are antioxidants that protect against free radical damage. They are difficult to obtain in sufficient amounts solely from food sources.

supportive nutrients
& foods that contain them

quick LIST

proteins

Chicken
Herring
Liver
Mackerel
Oysters
Salmon
Shellfish
Tuna
Turkey

fats

Coconut oil
Red palm oil
Walnuts
Pecans

vegetables

Beets
Broccoli
Brussels sprouts
Butternut squash
Cauliflower
Daikon radish
Okra
Squash
Sweet potatoes
Swiss chard

fruits

Berries
Citrus
Melon
Tropical fruit

superfoods

Bone broth
Fermented cod liver oil/
butter oil blend
Sauerkraut

spices

Basil
Cilantro
Cinnamon
Cumin
Garlic
Ginger
Oregano
Parsley
Turmeric

VITAMIN A (RETINOL)
» Liver, eel, grass-fed butter, clarified butter, or ghee

VITAMIN C
» Adrenal glands, beets, bell peppers, garlic, lemons, Brussels sprouts, cauliflower, collard greens, broccoli, daikon radish, kale, mustard greens, parsley, spinach, strawberries

CAROTENOIDS
» Alpha-carotene: pumpkin, carrots
» Cryptoxanthin: citrus, peaches, apricots
» Lycopene: tomato, guava, watermelon, pink grapefruit
» Lutein: kale, spinach, collard greens, beet greens
» Zeaxanthin: green vegetables, citrus
» Beta carotene: kale, broccoli, sweet potatoes, carrots, red pepper, mango, apricots, peaches, persimmons, cantaloupe

CURCUMIN
» Turmeric - dried or fresh

DIINDOLYLMETHANE (DIM)
» Broccoli, Brussels sprouts, cauliflower, kale, chard, collards

VITAMIN D
A potent immune system modulator and is most available via sun exposure.
» Egg yolks, cold water fish (salmon, herring, mackerel, etc.)
» Grass-fed butter or ghee
» Fermented cod liver oil (Green Pasture brand only)

VITAMIN E
» Extra-virgin olive oil
» Pecans, spinach
» Broccoli, Brussels sprouts

FLAVANOIDS
» Green tea

LIMONENE
It may have anti-angiogenic effects.
» Citrus

MAGNESIUM
Magnesium is critical to cellular energy production in order to battle fatigue and maintain proper calcium metabolism for vascular health.
» Kale, green leafy vegetables
» Beets
» Pumpkin seeds/pepitas

OMEGA-3 FATS
An anti-inflammatory essential fatty acid that comes from limited food sources.
» Cold water fish (salmon, herring, mackerel, etc.), fermented cod liver oil (Green Pasture brand only)
» Walnuts, pecans

POLYPHENOLS
They may help to inhibit the growth of oral, colon, and prostate cancer cells.
» Pomegranate, strawberries, cherries, blueberries

PROTEOLYTIC ENZYMES
» Papaya, pineapple

cancer recovery

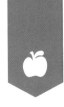

DAY	BREAKFAST	LUNCH	DINNER
1 ●■◆	Swirly Crustless Quiche (240)	Mustard Glazed Chicken Thighs (266), Green Salad*, Balsamic Vinaigrette (378)	Simple Shrimp Ceviche (316), Lemon Roasted Romanesco (346)
2 ●◆■	*left-over* Swirly Crustless Quiche, *left-over* Lemon Roasted Romanesco	Wild Canned Salmon with Olives, Avocado, Lemon Juice, Tomato, EVOO	Sage Roasted Turkey Legs (276), Sweet Potato Pancakes (298), Steamed Spinach*
3 ■■●	*left-over* Sweet Potato Pancakes, *left-over* Mustard-Glazed Chicken Thighs	*left-over* Sage Roasted Turkey Legs, Persimmon, Asparagus & Fennel Salad (380)	Lemony Lamb Dolmas (318), Cilantro Cauli-Rice (340)
4 ●●◆	Pesto Scrambled Eggs (252), *left-over* Cilantro Cauli-Rice	*left-over* Lemony Lamb Dolmas, Spinach Salad with Walnuts & Artichokes (380)	Citrus Macadamia Nut Sole (314), Butternut Squash**
5 ◆◆■	*left-over* Citrus Macadamia Nut Sole, Butternut Squash**	Nori Salmon Handrolls (316)	Savory Baked Chicken Legs (264), Baked Beets with Fennel**(362)
6 ■■●	Pumpkin Pancakes (242), Chicken Thighs or Breast	*left-over* Savory Baked Chicken Legs, *left-over* Baked Beets with Fennel	Lamb Lettuce Boats with Avo-Ziki Sauce (322)
7 ●◆■	Pesto Scrambled Eggs (252), Kale*, Blueberries	Mixed Greens with Wild Canned Salmon, Asparagus*, Lemon Juice, EVOO	Citrus & Herb Whole Roasted Chicken (256), Roasted Rosemary Roots (350), Kale Chips*(356)
8 ■■■	Grain-Free Porridge (252), Berries, *left-over* Citrus & Herb Whole Roasted Chicken	Spinach Salad with Walnuts & Artichokes (380), *left-over* Citrus & Herb Whole Roasted Chicken	Chinese 5-Spice Lettuce Cups (272)
9 ●■◆	Swirly Crustless Quiche (240), Steamed Broccoli*	Indian-Spiced Turkey Burgers (268), Steamed Broccoli*	Pesto Shrimp & Squash Fettuccine (308)
10 ●◆○	Omelet or Pesto Scrambled Eggs, *left-over* Shrimp & Avocado	Simple Shrimp Ceviche (316), Mixed Greens*, EVOO	Cumin Spiced Pork Tenderloin with Root Vegetables**(328)

» *A complete shopping list for this meal plan can be found on balancedbites.com*

KEY
- ◆ **Red-Meat**
- ■ **Poultry**
- ● **Eggs**
- ● **Pork**
- ● **Lamb**
- ◆ **Seafood**

NOTES

EVOO   Extra-virgin olive oil

CO   Coconut oil

*   or other non-starchy vegetable

**   or other starchy vegetable (refer to page 110)

If no page number is listed, simply prepare the items as noted or any way you like.

For additional protein, vegetable, and fat recommendations, refer to the QUICK LIST that is associated with your meal plan!

DAY	BREAKFAST	LUNCH	DINNER
11 ● ● ◆	Swirly Crustless Quiche (240), *left-over* Root Vegetables**	*left-over* Cumin Spiced Pork Tenderloin, Rainbow Red Cabbage Salad*(372)	Asian Orange Pan-Seared Scallops (304), Tomatillo Shrimp Cocktail (312), Spinach*
12 ● ◆ ■	Eggs, *left-over* Rainbow Red Cabbage Salad	Wild Salmon over a Green Salad*, Orange Vinaigrette (382)	Savory Baked Chicken Legs (264), Brussels Sprouts with Fennel*(350), Berries
13 ● ■ ◆	Zucchini Pancakes (248), Berries	*left-over* Savory Baked Chicken Legs, *left-over* Brussels Sprouts with Fennel*	Lemon Rosemary Broiled Salmon (306), Asparagus with Lemon & Olives (338), Sweet Potato**
14 ◆ ■ ◆	*left-over* Lemon Rosemary Broiled Salmon, *left-over* Asparagus with Lemon & Olives*	Buffalo Chicken Lettuce Wraps (270), Orange	Red Palm & Coriander Tuna Over Daikon Noodle Salad (302), Green Salad*
15 ● ◆ ◆	Scrambled Eggs with Olives, Steamed Spinach*, Avocado	Spinach Salad with EVOO, *left-over* Red Palm & Coriander Tuna, Avocado, Lemon Juice	Italian-Style Stuffed Peppers (300), Green Salad* with Balsamic Vinaigrette (378)
16 ● ◆ ■	Apple Streusel Egg Muffins (254), Broccoli*	*left-over* Italian-Style Stuffed Peppers (300), Green Salad*	Mustard Glazed Chicken Thighs (266), Mixed Greens Salad with Beets & Blood Oranges (376)
17 ● ■ ■	*left-over* Apple Streusel Egg Muffins, Broccoli*, Orange	*left-over* Mustard Glazed Chicken Thighs, Green Salad*	Lemon & Artichoke Chicken (260), Broc-Cauli Chowder with Bacon (336), Berries
18 ■ ■ ●	*left-over* Mustard Glazed Chicken Thighs, Pumpkin Pancakes (242), Berries	*left-over* Lemon & Artichoke Chicken, Spinach*	Thanksgiving Stuffing Meatballs (334), Mashed Faux-Tatoes (344)
19 ● ● ◆	Scrambled Eggs, Avocado, Spinach or Kale*	*left-over* Thanksgiving Stuffing Meatballs, *left-over* Mashed Faux-Tatoes, Orange	Citrus Macadamia Nut Sole (314), Roasted Romanesco*(346), Sweet & Savory Potatoes**(362)
20 ● ◆ ■	Bacon & Egg Salad (248), Sweet Potato or Beets**, Orange	*left-over* Citrus Macadamia Nut Sole, *left-over* Lemon Roasted Romanesco*	Roasted Duck with Cherry Sauce (274), Sautéed Red Cabbage with Onions and Apples*(352)

»   *A complete shopping list for this meal plan can be found on balancedbites.com*

KEY

◆ Red-Meat
■ Poultry
● Eggs
● Pork
● Lamb
◆ Seafood

NOTES

EVOO   Extra-virgin olive oil
CO   Coconut oil
*   or other non-starchy vegetable
**   or other starchy vegetable (refer to page 110)

If no page number is listed, simply prepare the items as noted or any way you like.

For additional protein, vegetable, and fat recommendations, refer to the QUICK LIST that is associated with your meal plan!

cancer recovery

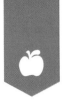

DAY	BREAKFAST	LUNCH	DINNER
21 ●◆●	Scrambled Eggs, *left-over* Sautéed Red Cabbage with Onions and Apples*	Nori Salmon Handrolls (316), Apple	Lamb Chops with Olive Tapenade (326), Greek Salad with Avo-Ziki (374)
22 ●●◆	Swirly Crustless Quiche (240), Breakfast Sausage, Melon	*left-over* Lamb Chops with Olive Tapenade, *left-over* Greek Salad with Avo-Ziki	Orange Braised Beef Shanks (284), Butternut Sage Soup**(348)
23 ●◆■	*left-over* Swirly Crustless Quiche, Melon	*left-over* Orange Braised Beef Shanks, *left-over* Butternut Sage Soup**	Buffalo Chicken Lettuce Wraps (270), Asparagus*, Berries
24 ●◆■	Eggs, Acorn Squash with Cinnamon & Coconut Butter (358)	Tangy Taco Salad (296), Salsa (296)	Indian-Spiced Turkey Burgers (268), Steamed Broccoli*, Red Roasted Garlic (370)
25 ●◆◆	Sweet Potato Pancakes (298), Eggs, Avocado, Orange	Quick & Easy Salmon Cakes (310), Green Salad*, Avocado, Olives	Asian Orange Pan-Seared Scallops (304), Tomatillo Shrimp Cocktail (312), Zucchini*
26 ●◆●	Zucchini Pancakes (248), Melon	Tuna, Mixed Greens Salad with Persimmons, Asparagus & Fennel (380), Orange Vinaigrette (382)	Grandma Barbara's Stuffed Mushrooms (332), Roasted Marrow Bones (288), Spinach*
27 ●●●	Pesto Scrambled Eggs (252), Melon, Broccoli*	*left-over* Grandma Barbara's Stuffed Mushrooms, Mixed Greens Salad*, Balsamic Vinaigrette (378)	Spiced Lamb Meatballs with Balsamic-Fig Compote (324), Green Beans with Shallots*(358)
28 ●◆■	*left-over* Spiced Lamb Meatballs, Spinach or Cabbage*, Apple	Wild Canned Salmon with Olives, Avocado, Lemon Juice, Tomato, EVOO	Lemon & Artichoke Chicken (260), Broc-Cauli Chowder with Bacon (336)
29 ●■◆	Apple Streusel Egg Muffins (254), Broccoli*	*left-over* Lemon & Artichoke Chicken, Kale & Carrot Salad with Lemon-Tahini Dressing (376)	Mom's Stuffed Cabbage Rolls with Tomato Cranberry Sauce (290), Green Salad*
30 ●●●	*left-over* Apple Streusel Egg Muffins (254), Cauliflower*	Chorizo Meatballs (330), Mixed Greens Salad* with Avocado, Lemon Juice, and EVOO	Mediterranean Lamb Roast (320), Sautéed Spinach with Pine Nuts & Currants*(366)

» *A complete shopping list for this meal plan can be found on balancedbites.com*

KEY
- ◆ **Red-Meat**
- ■ **Poultry**
- ● **Eggs**
- ● **Pork**
- ● **Lamb**
- ◆ **Seafood**

NOTES

EVOO	Extra-virgin olive oil
CO	Coconut oil
*	or other non-starchy vegetable
**	or other starchy vegetable (refer to page 110)

If no page number is listed, simply prepare the items as noted or any way you like.

For additional protein, vegetable, and fat recommendations, refer to the QUICK LIST that is associated with your meal plan!

30-DAY MEAL PLANS

ATHLETIC PERFORMANCE

While fueling needs can vary greatly from athlete to athlete, there are basic guidelines that will get you started in the right direction. This plan will provide an overall higher carbohydrate intake, as well as focus on nutrient-dense foods and superfoods. The best way to figure out how well this or any other meal plan works for your own performance needs and goals is to keep records of your diet and activities on a daily basis. By keeping records, you can analyze and assess where changes may need to be made. Detailed records will also be helpful when approaching a practitioner for assistance on modifying your approach in any way, as information is king for your needs.

Refer to the book resources page on balancedbites.com for a handy nutrition and performance tracking form PDF download.

Disclaimer: The information in this book is not intended to be a replacement for professional medical diagnosis or treatment for a medical condition. It consists solely of nutritional and lifestyle recommendations to support a healthier body.

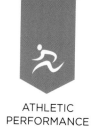

diet & lifestyle recommendations

add [+]

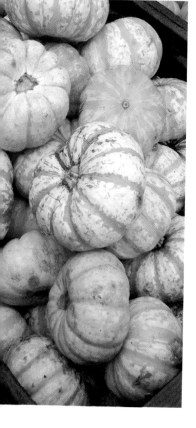

SUPERFOODS & PROBIOTICS

Eat as often as possible (see page 29 for the Guide to Paleo Foods). Eat raw sauerkraut (recipe on page 238) or other fermented vegetables daily (1/4 cup), especially with breakfast.

PROTEIN

Eat protein to satisfy the appetite for longer periods of time (meals focused on both fat and protein will help.)

NUTRIENT-DENSE FOODS

Replenish depleted nutrient stores from eating excess refined foods over time.

STARCHY CARBOHYDRATES BEFORE & AFTER EXERCISE

(see page 110 for dense carb sources); eat approximately 50-75g+ of carbohydrates in meals pre and post-workout depending on the length of exercise. Track how you feel, and add/subtract if you are not making progress or don't feel well-fueled for your training.

SMART TRAINING

Listen to your body; take rest and recovery days when necessary.

SLEEP

Sleep at least eight hours every night in a dark room in order to recover from exercise and have healthy hormonal balance.

MASSAGE

Be sure you are taking care of your body with regular sports massage, chiropractic care and/or ART (Active Release Techniques).

avoid [-]

GLUTEN

Gluten 100% of the time. See the "Guide to Gluten" on page 89 to keep systemic inflammation low and allow for optimal recovery times.

OVER-TRAINING

Be smart and rest when you are in pain; allowing an inflammatory process in your body to do its job will bring you back to training much stronger than if you push through pain on a regular basis (meaning pain from injury, not just from a hard workout).

EXCESSIVE SUPPLEMENTATION

Eat real food to obtain nutrients as your body knows how to use real, whole foods better than any supplement. Try some of the recommended supplements in this plan, however, if you do not think you need them all, you certainly don't need to be taking them all in supplemental form.

LOW-QUALITY PROTEIN POWDERS

Post-workout recovery from liquid food in the form of a protein shake can be useful and effective, but beware low-quality or powders with too many additives. Seek out a grass-fed whey source or egg white protein if you tolerate them. Monitor your digestion and signs of chronic inflammation carefully and eliminate powders at any sign of intolerance.

DISCLAIMER:

The information in this book is not intended to be a replacement for professional medical diagnosis or treatment for a medical condition. It consists solely of nutritional and lifestyle recommendations to support a healthier body.

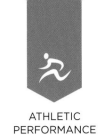

nutritional supplements & herbs to consider

These recommendations are made as a starting point. Do your own research and determine which supplements may serve you best. It's best to get as many of your nutrients from food as possible. See the next page for specific food-based nutrients on which to focus. The items below are listed in no particular order.

» **VITAMIN A (retinol)** helps to maintain the integrity of the mucosal lining of the gut. It is also helpful in maintaining immunity when balanced with vitamin D, and it is necessary for the assimilation of dietary minerals. Vitamin A is depleted by stress and strenuous physical exercise.

» **FERMENTED COD LIVER OIL/ BUTTER OIL BLEND** for fat-soluble vitamins A, D, E, and K2 as well as some omega 3 fats. I only recommend Green Pasture brand.

» **B VITAMINS (especially B1, B7, B12)** are critical in assisting neurotransmitters for improved brain health, as well as nerve and muscular activities.

» **VITAMIN B1 (thiamin)** is beneficial in nerve and muscular activity. Magnesium is required to activate thiamin.

» **VITAMIN B7 (biotin)** is a coenzyme required for the metabolism of glucose, amino acids, and lipids.

» **VITAMIN B12 (cobalamin)** supports homocysteine metabolism, energy metabolism, and immune and nerve function.

» **VITAMIN C** is a potent antioxidant with anti-inflammatory properties; promotes collagen production and supports carnitine synthesis. It is a potent antioxidant with anti-inflammatory properties that helps to regenerate vitamin E and improves iron absorption.

» **CARNITINE / L-CARNITINE** can help to improve insulin sensitivity and glucose storage, and it optimizes fat and carbohydrate metabolism. It may also improve the utilization of fat as an energy source. Cofactors include iron, vitamin C, vitamin B3 (niacin), and vitamin B6.

» **COENZYME Q10 (CoQ10)** enhances mitochondrial (cellular) energy production and can help alleviate fatigue.

» **VITAMIN E** is an antioxidant that benefits neurological function, smooth muscle growth, and cellular communication.

» **L-GLUTAMINE** aids in the healing of the epithelial cells that line the small intestine; also aids in general cellular repair and recovery.

» **LIPOIC ACID (alpha-lipoic acid/ ALA)** has antioxidant properties and may motivate greater glucose uptake from the bloodstream by promoting the conversion of carbohydrates into energy.

» **MAGNESIUM** is required for more than 300 enzymatic processes in the body, and most people are deficient in it. Look for magnesium glycinate or magnesium malate forms.

» **OMEGA-3 FATS** are anti-inflammatory essential fatty acids. I only recommend Green Pasture brand fermented cod liver oil.

» **ZINC** is a potent antioxidant that aids in vitamin A metabolism. May be taken as ZMA (zinc and magnesium).

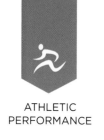

supportive nutrients & foods that contain them

quick LIST

proteins

Beef
Bison
Chicken
Eel
Lamb
Liver
Salmon
Scallops
Swordfish

fats

Coconut oil
Extra-virgin olive oil
Grass-fed butter/ghee
Red palm oil

vegetables

Beets
Broccoli
Brussels sprouts
Butternut squash
Cauliflower
Kale
Daikon radish
Okra
Sweet potatoes
Squash

fruits

Berries
Citrus
Melons
Tropical fruits

superfoods

Bone broth
Fermented cod liver oil/
butter oil blend
Liver

spices

Basil
Cilantro
Cinnamon
Cumin
Garlic
Ginger
Oregano
Parsley
Turmeric

VITAMIN A (RETINOL)

» Liver, eel, grass-fed butter, clarified butter, or ghee

VITAMIN B1

» Brewer's yeast (Lewis Labs brand only)
» Trace amounts: sunflower seeds, Brazil nuts, hazelnuts, walnuts, garlic, almonds

VITAMIN B7

» Liver, brewer's yeast (Lewis Labs brand only)
» Trace amounts: Swiss chard, Walnuts, pecans, almonds

VITAMIN B12

» Liver, clams, kidney, lamb, beef, eggs
» Oysters, sardines, trout, salmon, tuna, haddock, flounder, scallops, halibut, swordfish
» Cheeses (raw/grass-fed)

VITAMIN C

» Adrenal glands, beets, bell peppers, garlic, lemons, Brussels sprouts, cauliflower, collard greens, broccoli, daikon radish, kale, mustard greens, parsley, spinach, strawberries

CARNITINE

» Red meat (darker will contain more)

CONJUGATED LINOLEIC ACID (CLA)

A potent antioxidant that supports fat loss.
» Grass-fed beef and lamb

VITAMIN D

A potent immune system modulator and is most available via sun exposure.
» Egg yolks, cold water fish (salmon, herring, mackerel, etc.)
» Grass-fed butter or ghee
» Fermented cod liver oil (Green Pasture brand only)

VITAMIN E

» Extra-virgin olive oil
» Pecans, broccoli, Brussels sprouts, spinach

IRON

» Beef, bison
» Lamb, liver

LIPOIC ACID

» Red meat, organ meats
» Trace amounts: spinach

OMEGA-3 FATS

An anti-inflammatory essential fatty acid that comes from limited food sources.
» Cold water fish (salmon, herring, mackerel, etc.), fermented cod liver oil (Green Pasture brand only)
» Walnuts, pecans

ZINC

» Oysters, shellfish
» Lamb, red meat
» Pumpkin seeds (pepitas)

athletic performance

DAY	BREAKFAST	LUNCH	DINNER
1 ●■◆	Swirly Crustless Quiche (240), Perfectly Baked Bacon (236), Sweet Potato**	Mustard Glazed Chicken Thighs (266), Green Salad*, Balsamic Vinaigrette (378)	Grilled Garlic Flank Steak with Peppers & Onions (294), Baked Beets with Fennel**(362)
2 ●◆■	*left-over* Swirly Crustless Quiche, *left-over* Garlic Flank Steak with Peppers & Onions	Wild Canned Salmon with Olives, Avocado, Lemon Juice, Tomato, EVOO	Sage Roasted Turkey Legs (276), Sweet Potato Pancakes (298), Steamed Spinach*
3 ■■●	*left-over* Sweet Potato Pancakes, *left-over* Mustard-Glazed Chicken Thighs	*left-over* Sage Roasted Turkey Legs, Persimmon, Asparagus & Fennel Salad (380)	Lemony Lamb Dolmas (318), Cilantro Cauli-Rice (340), Banana
4 ●●◆	Pesto Scrambled Eggs (252), *left-over* Cilantro Cauli-Rice, Apple	*left-over* Lemony Lamb Dolmas, Spinach Salad with Walnuts & Artichokes (380)	Citrus Macadamia Nut Sole (314), Butternut Squash**, Berries
5 ◆◆◆	*left-over* Citrus Macadamia Nut Sole, Plantains in CO**	Nori Salmon Handrolls (316), Berries or other fruit	Beef & Mixed Veggie Stir Fry (286), Winter Squash**
6 ●◆●	Pumpkin Pancakes (242), Breakfast Sausage using Italian Sausage Spice Blend (233)	*left-over* Beef Stir Fry with Mixed Veggies, Sweet Potato**	Lamb Lettuce Boats with Avo-Ziki Sauce (322), Roasted Rosemary Roots**(350)
7 ●◆■	Eggs, Perfectly Baked Bacon (236), Crispy Curried Sweet Potato Coins (364)	Mixed Greens with Wild Canned Salmon, Asparagus*, Lemon Juice, EVOO	Citrus & Herb Whole Roasted Chicken (256), Roasted Rosemary Roots (350), Kale Chips*(356)
8 ■■■	Carrot Gingerbread Muffins (244), *left-over* Citrus & Herb Whole Roasted Chicken	Spinach Salad with Walnuts & Artichokes (380), *left-over* Citrus & Herb Whole Roasted Chicken	Chinese 5-Spice Lettuce Cups (272), Parsnips**
9 ●■■	Swirly Crustless Quiche (240), Sweet Potato**	Indian-Spiced Turkey Burgers (268), Steamed Broccoli*, Berries	Chicken Liver Pâté (384), Cucumber, Crispy Curried Sweet Potato Coins (364)
10 ●◆○	Omelet or Pesto Scrambled Eggs, *left-over* Shrimp & Avocado, Banana	Simple Shrimp Ceviche (316), Mixed Greens*, EVOO, *left-over* Chicken Liver Pâté, Cucumber	Cumin Spiced Pork Tenderloin with Root Vegetables**(328)

» *A complete shopping list for this meal plan can be found on balancedbites.com*

KEY
◆ Red-Meat
■ Poultry
● Eggs
○ Pork
● Lamb
◆ Seafood

NOTES
EVOO   Extra-virgin olive oil
CO   Coconut oil
*   or other non-starchy vegetable
**   or other starchy vegetable (refer to page 110)
If no page number is listed, simply prepare the items as noted or any way you like.
For additional protein, vegetable, and fat recommendations, refer to the QUICK LIST that is associated with your meal plan!

DAY	BREAKFAST	LUNCH	DINNER
11 ● ● ◆	Swirly Crustless Quiche (240) Perfectly Baked Bacon (236), *left-over* Root Vegetables	*left-over* Cumin Spiced Pork Tenderloin, Rainbow Red Cabbage Salad*(372)	Balsamic Braised Short Ribs (278), Candied Carrots (340), Spinach*
12 ● ◆ ■	Eggs, *left-over* Rainbow Red Cabbage Salad, Plantains in CO**	*left-over* Balsamic Braised Short Ribs, *left-over* Candied Carrots, Green Salad*	Savory Baked Chicken Legs (264), Brussels Sprouts with Fennel*(350), Berries
13 ● ■ ◆	Zucchini Pancakes (248), Perfectly Baked Bacon (236), Orange	*left-over* Savory Baked Chicken Legs, *left-over* Brussels Sprouts with Fennel*, Sweet Potato**	Lemon Rosemary Broiled Salmon (306), Asparagus with Lemon & Olives (338), Berries
14 ◆ ■ ◆	*left-over* Lemon Rosemary Broiled Salmon, *left-over* Asparagus with Lemon & Olives*	Buffalo Chicken Lettuce Wraps (270), Banana	Red Palm & Coriander Tuna Over Daikon Noodle Salad (302), Green Salad*
15 ● ◆ ◆	Scrambled Eggs with Olives, Steamed Spinach*, Avocado	Spinach Salad with EVOO, *left-over* Red Palm & Coriander Tuna, Avocado, Lemon Juice	Italian-Style Stuffed Peppers (300), Green Salad* with Balsamic Vinaigrette (378)
16 ● ◆ ■	Blueberry Lemon Muffins (246), Breakfast Sausage, Apple	*left-over* Italian-Style Stuffed Peppers (300), Green Salad*	Bacon-Wrapped Smoky Chicken Thighs (262), Mixed Greens Salad with Beets & Blood Oranges (376)
17 ● ■ ◆	Bacon & Egg Salad (248), Sweet Potato or Beets**	*left-over* Bacon-Wrapped Smoky Chicken Thighs, Green Salad*, Butternut Squash**	Spaghetti Squash Bolognese (280), Simple Baked Kale Chips (356)
18 ● ◆ ●	Pumpkin Pancakes (242), Breakfast Sausage or Bacon	*left-over* Spaghetti Squash Bolognese, Apple	Thanksgiving Stuffing Meatballs (334), Mashed Faux-Tatoes (344), Chicken Liver Pâté (384)
19 ● ● ◆	Scrambled Eggs, Avocado, Spinach or Kale*, Sweet Potato**	*left-over* Thanksgiving Stuffing Meatballs, *left-over* Mashed Faux-Tatoes, left-over Liver Pâté	Citrus Macadamia Nut Sole (314), Roasted Romanesco*(346), Sweet & Savory Potatoes**(362)
20 ● ◆ ■	Grain-Free Porridge (252), Berries, Hard Boiled Eggs	*left-over* Citrus Macadamia Nut Sole, *left-over* Lemon Roasted Romanesco*	Roasted Duck with Cherry Sauce (274), Sautéed Red Cabbage with Onions and Apples*(352)

» *A complete shopping list for this meal plan can be found on balancedbites.com*

KEY
◆ Red-Meat
■ Poultry
● Eggs
● Pork
● Lamb
◆ Seafood

NOTES

EVOO   Extra-virgin olive oil

CO   Coconut oil

*   or other non-starchy vegetable

**   or other starchy vegetable (refer to page 110)

If no page number is listed, simply prepare the items as noted or any way you like.

For additional protein, vegetable, and fat recommendations, refer to the QUICK LIST that is associated with your meal plan!

athletic performance

DAY	BREAKFAST	LUNCH	DINNER
21 ●◆●	Hard Boiled Eggs, Breakfast Sausage, Sweet Potato**	Nori Salmon Handrolls (316)	Lamb Chops with Olive Tapenade (326), Greek Salad with Avo-Ziki (374)
22 ●●◆	Swirly Crustless Quiche (240), Breakfast Sausage, Banana	*left-over* Lamb Chops with Olive Tapenade, *left-over* Greek Salad with Avo-Ziki	Orange Braised Beef Shanks (284), Butternut Sage Soup**(348)
23 ●◆◆	*left-over* Swirly Crustless Quiche, Perfectly Baked Bacon (236), Plantains in CO**	*left-over* Orange Braised Beef Shanks, *left-over* Butternut Sage Soup**	Hayley's Skirt Steak Tacos (292), Salsa (296), Grilled Squash & Pineapple (342)
24 ◆◆◆	Zucchini Pancakes (248), Perfectly Baked Bacon (236), Berries	Tangy Taco Salad (296), *left-over* Salsa	Fiery Jalapeño Burgers with Sweet Potato Pancakes (298), Red Roasted Garlic (370)
25 ●◆◆	*left-over* Sweet Potato Pancakes, Eggs, Avocado	Quick & Easy Salmon Cakes (310), Green Salad*, Avocado, Olives, Apple	Asian Orange Pan-Seared Scallops (304), Shrimp Cocktail (312), Acorn Squash (358)
26 ●◆●	*left-over* Acorn Squash with Cinnamon & Coconut Butter (358), Breakfast Sausage/Bacon	Tuna, Mixed Greens Salad with Persimmons, Asparagus & Fennel (380), Orange Vinaigrette (382)	Grandma Barbara's Stuffed Mushrooms (332), Roasted Marrow Bones (288), Spinach*
27 ●●●	Pumpkin Cranberry Muffins (246), Breakfast Sausage using Italian Sausage Spice Blend (233)	*left-over* Grandma Barbara's Stuffed Mushrooms, Mixed Greens Salad, Balsamic Vinaigrette (378)	Spiced Lamb Meatballs with Balsamic-Fig Compote (324), Green Beans with Shallots*(358)
28 ●◆■	*left-over* Spiced Lamb Meatballs, Spinach or Cabbage*, Apple	Wild Canned Salmon with Olives, Avocado, Lemon Juice, Tomato, EVOO, Sweet Potato**	Lemon & Artichoke Chicken (260), Broc-Cauli Chowder with Bacon (336)
29 ●■◆	Apple Streusel Egg Muffins (254), Bacon or Breakfast Sausage,	*left-over* Lemon & Artichoke Chicken, Kale & Carrot Salad with Lemon-Tahini Dressing* (376)	Mom's Stuffed Cabbage Rolls with Tomato Cranberry Sauce (290), Green Salad*
30 ●●●	*left-over* Apple Streusel Egg Muffins (254), Bacon or Breakfast Sausage	Chorizo Meatballs (330), Mixed Greens Salad* with Avocado, Lemon Juice, and EVOO	Mediterranean Lamb Roast (320), Sautéed Spinach with Pine Nuts & Currants*(366), Sweet Potato**

» *A complete shopping list for this meal plan can be found on balancedbites.com*

KEY
- ◆ **Red-Meat**
- ■ **Poultry**
- ● **Eggs**
- ● **Pork**
- ● **Lamb**
- ◆ **Seafood**

NOTES

EVOO   Extra-virgin olive oil
CO   Coconut oil
*   or other non-starchy vegetable
**   or other starchy vegetable (refer to page 110)

If no page number is listed, simply prepare the items as noted or any way you like.

For additional protein, vegetable, and fat recommendations, refer to the QUICK LIST that is associated with your meal plan!

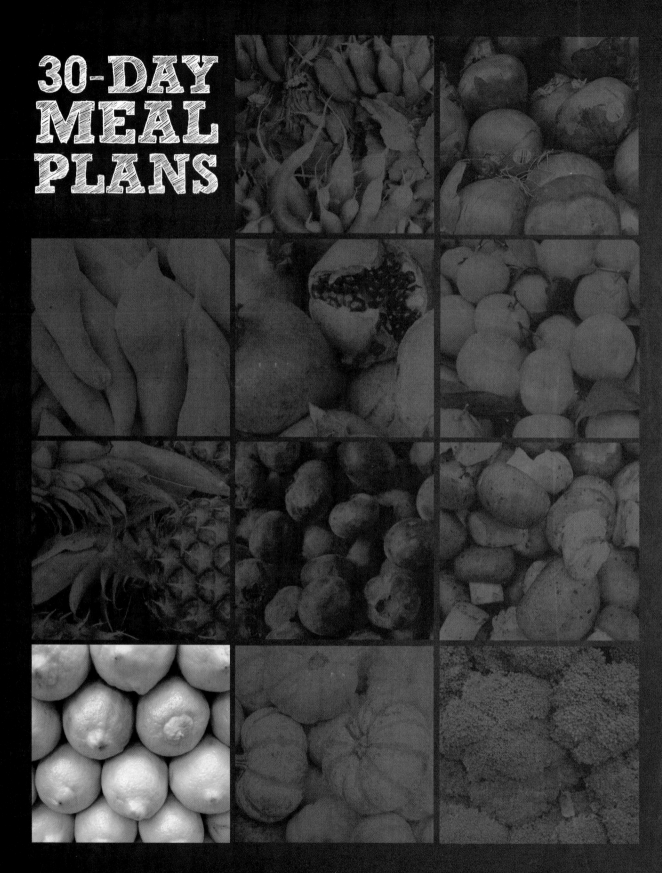

30-DAY MEAL PLANS

FAT LOSS

While the root causes of weight-gain and weight-loss resistance vary greatly from person to person, there are basic guidelines that will get you started in the right direction. This plan will keep your overall carbohydrate intake lower than it may have been before but will continue to fuel your body appropriately for exercise.

If you are completely new to the Paleo way of eating, you may want to try the Squeaky-Clean Paleo 30-Day Meal Plan or the Blood Sugar Regulation 30-Day Meal Plan first, as you may lose a sufficient amount of weight with those plans, which don't have the additional modifications that this one includes.

Others who may benefit from this meal plan include:

» PEOPLE WHO EXPERIENCE SUGAR AND CARBOHYDRATE CRAVINGS.
» PEOPLE THAT HAVE TROUBLE DIGESTING FRUIT OR SUSPECT BACTERIAL OR FUNGAL OVERGROWTH.

diet & lifestyle recommendations

add [+]

SUPERFOODS & PROBIOTICS

Eat these foods as often as possible (see page 29 for the Guide to Paleo Foods). Eat raw sauerkraut (recipe on page 238) or other fermented vegetables daily (1/4 cup), especially with breakfast.

PROTEIN

Eat protein to satisfy the appetite for longer periods of time (meals focused on both fat and protein will help).

NUTRIENT-DENSE FOODS

Replenish depleted nutrient stores from eating excess refined foods over time.

STARCHY CARBOHYDRATES AFTER EXERCISE

(see page 110 for dense carb sources); eat approximately 30-75g of carbohydrates only in a post-workout meal depending on the length of exercise. Track how you feel, and add/subtract if you are not making progress or don't feel well-fueled for exercise the next day.

STRESS MANAGEMENT

Keep systemic inflammation low and allow your body to let go of excess fat.

SLEEP

Sleep at least eight hours every night in a dark room in order to wake up refreshed and without cravings during the day.

MOVEMENT

Slowly introduce weight training with moderate to heavy loads, not excessively demanding in terms of stress response or cortisol output. If you are not fatigued, try high intensity exercise for 5-25 minutes a few times per week (not more than four). Take walks outside, or practice gentle yoga for movement without systemic stress.

avoid [-]

GLUTEN & DAIRY

Gluten 100% of the time. See the "Guide to Gluten" on page 89; avoid dairy for its potential growth-promotion effects. (Butter and ghee are okay.)

EXCESS DIETARY FAT

This does not mean to avoid fat, but eat the naturally occurring fat in your foods (meats, seafood, eggs, avocado) as opposed to adding a lot *extra* fat when cooking.

FRUIT

The sweet taste may trigger the desire for more sweet foods. Instead, opt for starch as a carbohydrate source. Eat fruit only in small amounts as a dessert, not a regular part of meals.

REFINED FOODS, SWEETENERS, & ALCOHOL

They will impair your liver's ability to detoxify and lose fat.

EXCESS CAFFEINE

Caffeine can be a stressor and may increase cortisol response and promote weight-loss resistance.

ENVIRONMENTAL TOXINS

Toxins and estrogens (xenoestrogens), including the excessive use of plastics, commercially raised meats, and non-organic foods can disrupt hormonal balance.

CHRONIC CARDIOVASCULAR EXERCISE

(meaning 30-60+ minutes at a steady-state of intensity like jogging or biking), as it can lead to low blood sugar episodes, as well as provoke a stress response.

nutritional supplements & herbs to consider

These recommendations are made as a starting point. Do your own research and determine which supplements may serve you best. It's best to get as many of your nutrients from food as possible. See the next page for specific food-based nutrients on which to focus. The items below are listed in no particular order.

» **VITAMIN A (RETINOL)** helps to maintain the integrity of the mucosal lining of the gut. It is also helpful in maintaining immunity when balanced with vitamin D, and it is necessary for the assimilation of dietary minerals. Vitamin A is depleted by stress, strenuous physical exercise, pregnancy, lactation, and infection.

» **FERMENTED COD LIVER OIL/ BUTTER OIL BLEND** for fat-soluble vitamins A, D, E, and K2 as well as some omega 3 fats. I only recommend Green Pasture brand.

» **CARNITINE / L-CARNITINE** can help to improve insulin sensitivity and glucose storage. It also optimizes fat and carbohydrate metabolism, and it may improve the utilization of fat as an energy source. Cofactors include iron, vitamin C, vitamin B3 (niacin), and vitamin B6.

» **CHROMIUM** may improve insulin sensitivity and reduce appetite. Look for chromium picolinate, polynicotinate, or chelavite.

» **L-GLUTAMINE** aids in the healing of the epithelial cells that line the small intestine.

» **LIPOIC ACID (ALPHA-LIPOIC ACID/ALA)** has antioxidant properties and may motivate greater glucose uptake from the bloodstream by promoting the conversion of carbohydrates into energy.

» **MAGNESIUM** is required for more than 300 enzymatic processes in the body, and most people are deficient in it. Look for magnesium glycinate or magnesium malate forms.

» **OMEGA-3 FATS** are anti-inflammatory essential fatty acids. I only recommend Green Pasture brand fermented cod liver oil.

» **PROBIOTICS** promote healthy gut flora, which is critical to proper digestion and elimination; use a supplement if necessary.

supportive nutrients & foods that contain them

quick LIST

proteins

Beef
Chicken
Eggs
Lamb
Oysters
Salmon
Sardines
Shellfish
Tuna

fats

Coconut oil
Eggs
Extra-virgin olive oil
Grass-fed butter/ghee

vegetables

Beets
Broccoli
Brussels sprouts
Cabbage
Carrots
Cauliflower
Daikon radish
Green bell pepper
Parsnips
Swiss chard

fruits

Green apple
Lemons
Limes

superfoods

Bone broth
Fermented cod liver oil/
butter oil blend
Liver

spices

Basil
Cilantro
Cinnamon
Cumin
Garlic
Ginger
Oregano
Parsley
Turmeric

VITAMIN A (RETINOL)

» Liver, eel, grass-fed butter, clarified butter, or ghee

VITAMIN B3

» Liver, chicken, tuna, lamb, salmon
» Brewer's yeast (Lewis Labs brand only)
» Trace amounts: sesame seed, sunflowers seeds, almond, mushrooms

VITAMIN B7

» Liver, brewer's yeast (Lewis Labs brand only)
» Trace amounts: Swiss chard, Walnuts, pecans, almonds

VITAMIN C

» Adrenal glands from pasture-raised animals, beets, bell peppers, garlic, lemons, Brussels sprouts, cauliflower, collard greens, broccoli, daikon radish, kale, mustard greens, parsley, spinach, strawberries

CHROMIUM

» Liver, grass-fed cheese
» Brewer's yeast (Lewis Labs brand only)
» Trace amounts: green pepper, apple, parsnips, spinach, carrots

CARNITINE

» Red meat (darker will contain more)

CONJUGATED LINOLEIC ACID (CLA)

A potent antioxidant that supports fat loss.
» Grass-fed beef and lamb

VITAMIN D

A potent immune system modulator and is most available via sun exposure.
» Egg yolks, cold water fish (salmon, herring, mackerel, etc.)
» Grass-fed butter or ghee
» Fermented cod liver oil (Green Pasture brand only)

MAGNESIUM

Magnesium is critical to cellular energy production in order to battle fatigue and maintain proper calcium metabolism for vascular health.
» Kale, green leafy vegetables
» Beets
» Pumpkin seeds/pepitas

MANGANESE

Manganese is beneficial to energy metabolism and thyroid hormone function. Intake should be balanced with magnesium, calcium, iron, copper, and zinc. Antacids may inhibit manganese absorption.
» Pecans, walnuts, turnip greens, rhubarb, beet greens
» Cloves, cinnamon, thyme, black pepper, turmeric

OMEGA-3 FATS

An anti-inflammatory essential fatty acid that comes from limited food sources.
» Cold water fish (salmon, herring, mackerel, etc.), Fermented cod liver oil (Green Pasture brand only)
» Walnuts, pecans

PROBIOTICS

Promote healthy gut flora, which is critical to proper digestion and elimination.
» Fermented vegetables: cabbage (sauerkraut/kimchi) carrots, beets, or other vegetables
» Kombucha (fermented tea)

fat loss

DAY	BREAKFAST	LUNCH	DINNER
1 ●■◆	Swirly Crustless Quiche (240), Perfectly Baked Bacon (236)	Mustard Glazed Chicken Thighs (266), Green Salad*, Balsamic Vinaigrette (378)	Grilled Garlic Flank Steak with Peppers & Onions (294), Spinach*
2 ●◆■	*left-over* Swirly Crustless Quiche, *left-over* Garlic Flank Steak with Peppers & Onions	Wild Canned Salmon with Olives, Lemon Juice, Tomato, EVOO	Sage Roasted Turkey Legs (276), Roasted Pearl Onions (370), Green Salad*
3 ■■●	*left-over* Mustard-Glazed Chicken Thighs, *left-over* Roasted Onions	*left-over* Sage Roasted Turkey Legs, Persimmon, Asparagus & Fennel Salad (380)	Lemony Lamb Dolmas (318), Cilantro Cauli-Rice (340)
4 ●●◆	Pesto Scrambled Eggs (252), *left-over* Cilantro Cauli-Rice	*left-over* Lemony Lamb Dolmas, Spinach Salad with Walnuts & Artichokes (380)	Citrus Macadamia Nut Sole (314), Green Beans with Shallots*(358)
5 ◆◆◆	*left-over* Citrus Macadamia Nut Sole, Brussels Sprouts*	Nori Salmon Handrolls (316)	Beef & Mixed Veggie Stir Fry (286)
6 ●◆●	Pumpkin Pancakes (242), Breakfast Sausage using Italian Sausage Spice Blend (233)	*left-over* Beef Stir Fry with Mixed Veggies	Lamb Lettuce Boats with Avo-Ziki Sauce (322)
7 ●◆■	Eggs, Perfectly Baked Bacon (236), Kale*	Mixed Greens with Wild Canned Salmon, Asparagus*, Lemon Juice, EVOO	Citrus & Herb Whole Roasted Chicken (256), Simple Baked Kale Chips*(356)
8 ■■■	Grain-Free Porridge (252), Berries, *left-over* Citrus & Herb Whole Roasted Chicken	Spinach Salad with Walnuts & Artichokes (380), *left-over* Citrus & Herb Whole Roasted Chicken	Chinese 5-Spice Lettuce Cups (272)
9 ●■◆	Swirly Crustless Quiche (240), Steamed Broccoli*	Indian-Spiced Turkey Burgers (268), Steamed Broccoli*	Pesto Shrimp & Squash Fettuccine (308)
10 ●◆○	Omelet or Pesto Scrambled Eggs, *left-over* Shrimp & Avocado	Simple Shrimp Ceviche (316), Mixed Greens*, EVOO	Cumin Spiced Pork Tenderloin with Root Vegetables**(328)

» *A complete shopping list for this meal plan can be found on balancedbites.com*

KEY
- ◆ Red-Meat
- ■ Poultry
- ● Eggs
- ○ Pork
- ● Lamb
- ◆ Seafood

NOTES

EVOO   Extra-virgin olive oil

CO   Coconut oil

*   or other non-starchy vegetable

**   or other starchy vegetable (refer to page 110)

If no page number is listed, simply prepare the items as noted or any way you like.

For additional protein, vegetable, and fat recommendations, refer to the QUICK LIST that is associated with your meal plan!

DAY	BREAKFAST	LUNCH	DINNER
11 ● ● ◆	Swirly Crustless Quiche (240)	*left-over* Cumin Spiced Pork Tenderloin, Rainbow Red Cabbage Salad*(372)	Balsamic Braised Short Ribs (278), Spinach*
12 ● ◆ ■	Eggs, *left-over* Rainbow Red Cabbage Salad	*left-over* Balsamic Braised Short Ribs, Green Salad*	Savory Baked Chicken Legs (264), Brussels Sprouts with Fennel*(350)
13 ● ■ ◆	Zucchini Pancakes (248), Perfectly Baked Bacon (236)	*left-over* Savory Baked Chicken Legs, *left-over* Brussels Sprouts with Fennel*	Lemon Rosemary Broiled Salmon (306), Asparagus with Lemon & Olives (338)
14 ◆ ■ ◆	*left-over* Lemon Rosemary Broiled Salmon, *left-over* Asparagus with Lemon & Olives*	Buffalo Chicken Lettuce Wraps (270)	Red Palm & Coriander Tuna Over Daikon Noodle Salad (302), Green Salad*
15 ● ◆ ◆	Scrambled Eggs with Olives, Steamed Spinach*, Avocado	Spinach Salad with EVOO, *left-over* Red Palm & Coriander Tuna, Avocado, Lemon Juice	Italian-Style Stuffed Peppers (300), Green Salad* with Balsamic Vinaigrette (378)
16 ● ◆ ■	Breakfast Sausage, Brussels Sprouts*	*left-over* Italian-Style Stuffed Peppers (300), Green Salad*	Bacon-Wrapped Smoky Chicken Thighs (262), Mixed Greens Salad with Beets & Blood Oranges (376)
17 ● ■ ◆	Bacon & Egg Salad (248), Broccoli*	*left-over* Bacon-Wrapped Smoky Chicken Thighs, Green Salad*	Spaghetti Squash Bolognese (280), Simple Baked Kale Chips* (356)
18 ● ◆ ●	*left-over* Bacon & Egg Salad Breakfast Sausage or Bacon	*left-over* Spaghetti Squash Bolognese	Thanksgiving Stuffing Meatballs (334), Mashed Faux-Tatoes (344)
19 ● ● ◆	Scrambled Eggs, Avocado, Spinach or Kale*	*left-over* Thanksgiving Stuffing Meatballs, *left-over* Mashed Faux-Tatoes	Citrus Macadamia Nut Sole (314), Lemon Roasted Romanesco*(346)
20 ● ◆ ■	Hard Boiled Eggs, Perfectly Baked Bacon (236)	*left-over* Citrus Macadamia Nut Sole, *left-over* Lemon Roasted Romanesco*	Roasted Duck with Cherry Sauce (274), Sautéed Red Cabbage with Onions and Apples*(352)

» *A complete shopping list for this meal plan can be found on balancedbites.com*

KEY
◆ Red-Meat
■ Poultry
● Eggs
● Pork
● Lamb
◆ Seafood

NOTES
EVOO   Extra-virgin olive oil
CO   Coconut oil
*   or other non-starchy vegetable
**   or other starchy vegetable (refer to page 110)
If no page number is listed, simply prepare the items as noted or any way you like.
For additional protein, vegetable, and fat recommendations, refer to the QUICK LIST that is associated with your meal plan!

fat loss

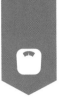

DAY	BREAKFAST	LUNCH	DINNER
21 ●◆●	Hard Boiled Eggs, Breakfast Sausage	Nori Salmon Handrolls (316)	Lamb Chops with Olive Tapenade (326), Greek Salad with Avo-Ziki (374)
22 ●●◆	Swirly Crustless Quiche (240), Breakfast Sausage	*left-over* Lamb Chops with Olive Tapenade, *left-over* Greek Salad with Avo-Ziki	Orange Braised Beef Shanks (284), Butternut Sage Soup**(348)
23 ●◆◆	*left-over* Swirly Crustless Quiche, Perfectly Baked Bacon (236)	*left-over* Orange Braised Beef Shanks, *left-over* Butternut Sage Soup**	Hayley's Skirt Steak Tacos (292), Salsa (296), Grilled Squash & Pineapple (342)
24 ●◆●	Pesto Scrambled Eggs (252), Breakfast Sausage or Bacon	Tangy Taco Salad (296), *left-over* Salsa	Fiery Jalapeño Burgers with Sweet Potato Pancakes (298), Red Roasted Garlic (370)
25 ●◆◆	*left-over* Sweet Potato Pancakes, Eggs, Avocado	Quick & Easy Salmon Cakes (310), Green Salad*, Avocado, Olives	Asian Orange Pan-Seared Scallops (304), Tomatillo Shrimp Cocktail (312), Zucchini*
26 ●◆○	Zucchini Pancakes (248), Savory Baked Chicken Legs (264)	Tuna, Mixed Greens Salad with Persimmons, Asparagus & Fennel (380), Orange Vinaigrette (382)	Grandma Barbara's Stuffed Mushrooms (332), Roasted Marrow Bones (288), Spinach*
27 ○●●	Grain-Free Porridge (252), Breakfast Sausage using Italian Sausage Spice Blend (233)	*left-over* Grandma Barbara's Stuffed Mushrooms, Mixed Greens Salad*, Balsamic Vinaigrette (378)	Spiced Lamb Meatballs with Balsamic-Fig Compote (324), Green Beans with Shallots*(358)
28 ●◆■	*left-over* Spiced Lamb Meatballs, Spinach or Cabbage*	Wild Canned Salmon with Olives, Avocado, Lemon Juice, Tomato, EVOO	Lemon & Artichoke Chicken (260), Broc-Cauli Chowder with Bacon (336)
29 ●■◆	Apple Streusel Egg Muffins (254), Bacon or Breakfast Sausage	*left-over* Lemon & Artichoke Chicken, Kale & Carrot Salad with Lemon-Tahini Dressing* (376)	Mom's Stuffed Cabbage Rolls with Tomato Cranberry Sauce (290), Green Salad*
30 ●○●	*left-over* Apple Streusel Egg Muffins (254), Bacon or Breakfast Sausage	Chorizo Meatballs (330), Mixed Greens Salad* with Avocado, Lemon Juice, and EVOO	Mediterranean Lamb Roast (320), Sautéed Spinach with Pine Nuts & Currants*(366)

» *A complete shopping list for this meal plan can be found on balancedbites.com*

KEY
◆ Red-Meat
■ Poultry
● Eggs
○ Pork
● Lamb
◆ Seafood

NOTES
EVOO   Extra-virgin olive oil
CO   Coconut oil
*   or other non-starchy vegetable
**   or other starchy vegetable (refer to page 110)
If no page number is listed, simply prepare the items as noted or any way you like.
For additional protein, vegetable, and fat recommendations, refer to the QUICK LIST that is associated with your meal plan!

30-DAY MEAL PLANS

SQUEAKY CLEAN PALEO

If you are not looking for help with a specific condition or goal but would rather simply take on what is known a strict or "clean" Paleo diet, this is the plan for you. You'll be eating only whole foods, without any grain-free "treat" options. This approach requires that you read labels especially closely to catch additives that sneak into your foods, especially hidden sugar and gluten.

There are no supplement recommendations for this plan specifically. If you have specific goals, please refer to the previous 30-Day Meal Plans to combine any supplement recommendations with the meals in this plan.

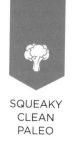

diet & lifestyle recommendations

add [+]

SUPERFOODS & PROBIOTICS

Eat as often as possible (see page 29 for the Guide to Paleo Foods). Eat raw sauerkraut (recipe on page 238) or other fermented vegetables daily (1/4 cup), especially with breakfast.

PROTEIN

Eat protein to satisfy the appetite for longer periods of time (meals focused on both fat and protein will help).

NUTRIENT-DENSE FOODS

Replenish depleted nutrient stores from eating excess refined foods over time.

STARCHY CARBOHYDRATES AFTER EXERCISE

(see page 110 for dense carb sources); eat approximately 30-75g of carbohydrates in meals pre and post-workout depending on the length of exercise. Track how you feel, and add/subtract if you are not making progress or don't feel well-fueled for your training.

SMART TRAINING

Listen to your body and take rest and recovery days when necessary.

STRESS MANAGEMENT

Manage stress to keep systemic inflammation low. Develop a guided meditation practice, or begin to practice Qi Gong. Practice meditation, biofeedback, Tai Chi, and/or guided imagery for deep relaxation.

SLEEP

Sleep at least eight hours every night in a dark room in order to wake up refreshed and without cravings during the day.

avoid [-]

GLUTEN & DAIRY

Gluten 100% of the time. See the "Guide to Gluten" on page 89; avoid dairy for its potentially gut-irritating or allergenic effects. (Butter and ghee are okay)

REFINED FOODS & SWEETENERS

Artificial sweeteners and caffeine, as they can provoke blood sugar fluctuations.

EXCESS CAFFEINE

Caffeine can be a stressor and may increase cortisol response and promote weight-loss resistance.

ALCOHOL

DISCLAIMER:

The information in this book is not intended to be a replacement for professional medical diagnosis or treatment for a medical condition. It consists solely of nutritional and lifestyle recommendations to support a healthier body.

squeaky clean paleo

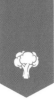

DAY	BREAKFAST	LUNCH	DINNER
1 ●■◆	Swirly Crustless Quiche (240), Perfectly Baked Bacon (236), Raw Sauerkraut (238)	Mustard Glazed Chicken Thighs (266), Green Salad*, Balsamic Vinaigrette (378)	Grilled Garlic Flank Steak with Peppers & Onions (294), Baked Beets with Fennel**(362)
2 ●◆■	*left-over* Swirly Crustless Quiche, *left-over* Garlic Flank Steak with Peppers & Onions	Wild Canned Salmon with Olives, Avocado, Lemon Juice, Tomato, EVOO	Sage Roasted Turkey Legs (276), Sweet Potato Pancakes (298), Steamed Spinach*
3 ■■●	*left-over* Sweet Potato Pancakes, Mustard-Glazed Chicken Thighs (266)	*left-over* Sage Roasted Turkey Legs, Persimmon, Asparagus & Fennel Salad (380)	Lemony Lamb Dolmas (318), Cilantro Cauli-Rice (340)
4 ●●◆	Pesto Scrambled Eggs (252), Cilantro Cauli-Rice (340), Raw Sauerkraut (238)	*left-over* Lemony Lamb Dolmas, Spinach Salad with Walnuts & Artichokes (380)	Citrus Macadamia Nut Sole (314), Butternut Squash**
5 ◆◆◆	*left-over* Citrus Macadamia Nut Sole, Butternut Squash**	Nori Salmon Handrolls (316)	Beef & Mixed Veggie Stir Fry (286)
6 ●◆●	Pumpkin Pancakes (242), Breakfast Sausage using Italian Sausage Spice Blend (233)	*left-over* Beef Stir Fry with Mixed Veggies	Lamb Lettuce Boats with Avo-Ziki Sauce (322)
7 ●◆■	Eggs, Perfectly Baked Bacon (236), Kale*, Raw Sauerkraut (238)	Mixed Greens with Wild Canned Salmon, Asparagus*, Lemon Juice, EVOO	Citrus & Herb Whole Roasted Chicken (256), Roasted Rosemary Roots (350), Kale Chips*(356)
8 ■■■	Grain-Free Porridge (252), Berries, *left-over* Citrus & Herb Whole Roasted Chicken	Spinach Salad with Walnuts & Artichokes (380), *left-over* Citrus & Herb Whole Roasted Chicken	Chinese 5-Spice Lettuce Cups (272)
9 ●■◆	Swirly Crustless Quiche (240), Steamed Broccoli*, Raw Sauerkraut (238)	Indian-Spiced Turkey Burgers (268), Steamed Broccoli*	Pesto Shrimp & Squash Fettuccine (308)
10 ●◆●	Omelet or Pesto Scrambled Eggs, *left-over* Shrimp & Avocado	Simple Shrimp Ceviche (316), Mixed Greens*, EVOO	Cumin Spiced Pork Tenderloin with Root Vegetables**(328)

» *A complete shopping list for this meal plan can be found on balancedbites.com*

KEY
◆ Red-Meat
■ Poultry
● Eggs
● Pork
● Lamb
◆ Seafood

NOTES
EVOO   Extra-virgin olive oil
CO   Coconut oil
*   or other non-starchy vegetable
**   or other starchy vegetable (refer to page 110)
If no page number is listed, simply prepare the items as noted or any way you like.
For additional protein, vegetable, and fat recommendations, refer to the QUICK LIST that is associated with your meal plan!

DAY	BREAKFAST	LUNCH	DINNER
11 ● ● ◆	Swirly Crustless Quiche (240), Perfectly Baked Bacon (236), *left-over* Root Vegetables	*left-over* Cumin Spiced Pork Tenderloin, Rainbow Red Cabbage Salad*(372)	Balsamic Braised Short Ribs (278), Candied Carrots (340), Spinach*
12 ● ◆ ■	Eggs, *left-over* Rainbow Red Cabbage Salad	*left-over* Balsamic Braised Short Ribs, *left-over* Candied Carrots, Green Salad*	Savory Baked Chicken Legs (264), Brussels Sprouts with Fennel*(350)
13 ● ■ ◆	Zucchini Pancakes (248), Perfectly Baked Bacon (236), Raw Sauerkraut (238)	*left-over* Savory Baked Chicken Legs, *left-over* Brussels Sprouts with Fennel*	Lemon Rosemary Broiled Salmon (306), Asparagus with Lemon & Olives (338), Sweet Potato**
14 ◆ ■ ◆	*left-over* Lemon Rosemary Broiled Salmon, *left-over* Asparagus with Lemon & Olives*	Buffalo Chicken Lettuce Wraps (270)	Red Palm & Coriander Tuna Over Daikon Noodle Salad (302), Green Salad*
15 ● ◆ ◆	Scrambled Eggs with Olives, Steamed Spinach*, Avocado	Spinach Salad with EVOO, *left-over* Red Palm & Coriander Tuna, Avocado, Lemon Juice	Italian-Style Stuffed Peppers (300), Green Salad* with Balsamic Vinaigrette (378)
16 ● ◆ ■	Grain-Free Porridge (252), Breakfast Sausage	*left-over* Italian-Style Stuffed Peppers (300), Green Salad*	Bacon-Wrapped Smoky Chicken Thighs (262), Mixed Greens Salad with Beets & Blood Oranges(376)
17 ● ■ ◆	Bacon & Egg Salad (248), Sweet Potato or Beets**	*left-over* Bacon-Wrapped Smoky Chicken Thighs, Green Salad*	Spaghetti Squash Bolognese (280), Kale Chips* (356)
18 ● ◆ ●	Pumpkin Pancakes (242), Breakfast Sausage or Bacon	*left-over* Spaghetti Squash Bolognese	Thanksgiving Stuffing Meatballs (334), Mashed Faux-Tatoes (344)
19 ● ● ◆	Scrambled Eggs, Avocado, Spinach or Kale*, Raw Sauerkraut (238)	*left-over* Thanksgiving Stuffing Meatballs, *left-over* Mashed Faux-Tatoes	Citrus Macadamia Nut Sole (314), Lemon Roasted Romanesco*(346), Sweet & Savory Potatoes**(362)
20 ● ◆ ■	Grain-Free Porridge (252), Hard Boiled Eggs	*left-over* Citrus Macadamia Nut Sole, *left-over* Lemon Roasted Romanesco*	Roasted Duck with Cherry Sauce (274), Sautéed Red Cabbage with Onions and Apples*(352)

» *A complete shopping list for this meal plan can be found on balancedbites.com*

KEY
◆ Red-Meat
■ Poultry
● Eggs
● Pork
● Lamb
◆ Seafood

NOTES

EVOO   Extra-virgin olive oil
CO   Coconut oil
*   or other non-starchy vegetable
**   or other starchy vegetable (refer to page 110)
If no page number is listed, simply prepare the items as noted or any way you like.
For additional protein, vegetable, and fat recommendations, refer to the QUICK LIST that is associated with your meal plan!

squeaky clean paleo

DAY	BREAKFAST	LUNCH	DINNER
21 ●◆●	Hard Boiled Eggs, Breakfast Sausage, Raw Sauerkraut (238)	Nori Salmon Handrolls (316)	Lamb Chops with Olive Tapenade (326), Greek Salad with Avo-Ziki (374)
22 ●●◆	Swirly Crustless Quiche (240), Breakfast Sausage	*left-over* Lamb Chops with Olive Tapenade, *left-over* Greek Salad with Avo-Ziki	Orange Braised Beef Shanks (284), Butternut Sage Soup**(348)
23 ●◆◆	*left-over* Swirly Crustless Quiche, Perfectly Baked Bacon (236)	*left-over* Orange Braised Beef Shanks, *left-over* Butternut Sage Soup**	Hayley's Skirt Steak Tacos (292), Salsa (296), Grilled Squash & Pineapple (342)
24 ●◆◆	Acorn Squash with Cinnamon & Coconut Butter (358), Breakfast Sausage or Bacon	Tangy Taco Salad (296), *left-over* Salsa	Fiery Jalapeño Burgers with Sweet Potato Pancakes (298), Red Roasted Garlic (370)
25 ●●◆	*left-over* Sweet Potato Pancakes, Eggs, Avocado	Quick & Easy Salmon Cakes (310), Green Salad*, Avocado, Olives	Asian Orange Pan-Seared Scallops (304), Tomatillo Shrimp Cocktail (312), Zucchini*
26 ●◆●	Zucchini Pancakes (248), Perfectly Baked Bacon (236)	Tuna, Mixed Greens Salad with Persimmons, Asparagus & Fennel (380), Orange Vinaigrette (382)	Grandma Barbara's Stuffed Mushrooms (332), Roasted Marrow Bones (288), Spinach
27 ●●●	Grain-Free Porridge (252), Breakfast Sausage using Italian Sausage Spice Blend (233)	*left-over* Grandma Barbara's Stuffed Mushrooms, Mixed Greens Salad, Balsamic Vinaigrette (378)	Spiced Lamb Meatballs with Balsamic-Fig Compote (324), Green Beans with Shallots*(358)
28 ●◆■	*left-over* Spiced Lamb Meatballs, Spinach or Cabbage*	Wild Canned Salmon with Olives, Avocado, Lemon Juice, Tomato, EVOO	Lemon & Artichoke Chicken (260), Broc-Cauli Chowder with Bacon (336)
29 ●■◆	Apple Streusel Egg Muffins (254), Bacon or Breakfast Sausage	*left-over* Lemon & Artichoke Chicken, Kale & Carrot Salad with Lemon-Tahini Dressing (376)	Mom's Stuffed Cabbage Rolls with Tomato Cranberry Sauce (290), Green Salad*
30 ●●●	*left-over* Apple Streusel Egg Muffins (254), Bacon or Breakfast Sausage	Chorizo Meatballs (330), Mixed Greens Salad* with Avocado, Lemon Juice, and EVOO	Mediterranean Lamb Roast (320), Sautéed Spinach with Pine Nuts & Currants*(366)

» *A complete shopping list for this meal plan can be found on balancedbites.com*

KEY

◆ Red-Meat
■ Poultry
● Eggs
● Pork
● Lamb
◆ Seafood

NOTES

EVOO   Extra-virgin olive oil

CO   Coconut oil

*   or other non-starchy vegetable

**   or other starchy vegetable (refer to page 110)

If no page number is listed, simply prepare the items as noted or any way you like.

For additional protein, vegetable, and fat recommendations, refer to the QUICK LIST that is associated with your meal plan!

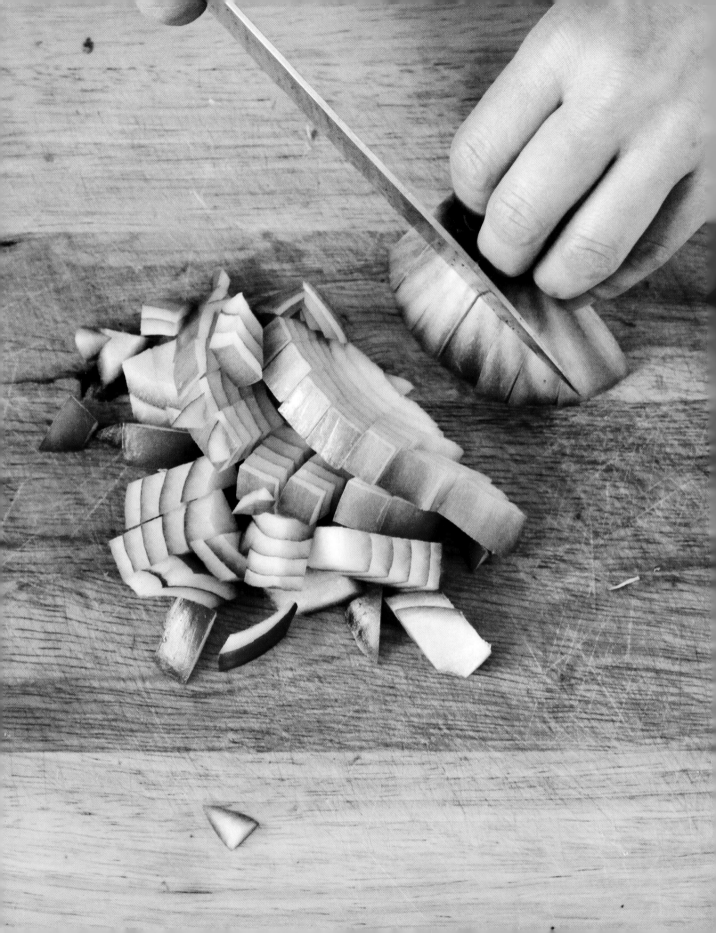

PART 3: RECIPES

how to: chop an onion

1. Pinch the base of the knife blade between your thumb and forefinger.

2. Extend your remaining fingers around the handle.

3. Grip the handle with your middle, ring, and little finger. Leave your thumb and forefinger pinching the knife blade.

4. Practice: Using a wood or composite surface cutting board, place the tip of the knife on the board and then rock the blade back and down, cutting your imaginary item. You can also place the back of the knife on the board and rock the blade forward and through the imaginary item.

5. Place the fingers of your free hand on the onion, making sure to curl your fingers slightly in to keep them safe. Next, place the blade of your knife on the onion.

6. Using the rocking motion previously practiced, cut off the end of onion. Notice how this provides you with a flat bottom to the onion.

7. Turn the onion over so that it is resting on the flat bottom you just created. Next, slice the onion in half, leaving part of the root intact on each side.

8. Separate the onion and work with one half at a time.

9. Peel the outer skin and the first layer of the onion if necessary/desired.

10. Slice down in 1/4-1/2 inch sections across, leaving the end of the onion intact.

11. Turn the onion forty-five degrees and slice across the previous cuts in 1/4-1/2 inch increments.

12. Continue to chop until you near the end of the onion.

13. Make the last chop about 1 inch from the end of the onion.

14. Turn the onion so that the root is now pointing upward.

15. Make one or two additional slices closer to the end.

16. Flip the onion back over one final time.

17. Finish chopping the remaining part.

18. Drop all chopped pieces into your bowl.

NO MORE TEARS
Keep onions in the refrigerator before chopping to prevent the tears that often accompany this task.

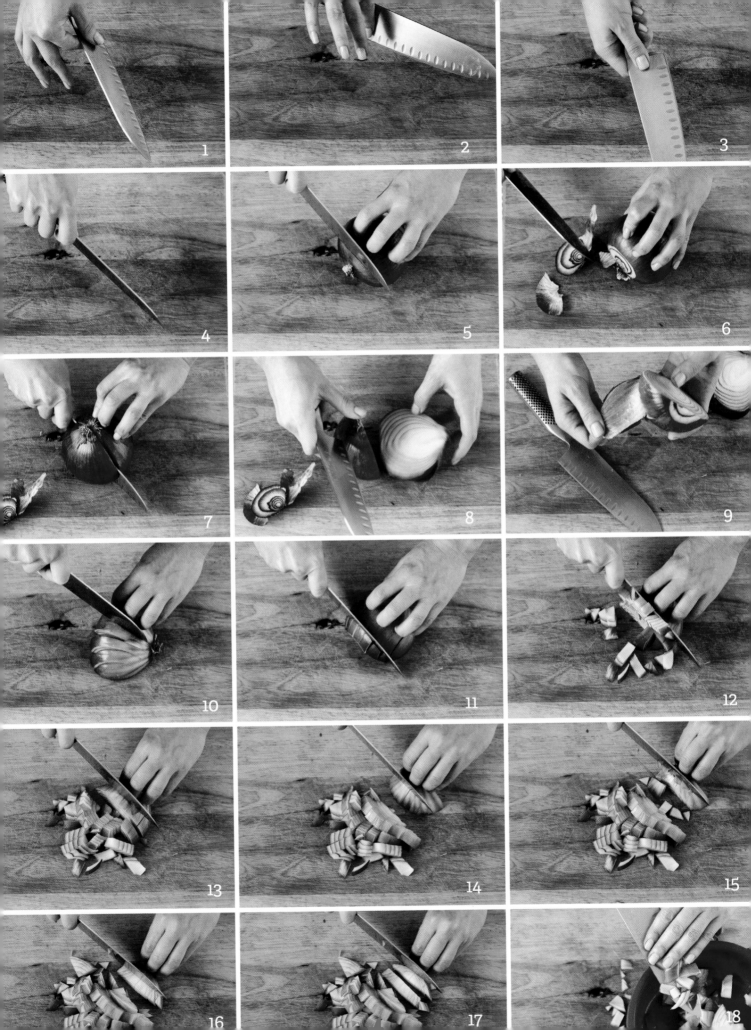

how to: chop a pepper

1. Pinch the base of the knife blade between your thumb and forefinger.

2. Extend your remaining fingers around the handle.

3. Grip the handle with your middle, ring, and little finger. Leave your thumb and forefinger pinching the knife blade.

4. Practice: Using a wood or composite surface cutting board, place the tip of the knife on the board and then rock the blade back and down, cutting your imaginary item. You can also place the back of the knife on the board and rock the blade forward and through the imaginary item.

5. Place the top of your pepper on your cutting board. Next, place the fingers of your free hand on the pepper, making sure to curl your fingers slightly in to keep them safe. Finally, place the blade of your knife across the center of the bottom of the pepper and slice using the rocking motion previously practiced.

6 & 7. Remove the white center and stem.

8. Chop the remaining pepper into sections along the ribs (white part).

9. Place the side of your knife into the pepper section, press down, and slide the blade sideways to begin removing the ribs.

10. To finish removing the ribs, pinch the opposite side of the pepper and continue to move the knife away from your hand.

11. Clean the remaining white ribs and seeds away from the pepper.

12-14. Slice the sections into 1/4 inch sticks.

15-17. Slice across the sticks evenly to create 1/4 inch cubes.

18. Drop all chopped pieces into your bowl.

HEY, HOT STUFF!

When working with hot peppers, remember that the heat is in the ribs (the white center part) and the seeds. Clear all of those away to reduce the overall heat of the pepper, then remember to wash your hands before touching your face!

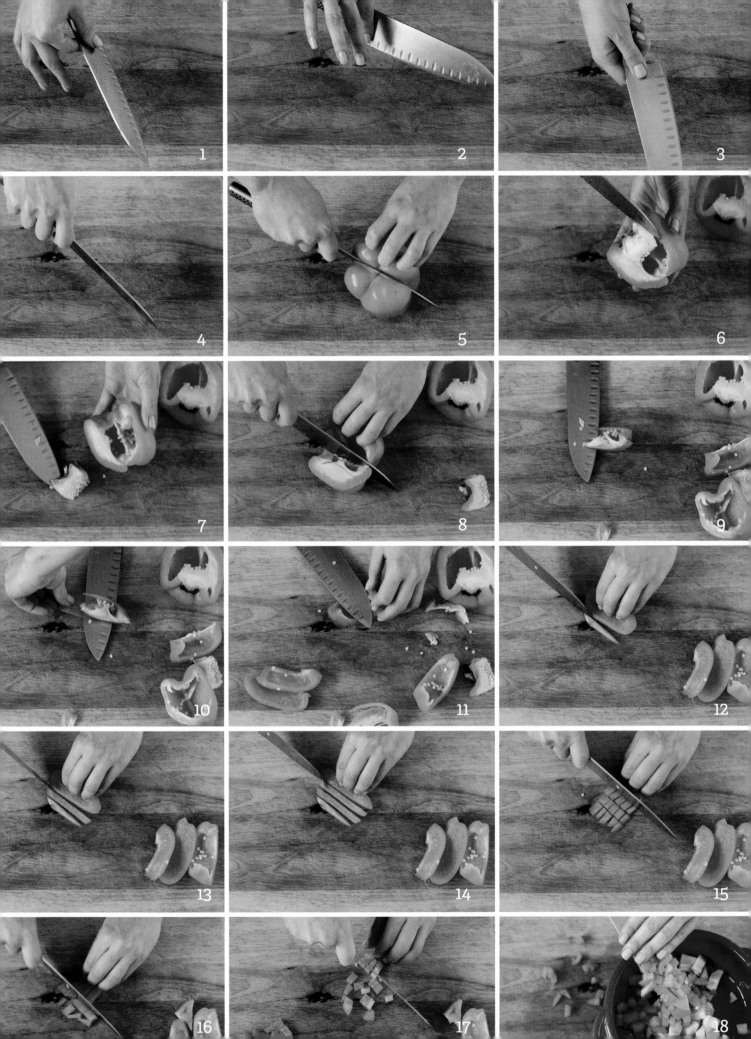

how to: chop anything

Follow instructions on the previous pages regarding how to hold the knife and your guide-hand.

All food can be chopped using the same principles:

You always create one of three "shapes" when chopping:

1) slices   2) sticks   3) cubes

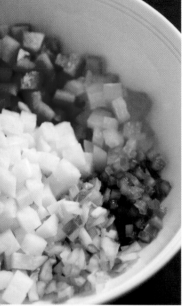

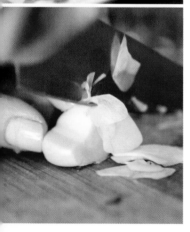

Slices: the first, basic cut made before it can be cut into sticks. The garlic to the left is being sliced very thinly!

Sticks: a slice, cut into even portions that are often longer than they are wide. The sweet potato on the top-left is being cut into sticks.

Diced (sometimes called "Chopped"): sticks that are cut into evenly-sized pieces, typically anywhere from 1-3 inches in size. The sweet potato on the top right is diced.

Julienne: a slice that is cut into matchstick-sized pieces—approximately 1/8 inch wide and anywhere from 1-3 inches long. The red bell pepper on the bottom-left is being julienned. You will julienne an item before you finely dice it.

Finely Diced: cut evenly into approximately 1/4 inch pieces. The red bell pepper on the bottom right and the bowl of ingredients on the top left of this page are examples of finely diced items.

Minced: cut into pieces smaller than 1/4 inch that may not be entirely even in size. Recipes often call for garlic to be minced.

Shredded: use a box grater or shredding disc on a food processor with items like carrots or zucchini to create short, thin pieces.

Grated: to make an ingredient's structure nearly indistinguishable in a recipe, use a fine box grater or zester to create a very finely minced (grated) result. Items like raw garlic can easily be grated into recipes.

HELPFUL TIP

It's useful to peel roots and tubers before chopping. Do this with a vegetable peeler.

This also applies to mangoes as I find they're easier to chop all at once if they're peeled first. However, they can be a bit slippery to hold for this part of the process.

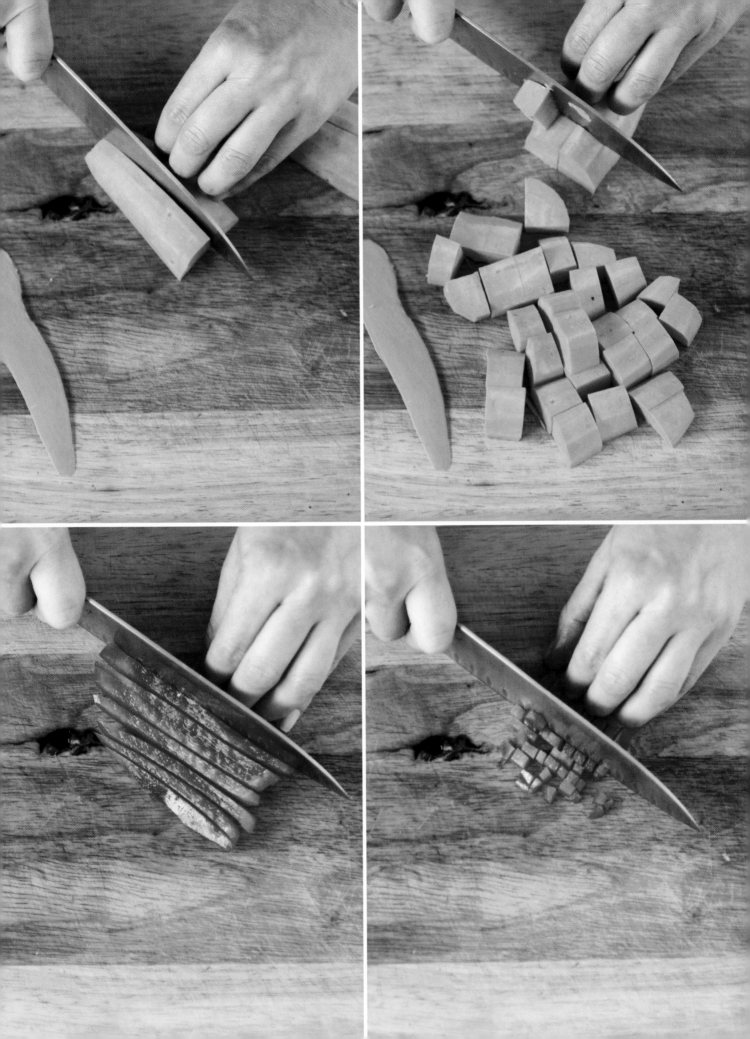

herb & lemon salt blends

PREP TIME
20 minutes

COOKING TIME
4 hours

YIELD
1/2 cup

Creating a blend of your favorite herbs with sea salt is an easy way to keep big flavor on-hand to add to any dish in a pinch (literally). Use a coarse, unrefined, mineral-rich salt (either white or grey). You can often find these salts in bulk at a grocery co-op, online, or even at your local grocery store.

1 cup fresh herbs (rosemary, sage,
    thyme, lemon peel, etc.)
1/2 cup coarse sea salt

SIDE NOTE
You can dehydrate your herbs overnight in a heated oven that's been turned off or even let them dry out for several hours on the lowest setting—just keep an eye on them so they don't burn. To fill your house with herbal aromas, allow the process to take longer at a lower temperature.

Preheat oven to 250°F or the lowest setting (a "warm" setting will work, too).

Spread individual herbs on their own baking sheets, and dry in the oven until they break apart when handled between your fingers. This takes roughly 4 hours.

Using a food processor or a mortar and pestle, grind dried herbs and salt to your desired consistency. Re-dry the herb salt in the oven if there is any remaining moisture.

Store the herb salt in glass jars in cool, dry place.

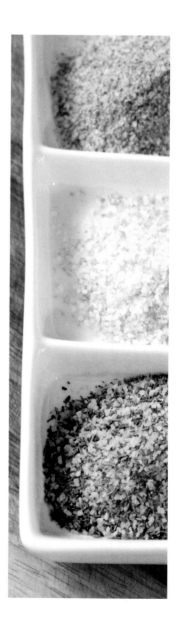

NUTS

EGGS

NIGHTSHADES

FODMAPS

Note: If a recipe calls for one of these salt blends and you do not have them prepared, simply use a 1:1 ratio of a dried herb or lemon peel to coarse sea salt.

I highly recommend that you make both a rosemary and a sage salt blend to keep on-hand for use on their own as well as in recipes later in this book!

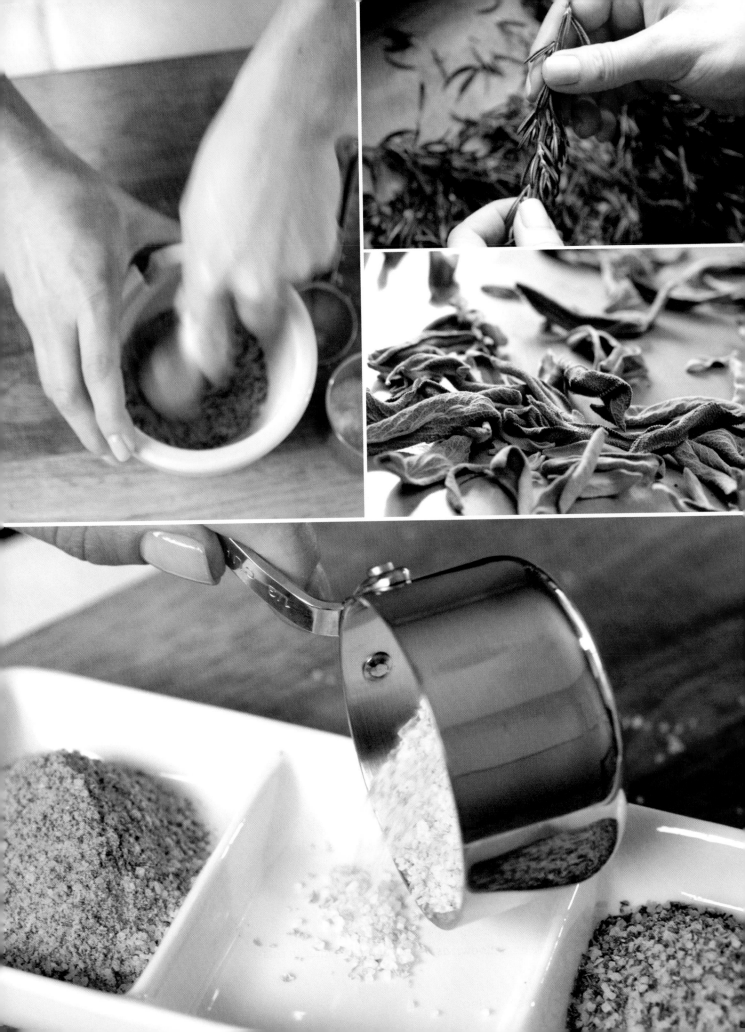

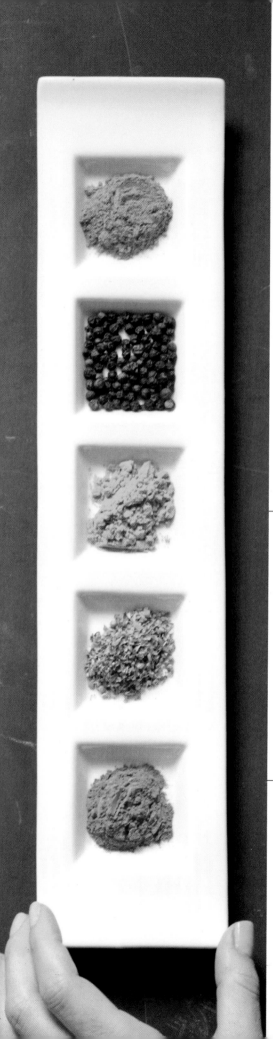

spice blends

NIGHTSHADE FREE?
Do not make recipes containing paprika, chili powder, chipotle powder, or red pepper flakes.

FODMAP FREE?
Eliminate the onion and garlic powders.

Unless otherwise noted, the preparation is the same for all spice blends: Combine all spices in a bowl, and store them in a small container. Use these blends as they appear in recipes throughout the book—or use them anytime!

SMOKY SPICE BLEND
1 tablespoon chipotle powder
1 tablespoon smoked paprika
1 tablespoon onion powder
1/2 tablespoon cinnamon
1 tablespoon sea salt
1/2 tablespoon black pepper

YIELD
5 tablespoons

CHORIZO SPICE BLEND
2 tablespoons chipotle powder
1 tablespoon smoked paprika
1 tablespoon onion powder
1 tablespoon garlic powder
1/2 tablespoon sea salt
1 teaspoon black pepper

YIELD
~6 tablespoons

When you want to add the blend to meat, combine 1/2 tablespoon of apple cider vinegar with each tablespoon of spice mix. Use 2 tablespoons of chorizo spice blend per pound of meat.

COOLING SPICE BLEND
1 tablespoon turmeric
1 tablespoon cinnamon
1 tablespoon cumin
1 tablespoon dried oregano
1 teaspoon black pepper
1 tablespoon onion powder
1 tablespoon garlic powder

YIELD
~6 tablespoons

INDIAN SPICE BLEND

2 tablespoons onion powder
2 teaspoons garam masala
2 teaspoons coriander
1 teaspoon sea salt
1 teaspoon black pepper
1/2 teaspoon cinnamon
1/2 teaspoon red pepper flakes

YIELD
4 1/2 tablespoons

ITALIAN SAUSAGE SPICE BLEND

1 teaspoon sea salt
1 tablespoon fennel seeds, ground
1 tablespoon ground sage
1 tablespoon garlic powder
1 tablespoon onion powder
¼ teaspoon white pepper
(or 1 teaspoon black pepper)
2 teaspoons dried parsley (optional)

YIELD
~5 tablespoons

Use 2 tablespoons per pound of meat to make sausage.

CURRY SPICE BLEND

1 tablespoon curry powder
1 tablespoon onion powder
1 tablespoon paprika
1/2 tablespoon cinnamon
1 tablespoon sea salt

YIELD
4 1/2 tablespoons

SAVORY SPICE BLEND

2 tablespoons Rosemary-Sage Salt
   (recipe on page 230)
1 tablespoon garlic powder
1 tablespoon onion powder
1/2 tablespoon paprika
1 teaspoon black pepper

YIELD
5 1/2 tablespoons

GREEK SPICE BLEND

2 tablespoons Lemon Salt (recipe on
   page 230)
2 tablespoons dried oregano
1 tablespoon garlic powder
2 teaspoons black pepper

YIELD
5 tablespoons

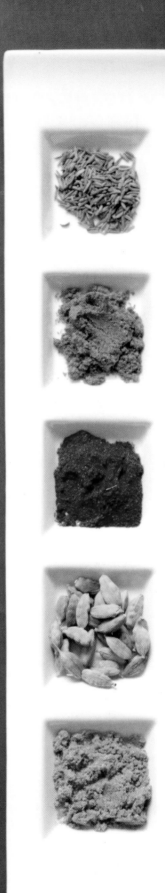

mineral-rich bone broth

There is nothing easier than making broth. It's as simple as boiling water, and making your own allows you to avoid food additives. With this recipe, you'll never buy boxed or canned broth/soup stock again.

PREP TIME
5 minutes

COOKING TIME
8-24 hours

YIELD
64 ounces of stock

SIDE NOTE

If you don't have a slow-cooker, you can use an enameled cast iron pot in a 300˚F oven or simmer in a pot on the stovetop on the lowest possible flame that allows a tiny bubble to consistently appear in the broth after you have brought it to a boil.

FODMAP FREE?

Make yours without the garlic.

NUTS

EGGS

NIGHTSHADES

FODMAPS

4 quarts filtered water
1 1/2 -2 lbs of bones (beef knuckle bones, marrow bones, meaty bones, chicken or turkey necks, chicken or turkey carcass bones, or any bones you have around)

2 tablespoons apple cider vinegar (organic, unfiltered such as Bragg's brand)
2 teaspoons (or to taste) unrefined sea salt (optional). I recommend Redmond Real Salt.
Cloves from 1 whole head of fresh garlic, peeled and smashed (optional)

Place all ingredients in a 6-quart slow-cooker and set heat to high. Bring the stock to a boil. Then, reduce the heat setting to low. Allow the stock to cook for a minimum of 8 hours and up to 24 hours. The longer it cooks, the better.

Turn off the crockpot and allow the stock to cool. Strain the stock through a fine mesh metal strainer or cheese cloth. Place the cooled stock into glass jars for storage in the refrigerator for a few days or the freezer for later use.

Before using the stock, chip away at the top and discard any fat that has solidified. You can drink the broth or use it as a base for soups, stews, or any recipe that calls for soup stock.

CHANGE IT UP

To make vegetable broth, combine 1 onion, 4 carrots, 2 stalks of celery, and 4 cloves of garlic chopped into ½-inch pieces, and boil, then simmer for 6 hours. Do not overcook vegetable broth, as it may become bitter.

herbal tea-infused gelatin cubes

If you're looking for some of the amazing gut-healing benefits of gelatin but want a change of pace from savory broth, make some herbal tea-infused gelatin. Use any tea you like with standard gelatin from the store, it's quite simple!

PREP TIME
10 minutes

COOKING TIME
10 minutes + set time

YIELD
Will vary with your gelatin.

TO YOUR TASTE

Make this with any kind of tea you like. Fruit teas may be an especially fun way to prepare this gelatin treat for kids!

NUTS

EGGS

NIGHTSHADES

FODMAPS

Water as noted on the package of your gelatin
1-2 tablespoons of herbal tea (or about 3-4 bags)

1 tablespoon honey (optional)
1 box of gelatin

Prepare water as called for on your package of gelatin mixture.

Steep your tea strainer (as pictured) or bags in the hot water along with the honey, then continue to prepare the gelatin as indicated.

Allow the gelatin to set in the refrigerator before cutting into cubes to serve.

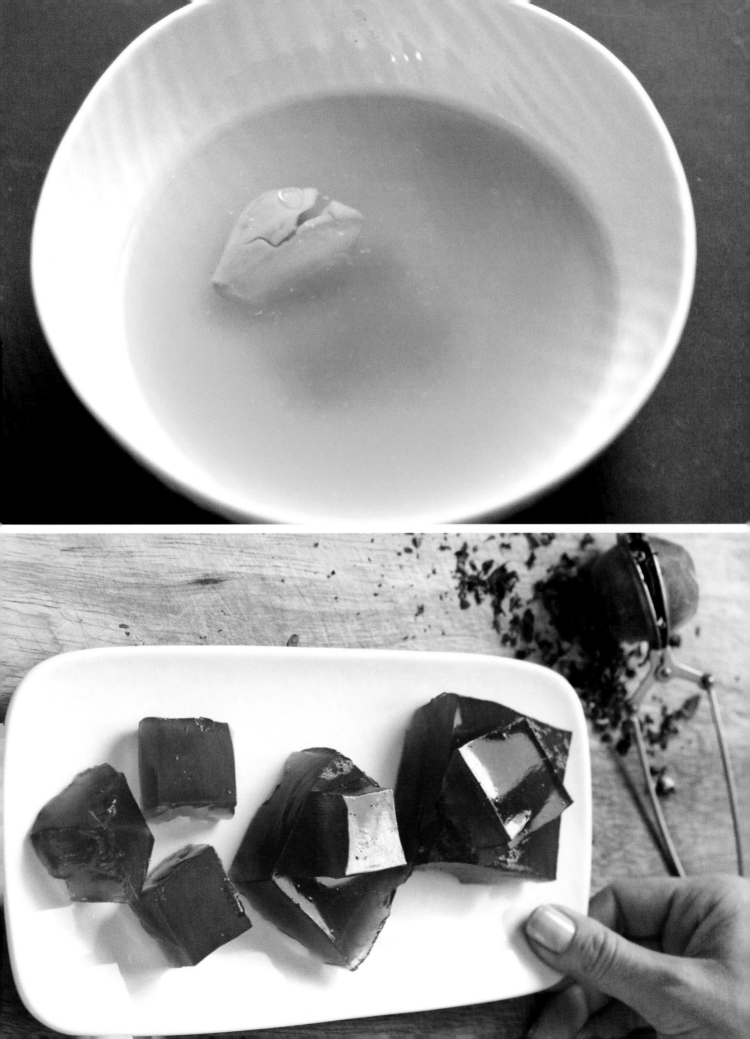

PREP TIME
5 minutes

COOKING TIME
20-30 minutes

YIELD
1 lb of bacon

QUALITY MATTERS

Try to buy bacon from a local farmer who pasture-raises pigs. Ask what the animals are being fed, and visit if you can to see their living conditions. Bacon is not inherently unhealthy, but copious amounts of feedlot pork are not good for you. See page 31 for more information on choosing quality meats.

NUTS

EGGS

NIGHTSHADES

FODMAPS

perfectly baked bacon

You may be surprised by the sparse appearance of bacon in the recipes in this book. I generally only bake it and serve it with sunny-side-up eggs and raw sauerkraut in the morning. It's worth the wait.

1 lb of pastured pork bacon
    (Use beef or lamb if you prefer;
    turkey bacon is not bacon.)

Preheat oven to 350° F. Place strips of bacon evenly onto an oven-safe baking rack positioned over a baking sheet (see photo). Bake until the strips are cooked to your liking, approximately 20-30 minutes depending on the thickness of the bacon.

If you are baking pastured pork bacon, it's a good idea to save the fat. Allow it to cool slightly, then pour it into a glass or ceramic container to store in the refrigerator for later use in recipes and as cooking fat.

CHANGE IT UP

You may also make this recipe in a toaster oven with a baking rack and tray if you're cooking a smaller portion at a time.

PREP TIME
-

COOKING TIME
20-30 minutes

YIELD
2 lbs of clarified butter
or ghee

BETTER BUTTER

There are several sources of grass-fed butter available in most grocery stores nationwide. Kerrygold is one brand that's pretty easy to find.

NUTS

EGGS

NIGHTSHADES

FODMAPS

clarified butter and ghee

Butter is an extremely nutrient-dense food that is loaded with vitamin D, vitamin A, and even vitamin K2. Still, many people cannot tolerate lactose, so clarifying grass-fed butter is a fantastic way to allow the nutrients to remain while the potentially irritating milk sugars and proteins are skimmed away.

2 lbs grass-fed/pastured butter

Place the butter in a medium-sized, heavy weight saucepan, and melt it slowly over low heat.

Allow the butter to simmer, and the milk solids will begin to float and become foamy at the top of the oil. Skim these milk solids off, and remove the butter from the heat. It is now clarified butter. Pour it through a cheese cloth to strain out the milk solids, and store it in a glass jar in the refrigerator for up to a month.

If you'd like to turn the clarified butter into ghee, allow the milk solids to continue to cook slowly until they become browned and begin to sink to the bottom of the pan. When there is no longer any material waiting to brown and sink to the bottom of the oil, the ghee is finished. Pour it through a cheese cloth to strain out the browned milk solids, and store it in a glass jar in the refrigerator for up to a month.

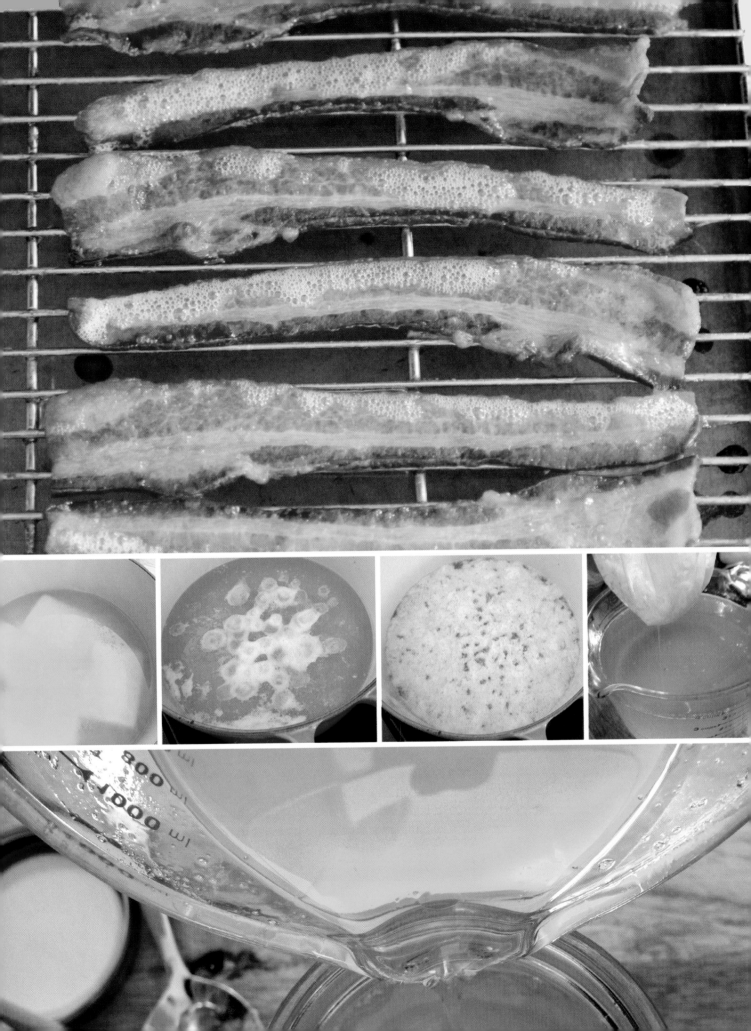

roasted jalapeño & garlic raw sauerkraut (probiotic)

PREP TIME
30 minutes

FERMENTING TIME
2-3 weeks

YIELD
Approximately
2, 32 ounce jars

CHANGE IT UP
Change the flavors by adding ginger or leave out the garlic and jalapeño and make a simple version with the addition of just 1 tablespoon of caraway seeds.

NIGHTSHADE FREE?
Make this recipe without the jalapeño pepper.

FODMAP FREE?
Make this recipe using shredded carrots only instead of the cabbage.

NUTS
EGGS
NIGHTSHADES
FODMAPS

Fermented foods are a must-have addition to your regular daily diet. The instructions here are detailed and seem complicated, but it's actually quite a simple process. Once you make this recipe, repeating it with your own twist will be a cinch! You'll need two, 32 ounce glass mason jars for the finished product.

1 large head of green cabbage,
   sliced into thin strips
   (set large outer leaves aside)
1-2 tablespoons of sea salt
2 large carrots, shredded

2-4 cloves of garlic, finely sliced
   (2 if large, 4 if smaller)
1-2 jalapeño peppers, roasted (see
   page 298 for instruction)
Black pepper to taste

Place 1/3 of your sliced cabbage into your large bowl and sprinkle 1 tablespoon of the salt over it. Using your hands, squeeze the cabbage until water begins to come out of it.

Repeat this process, adding the remaining cabbage and salt 1/3 at a time to the bowl. This will take time and elbow-grease, so be ready to get your hands involved.

Add the shredded carrots, garlic, jalapeños, and black pepper to the mixture and combine with your hands.

Fill two 32-ounce mason jars evenly, pressing the mixture down so that water releases and raises above the line of the vegetables with 2 inches of air-space remaining at the top.

Wedge the large outer leaves you had set aside into the top of the jars so that the mixture is pressed below and the water level raises above the leaf. A shot glass or ceramic or glass pinch-bowl serves nicely as additional weight to keep the mixture held securely down.

Set the filled jars aside in flat pan or dish with an edge so that if there is any spillover you keep it contained.

Store the jars in a secure, cool, dark-ish place where they will not be disturbed.

Check on your raw sauerkraut every day or two to make sure that the water level has remained above the vegetables and that no vegetables are coming into contact with air. The fermentation process happens under water, so if you see anything touching the surface, use a clean spoon to remove it. You may also see some growth or mold form around the top of the liquid—this is normal, but it's best to remove it when you see it. If you need to add liquid to the jars, add some fresh water to make sure that everything is below the water line. The weights should help a lot with this.

Allow the sauerkraut to sit for at least 2 weeks and taste it periodically.

Once the sauerkraut tastes as you like it, place the lid on the jar and store it in the refrigerator. It will last for several months while refrigerated and will not continue to ferment further.

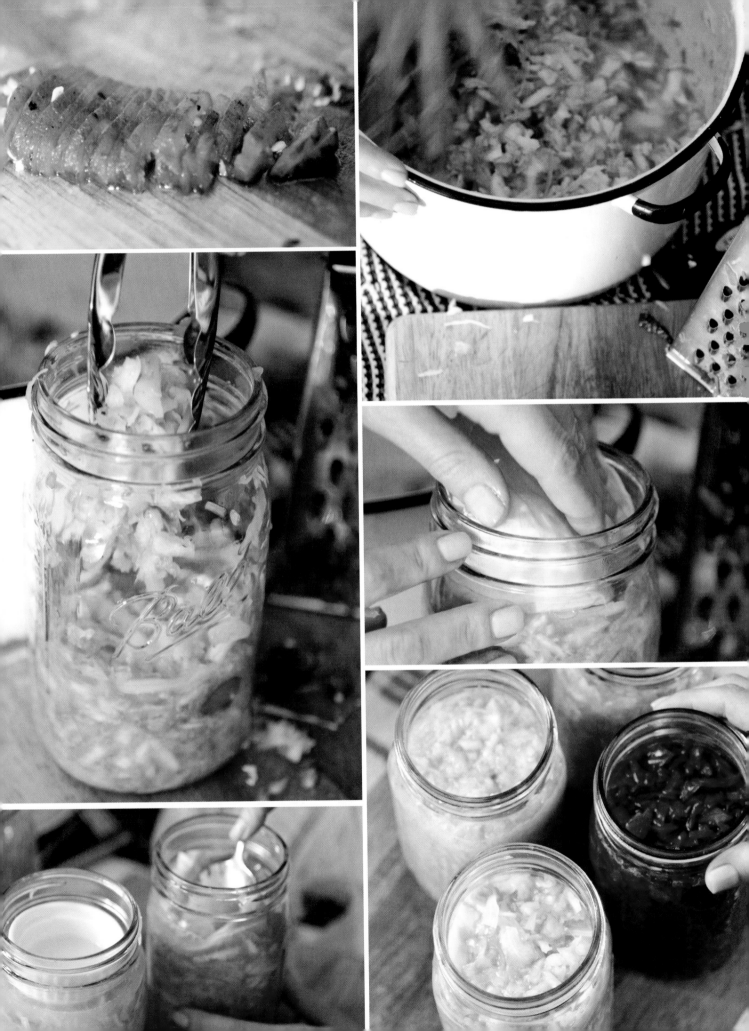

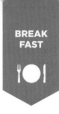
swirly crustless quiche

PREP TIME
20 minutes

COOKING TIME
45 minutes

YIELD
Makes 6 servings

CHANGE IT UP
For the athletes out there, try adding shredded sweet potato to this recipe for an added kick of "Good Carbs."

NUTS
EGGS
NIGHTSHADES
FODMAPS

This is a great go-to recipe that you can freeze and reheat in a toaster oven. Try using different types of vegetables and spices to change the flavors each time you make it. If you have ground meat on hand, turn it into Italian Sausage using the Spice Blend recipe on page 232, and mix it into this recipe.

1 large zucchini, shredded or grated
   and strained
2 large carrots, shredded or grated
1 teaspoon Rosemary-Sage Salt
   (recipe on page 230) (optional)

12 eggs, beaten
1 tablespoon butter, bacon grease,
   or coconut oil

Preheat oven to 375°F.

Strain the zucchini with a cheese cloth or strainer bag. (This step isn't absolutely necessary, but will help to yield a better consistency in your quiche.)

Mix together the zucchini, carrots, Rosemary-Sage Salt, and eggs in a large bowl, and then set aside.

Grease a 9 inch x 13 inch baking dish with butter, and pour the egg mixture into the pan. For a swirled effect, use a fork to create a circular pattern before baking.

Bake for approximately 45 minutes or until the edges are brown. The quiche will puff up while baking and then deflate when removed from the oven.

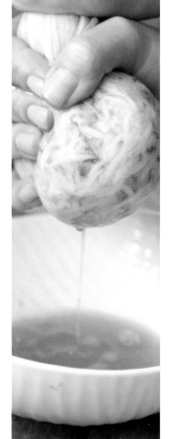

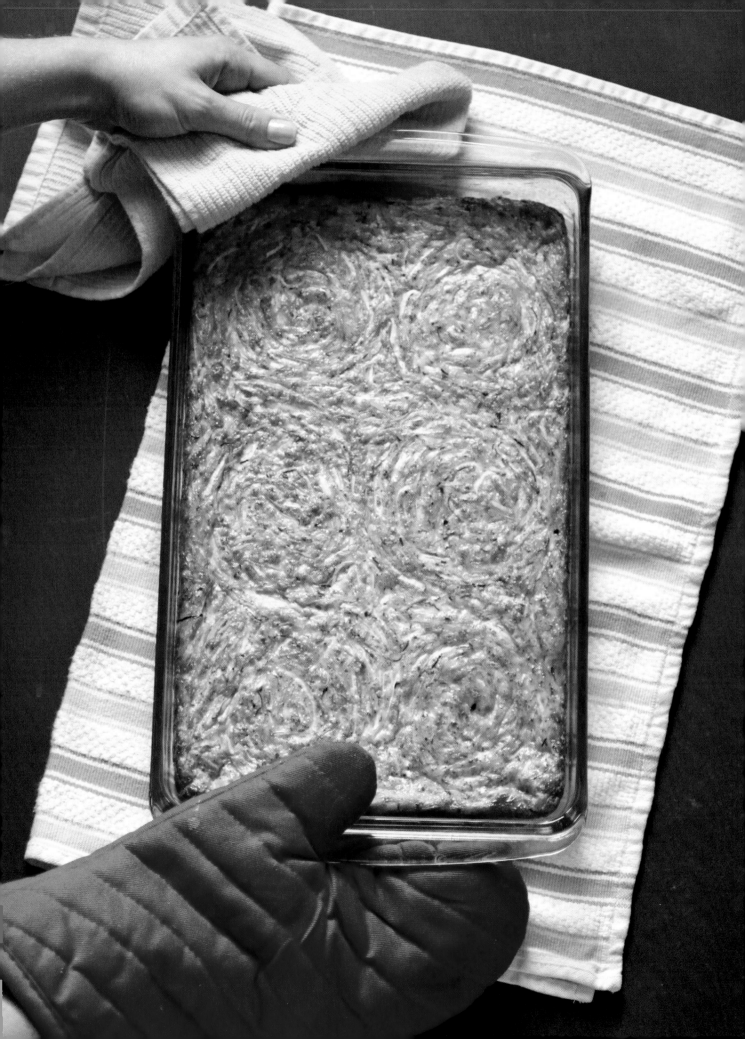

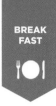
pumpkin pancakes

PREP TIME
10 minutes

COOKING TIME
20 minutes

YIELD
Approximately 8 small
pancakes or 2 servings

When fall rolls around, it seems only natural to want to make as many recipes as possible that use pumpkin! This is a quick and easy way to take an inexpensive ingredient (canned pumpkin) and turn it into something delicious.

CHANGE IT UP

Instead of adding maple syrup to sweeten this recipe, try adding a mashed, whole ripe banana to the mixture. If you add a banana, the yield will increase.

4 eggs
1/2 cup canned pumpkin
1 teaspoon pure vanilla extract
2 tablespoons pure maple syrup
   (optional)

1 teaspoon pumpkin pie spice
1 teaspoon cinnamon
1/4 teaspoon baking soda
2 tablespoons butter or coconut oil
   (plus extra for pan frying)

Whisk the eggs, canned pumpkin, pure vanilla extract, and pure maple syrup together. Sift the pumpkin pie spice, cinnamon, and baking soda into the wet ingredients.

Melt 2 tablespoons of butter in a large skillet over medium heat. Then, mix the butter into the batter.

Grease the skillet and spoon the batter into the skillet to make pancakes of your desired size. When a few bubbles appear, flip the pancakes once to finish cooking.

Serve with grass-fed butter and cinnamon or sliced bananas.

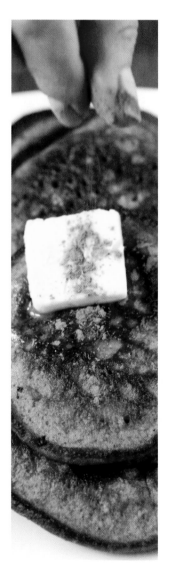

NUTS
EGGS
NIGHTSHADES
FODMAPS

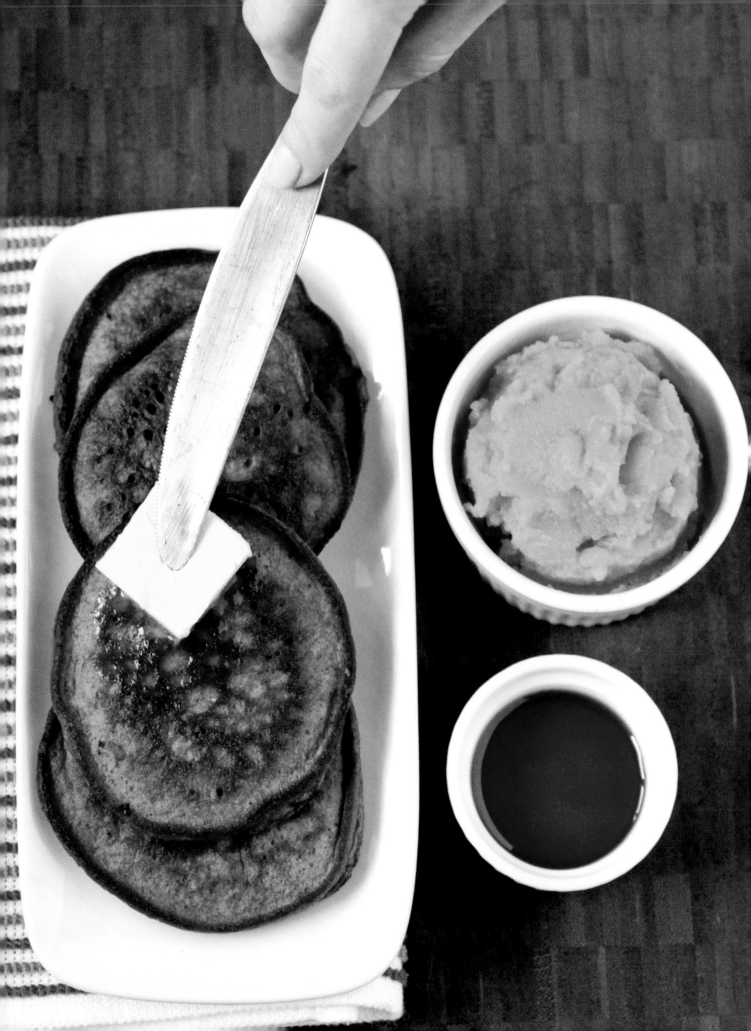

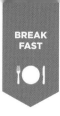
carrot gingerbread muffins

PREP TIME
20 minutes

COOKING TIME
35-40 minutes

YIELD
12-18 muffins

CHANGE IT UP
*The frosting recipe can
be modified and used
for other muffins as
well. Use lemon zest
instead of orange and
top the Blueberry Lemon
Muffins on page 246;
or, leave it as-is and top
the Pumpkin Cranberry
Muffins with it.*

NUTS
EGGS
NIGHTSHADES
FODMAPS

These muffins are a fantastic way to sneak some veggies into a treat. Each one contains about 1/4 cup of carrots, while the spiciness of the gingerbread is an indulgence.

6 eggs
1/2 cup butter or coconut oil
1 teaspoon pure vanilla extract
1/2 cup blackstrap molasses
1/4 cup grade B maple syrup
1/2 cup coconut flour
1/2 teaspoon sea salt
1/4 teaspoon baking soda
1 teaspoon cinnamon
1 teaspoon ginger
1/2 teaspoon ground cloves
3 cups carrots, shredded
1/2 cup raisins (optional)

FROSTING (OPTIONAL)
1/4 cup coconut butter
1/4 cup coconut oil
1/4 teaspoon of freshly grated
    ginger
1 tablespoon orange zest
1 tablespoon shredded coconut
1 tablespoon maple syrup

Preheat oven to 350°F.

Whisk the eggs, butter or coconut oil, pure vanilla extract, molasses, and maple syrup together in a large mixing bowl. Sift in the coconut flour, sea salt, baking soda, cinnamon, ginger, and ground cloves. Next add in the carrots and raisins (if using) and combine together.

In a muffin tin, scoop 1/4 cup of the batter into each lined muffin container (natural parchment muffin papers work best for lining), and bake for 35-40 minutes.

Combine all frosting ingredients until smooth. Allow the muffins to cool slightly before frosting.

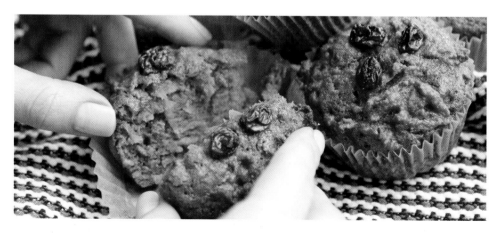

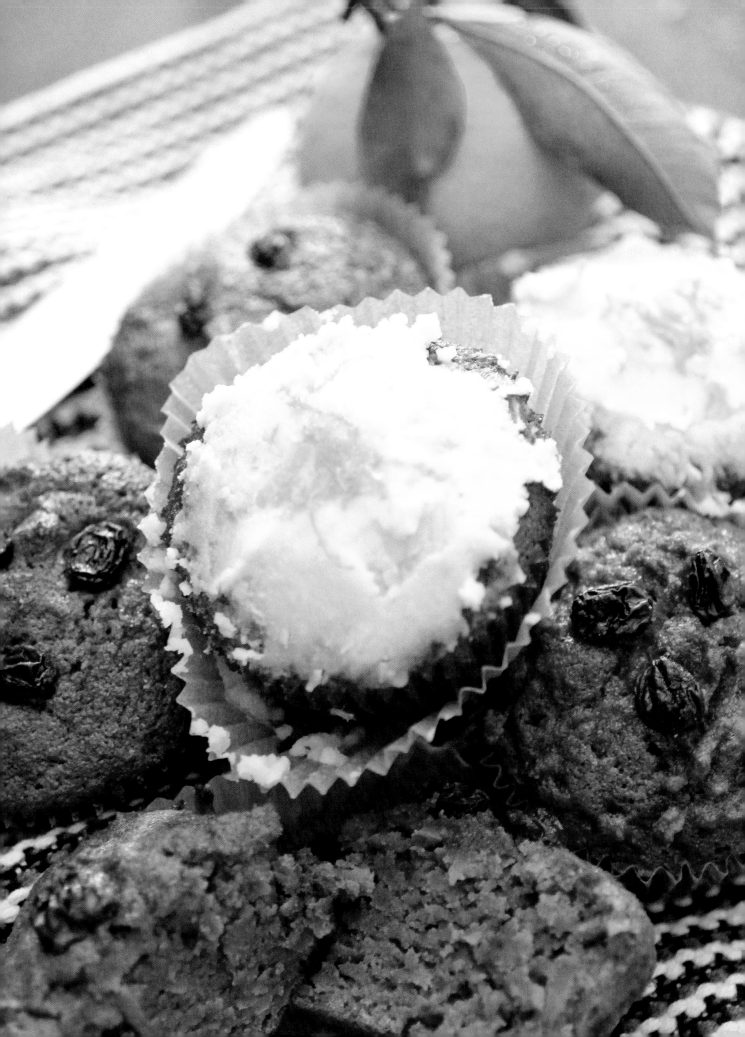

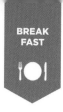
blueberry lemon muffins

If you love blueberries, these are the treat for you—they're packed with a fresh burst of the blue gems!

PREP TIME
15 minutes

COOKING TIME
35-40 minutes

YIELD
12 muffins

CHANGE IT UP
For standard blueberry muffins, leave out the lemon juice & zest.

NUTS

EGGS

NIGHTSHADES

FODMAPS

6 eggs
1/2 cup butter or coconut oil, melted
1 teaspoon pure vanilla extract
1/4 cup grade B maple syrup
1 lemon, juice and zest

1/2 cup coconut flour
1/2 teaspoon sea salt
1/4 teaspoon baking soda
1 cup fresh blueberries

Preheat oven to 350˚F.

Whisk the eggs, butter or coconut oil, pure vanilla extract, maple syrup, lemon juice, and lemon zest together in a large mixing bowl. Sift in the coconut flour, sea salt, and baking soda, and stir until well combined. Gently fold in the blueberries.

In a muffin tin, scoop 1/4 cup of the batter into each lined muffin cup (natural parchment muffin papers work best for lining), and bake for 35-40 minutes.

pumpkin cranberry muffins

This recipe is sure to be a fall-favorite in your house, and it's a great way to use up canned pumpkin. For an extra cranberry pop, spread Simple Cranberry Sauce (recipe on page 388) on top.

PREP TIME
15 minutes

COOKING TIME
35-40 minutes

YIELD
12 muffins

CHANGE IT UP
If fresh cranberries aren't in season, add chopped walnuts instead.

NUTS

EGGS

NIGHTSHADES

FODMAPS

6 eggs
1/4 cup canned pumpkin
1/2 cup butter or coconut oil, melted
1 teaspoon pure vanilla extract
1/4 cup grade B maple syrup

1/2 cup coconut flour
1/2 teaspoon sea salt
1/4 teaspoon baking soda
1 tablespoon pumpkin pie spice
1/2 cup fresh cranberries

Preheat oven to 350˚F.

Whisk the eggs, pumpkin, butter or coconut oil, pure vanilla extract, and maple syrup together in a large mixing bowl. Sift in the coconut flour, sea salt, baking soda, and pumpkin pie spice and stir until well combined. Gently fold in the cranberries.

In a muffin tin, scoop 1/4 cup of the batter into each lined muffin cup (natural parchment muffin papers work best for lining), and bake for 35-40 minutes.

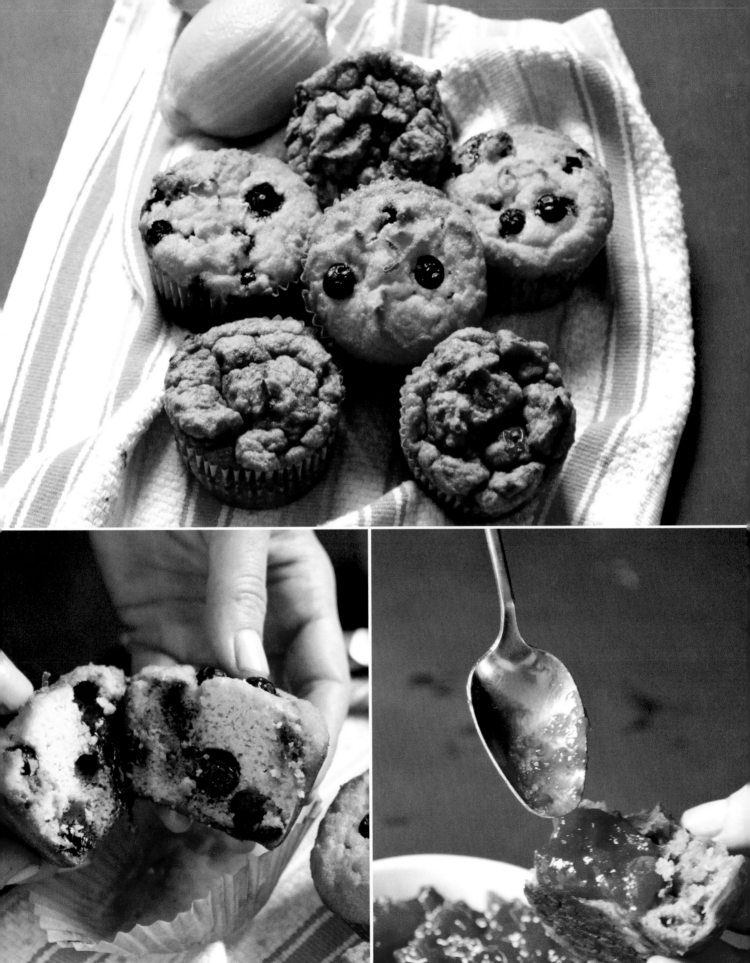

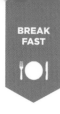

PREP TIME
20 minutes

COOKING TIME
20 minutes

YIELD
4 servings

SERVE IT UP

*With sliced cucumber
or celery sticks.*

NUTS
EGGS
NIGHTSHADES
FODMAPS

bacon & egg salad

*Egg salad is an old favorite of mine, but commercial mayonnaise is out of the
question when you're avoiding refined seed oils. This take on a classic uses
Baconnaise (recipe on page 390) and gets that bacon-y taste right into the dish.*

12 eggs
1/4 cup Baconnaise
    (recipe on page 390)
Sea salt and black pepper to taste

12 slices of bacon, chopped
2 tablespoons fresh chives,
    chopped (optional)

Take eggs out of the refrigerator, and allow them to come to room temperature.
Fill a large pot with 8 cups of water, and bring it to a boil.

Place the eggs in the boiling water for 10 minutes. Remove the eggs, and place
them in a large bowl with ice water for 10 minutes. This will keep them from
turning green around the yolk.

Peel the eggs, place them in a bowl, and mash them with a potato masher or
large fork. Mix in the Baconnaise, sea salt, black pepper, chopped bacon, and
chopped chives.

PREP TIME
10 minutes

COOKING TIME
20 minutes

YIELD
Approximately 8 small
pancakes or 2 servings

SIDE NOTE

*A food processor makes
this recipe super quick
and easy.*

NUTS
EGGS
NIGHTSHADES
FODMAPS

zucchini pancakes

*Looking for a pancake recipe that's savory instead of sweet? Look no further!
Make extra to reheat anytime or eat them cold the next day.*

3 eggs
1 tablespoon coconut flour
Sea salt and black pepper to taste
2 cups shredded zucchini (using
    a food processor with a shred-
    ding disc is ideal, or by hand)

Coconut oil or bacon grease for
    pan frying (amount will vary)

Beat the eggs with the coconut flour, sea salt, and black pepper. Mix in the
shredded zucchini until well combined.

Add about 1/8 inch of coconut oil to a large skillet over medium-low heat. Spoon
the mixture into the skillet in "cakes" that are approximately 4-6 inches in diameter.

Cook until they hold together, flipping once as you would a standard pancake.

Serve warm or at room temperature.

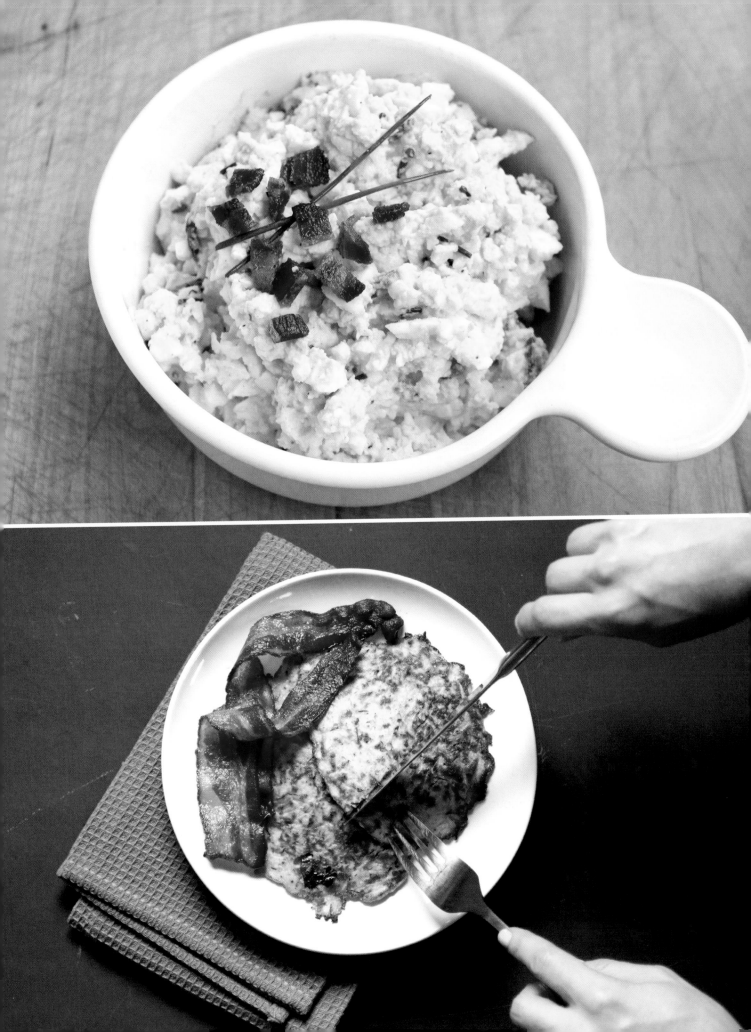

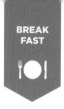
vanilla-almond sponge bread

PREP TIME
10 minutes

COOKING TIME
40 minutes

YIELD
6 servings

If you're looking for a basic morning bread replacement, this might be for you! Eat it plain, fresh out of the oven, or toast it with some extra butter and cinnamon. You can also use it to make a grain-free French toast. This pan-bread can also be flavored easily with the juice and zest of a lemon or orange.

SERVE IT UP

With berries, sliced bananas, or some almond butter smeared on top.

CHANGE IT UP

Try making this a more savory loaf by adding some Rosemary or Sage Salt to the mixture—about 1 teaspoon should do the trick!

6 eggs
Seeds from 1/4 pod of vanilla bean
1 teaspoon vanilla extract
2 tablespoons butter, melted
2 tablespoons full-fat coconut milk

1/4 cup coconut flour
Pinch of nutmeg
Pinch of sea salt
1/2 teaspoon baking soda
2 tablespoons sliced almonds

Preheat oven to 350°F.

Whisk eggs, vanilla bean, vanilla extract, butter, and coconut milk in a large mixing bowl. Sift coconut flour, nutmeg, salt, and baking soda into the egg mixture, and continue whisking until combined.

Pour the egg mixture into a 9 inch x 9 inch baking dish lined with parchment paper. Top with sliced almonds, and bake for approximately 40 minutes or until the edges are brown and a toothpick wipes clean when testing the center.

NUTS
EGGS
NIGHTSHADES
FODMAPS

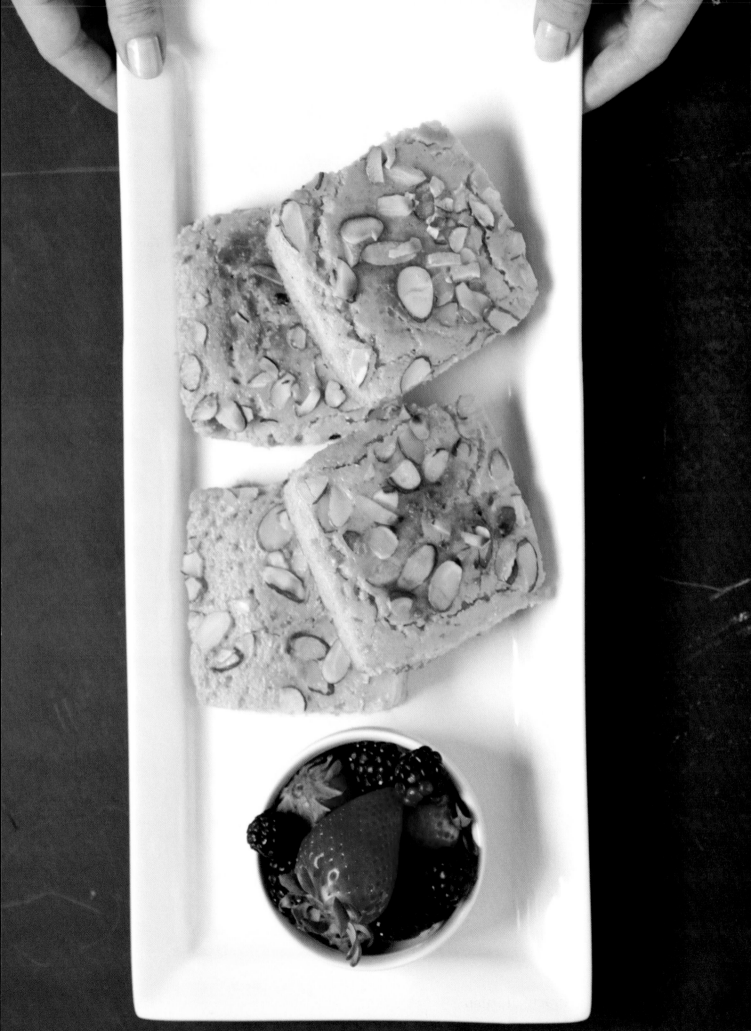

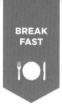
grain-free porridge, 2-ways

If you miss having a warm bowl of cereal in the morning, try these alternatives.

PREP TIME
10 minutes

COOKING TIME
10 minutes

YIELD
One large serving

SIDE NOTE
Play with combining different types of nut butter in this recipe!

NUTS
EGGS
NIGHTSHADES
FODMAPS

COCO-NUTTY
2 tablespoons almond butter
1/4 cup shredded coconut
6 tablespoons warm water
  or coconut milk (full-fat)
1/4 teaspoon vanilla extract
1/2 teaspoon cinnamon
1 teaspoon raw honey or maple
  syrup (optional)

PUMPKIN TAHINI (NUT-FREE)
1 tablespoon tahini
  (raw or roasted)
1/2 cup canned pumpkin
1/4 cup warm water
1/4 teaspoon vanilla extract
1/4 teaspoon cinnamon
1 tablespoon shredded coconut
1 tablespoon raisins
1 teaspoon raw honey or maple

Combine all ingredients in a small mixing bowl.

Transfer to a sauce pan, and heat over a low flame until it reaches your desired temperature.

pesto scrambled eggs

Spruce up your basic scrambled eggs with some pesto (recipe on page 308).

PREP TIME
5 minutes

COOKING TIME
3 minutes

YIELD
4 scrambled eggs

SIDE NOTE
You can also top fried or hard boiled eggs with pesto—yum!

NUTS
EGGS
NIGHTSHADES
FODMAPS

1 tablespoon of butter
  or coconut oil
4 eggs

1-2 tablespoons of pesto
  (recipe on page 308)

Melt the butter in a skillet over medium heat.

Crack the eggs directly into the pan, then scramble them slowly—combining the yolks and white loosely so that the color variation is still visible between the two. I recommend a heat-resistant silicone spatula for this process.

About one minute into cooking, add the pesto to the pan and continue to scramble the eggs, mixing the pesto in gently.

Once the eggs are no longer runny, they are done.

Serve with extra pesto and a side of Perfectly Baked Bacon (recipe on page 236).

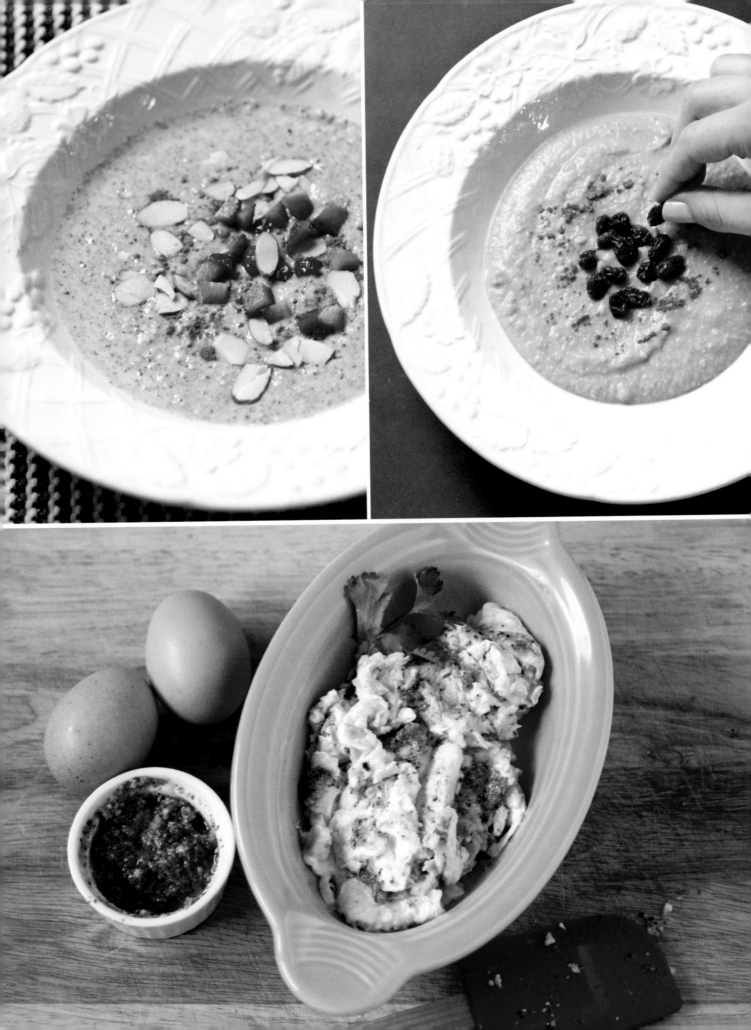

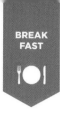
apple streusel egg muffins

PREP TIME
15 minutes

COOKING TIME
40 minutes

YIELD
12 muffins

SIDE NOTE
For more sweetness, add a couple of chopped, dried medjool dates to the apples as they cook.

FODMAP FREE?
Make this recipe with 2 chopped bananas instead of apples!

I wanted a breakfast made only from whole ingredients, yet still felt like a treat—the result was Apple Streusel Egg Muffins. You can easily make a savory version of egg muffins by using the recipe and ingredients for my Swirly Crustless Quiche (recipe on page 240) and baking them as noted here.

3 large green apples, chopped into 1/2 inch pieces (approximately 2 cups)
3 tablespoons warm water
2 teaspoons cinnamon, divided
9 eggs

1 1/2 tablespoon butter or coconut oil, melted
3 tablespoons coconut milk
1 1/2 tablespoons coconut flour
1/4 teaspoon baking soda
Pinch of sea salt

Preheat oven to 350˚F.

In a medium skillet, sauté the apples, water, and 1 1/2 teaspoon of the cinnamon until the apples are the consistency of chunky applesauce or apple pie filling. Allow the mixture to cool before combining with the egg mixture.

CHANGE IT UP
Substitute lightly cooked pears or bananas instead of apples.

Add 1/4 cup of chopped nuts or coconut for texture and healthy fats.

In a medium-sized mixing bowl, whisk the eggs, butter, coconut milk, coconut flour, 1/2 teaspoon of cinnamon, baking soda, and salt until well combined. Add the cooled apples, reserving 1/4 cup for a garnish.

Spoon egg and apple mixture into lined muffin tins—1/4 cup each. Gently spoon about one teaspoon of the remaining apple mixture onto the top of each muffin.

Bake for 40 minutes.

NUTS
EGGS
NIGHTSHADES
FODMAPS

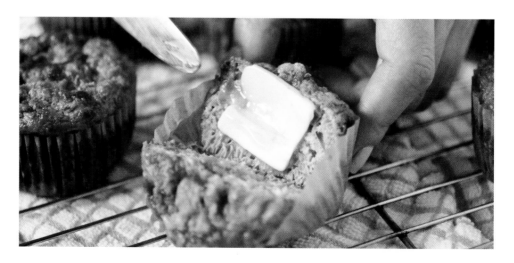

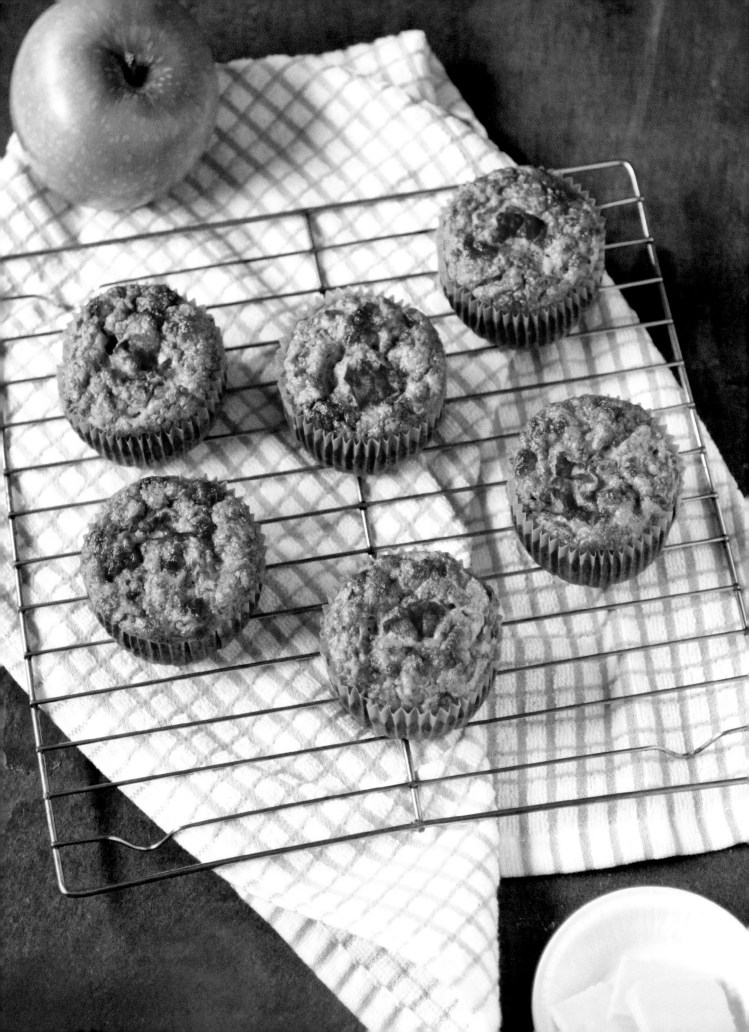

citrus & herb
whole roasted chicken

PREP TIME
10 minutes

COOKING TIME
60-120 minutes

YIELD
4-6 servings depending
on portion sizes

One of the easiest ways to save money on protein is to buy whole animals, and chickens are no exception. Several people can eat a whole chicken for dinner, and the carcass can be used to make bone broth.

CHANGE IT UP
Use any of the spice blends on pages 232-233 to make a totally new kind of bird.

1/4 cup melted butter, coconut oil, bacon grease, or duck fat
1 whole chicken
1 onion, cut into large chunks
4-6 cloves of garlic, smashed
1 orange or lemon, cut into 6 pieces

2-4 large carrots, cut into large chunks
1 tablespoon Herb Salt Blend (recipe on page 230)
Black pepper to taste

FODMAP FREE?
Leave out the garlic and onion.

Preheat the oven to 375°F.

Brush the bottom of a large roasting pan with some of the melted butter.

Remove any gizzards or organs (sometimes in a paper or plastic wrapping) from the inside of the chicken. Stuff the chicken with the onions, garlic, and some of the citrus. Place the carrots around the chicken in the roasting pan. Brush the chicken with melted butter, and sprinkle it with the Herb Salt Blend and black pepper.

Roast until the chicken reaches 165°F when a thermometer is placed between the leg and breast.

Cooking time depends on the size of the bird but is approximately 20 minutes per pound.

NUTS
EGGS
NIGHTSHADES
FODMAPS

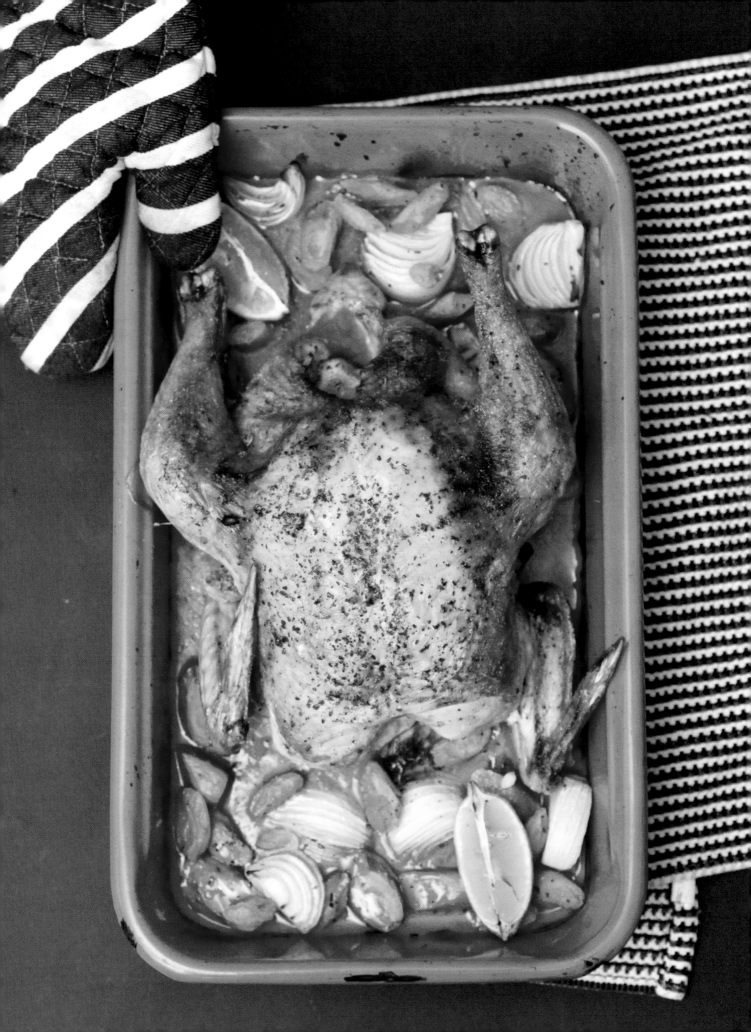

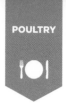

chicken wings, two-ways

You can still have perfect party foods without rolling them in flour and frying them. Instead, bake your chicken wings! You can even make them just one at a time. They're great on their own, but even better with dipping sauces.

PREP TIME
10 minutes

COOKING TIME
30 minutes

YIELD
2 dozen wings

NIGHTSHADE FREE?
Make only the Pineapple Teriyaki version.

NUTS
EGGS
NIGHTSHADES
FODMAPS

SMOKY WINGS
1 dozen chicken wings
2 tablespoons melted coconut oil, bacon fat, or palm oil
2 tablespoons Smoky Spice Blend (recipe on page 232)

Preheat oven to 375°F.

Divide the wings into two mixing bowls. Toss half of them in coconut oil and Smoky Spice Blend. Toss the other half in the Pineapple Teriyaki, onion powder, salt, and black pepper.

Place the chicken in an oven-safe dish, and bake for approximately 30 minutes or until the it reaches an internal temperature of 165°F

Serve the Smoky wings with Roasted Garlic Aioli, and serve the Pineapple Teriyaki with the remaining 1/4 cup of Teriyaki sauce.

FOR DIPPING
1/4 cup Roasted Garlic Aioli (recipe below)

PINEAPPLE TERIYAKI WINGS
1 dozen chicken wings
1/2 cup Pineapple Teriyaki Sauce divided, (recipe on page 390)
2 tablespoons onion powder
1/2 teaspoon sea salt
1/2 teaspoon black pepper

roasted garlic aioli

This is a combination of two recipes that makes a great dip or sauce.

PREP TIME
5 minutes

COOKING TIME
-

YIELD
1/2 cup

SIDE NOTE
Use this in place of plain mayonnaise in any recipe for a flavor-boost!

NUTS
EGGS
NIGHTSHADES
FODMAPS

1/2 cup Baconnaise (recipe on page 390)
6 cloves of Red Roasted Garlic (recipe on page 370)

Whisk the Baconnaise and Red Roasted Garlic together in a small mixing bowl.

Serve at room temperature or chilled.

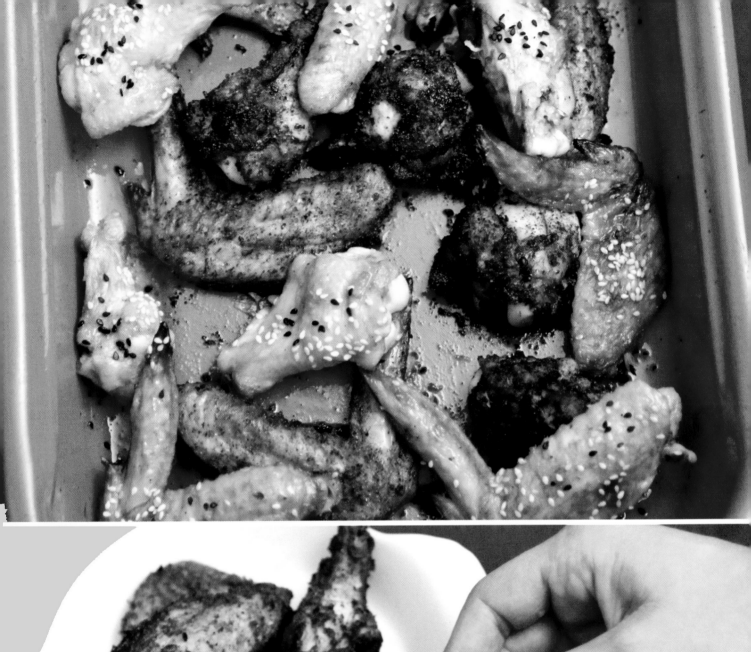
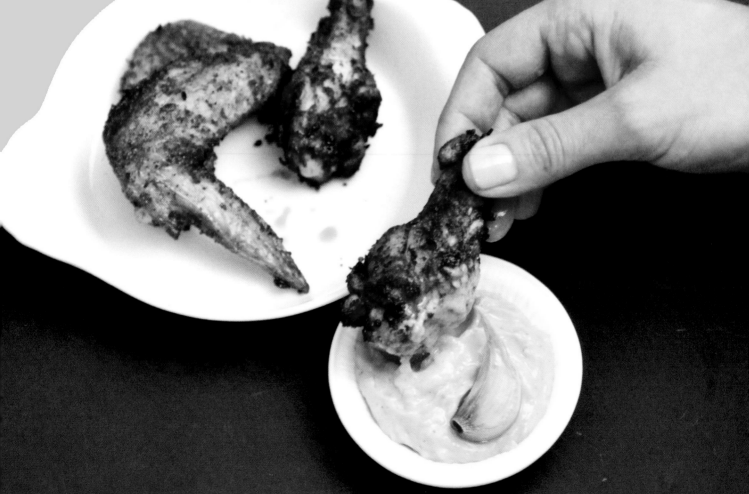

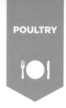
lemon & artichoke chicken

PREP TIME
10 minutes

COOKING TIME
50 minutes

YIELD
4 servings

FODMAP FREE?
Omit the shallots/onions, and replace the artichoke hearts with thinly sliced carrots or parsnips.

This is a twist on a classic chicken piccata using whole, bone-in, skin-on cuts, and it carries all of the flavor with none of the flour! This is sure to be a weeknight dinner go-to favorite for your family.

4 tablespoons butter, ghee, or coconut oil, divided
2 shallots or 1/4 of one onion, sliced
2 cups artichoke hearts, thawed and/or drained and rinsed

1/4 cup capers, drained
Juice of 2 lemons
2 lbs bone-in, skin-on chicken
Sea salt and black pepper to taste

Preheat oven to 375 ˚ F.

In a large, oven-safe skillet over medium heat, melt 2 tablespoons of butter. Add the shallots, and sauté them until they are translucent. Add the artichoke hearts, capers, and lemon juice. Stir to combine.

Place the chicken pieces in the skillet, and top each piece with a small pat of the remaining 2 tablespoons of butter. Place the entire skillet into the oven for 45 minutes or until the chicken reaches an internal temperature of 165 ˚ F.

CHANGE IT UP
You can make this recipe with whole chicken legs, bone-in, skin-on chicken breasts, or a whole chicken.

NUTS
EGGS
NIGHTSHADES
FODMAPS

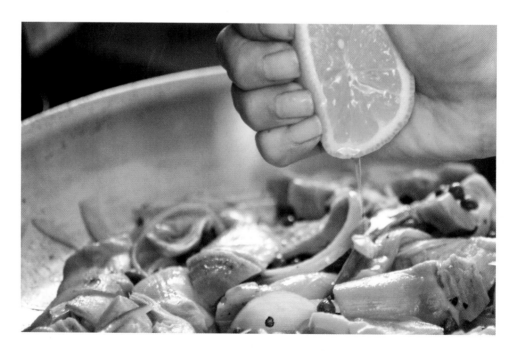

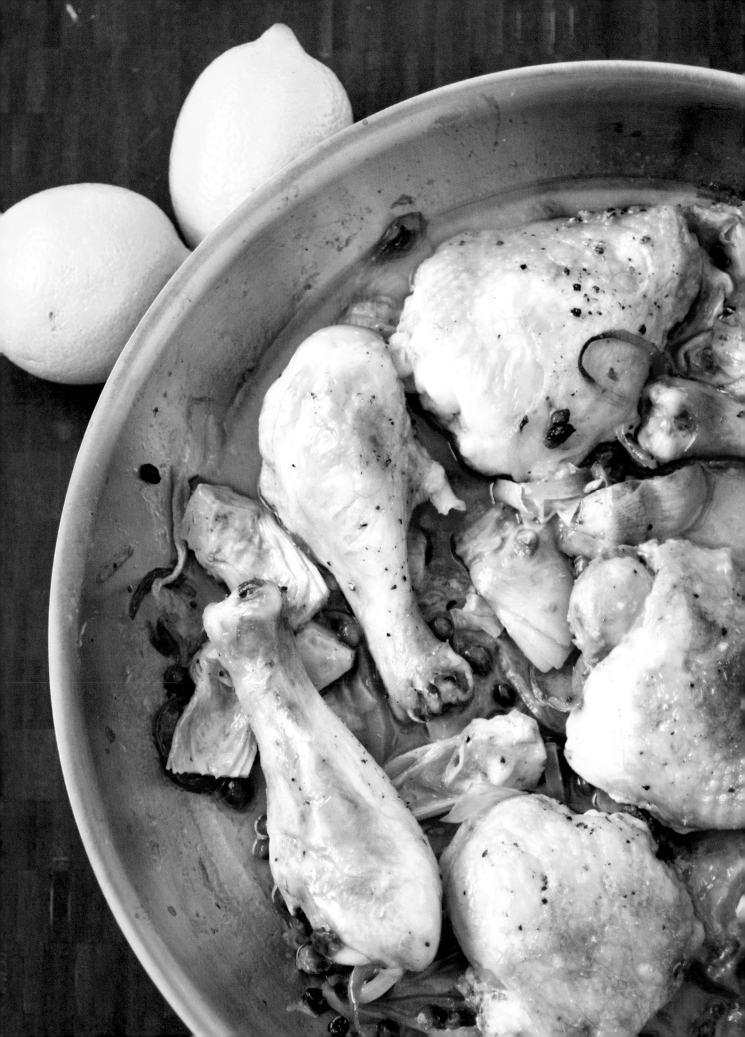

bacon-wrapped
smoky chicken thighs

PREP TIME
10 minutes

COOKING TIME
40 minutes

YIELD
4 chicken thighs
(2 servings)

What do you do when you get home with a pack of bone-in chicken thighs, only to discover that you accidentally bought the skinless ones? Wrap them in bacon! Add my Smoky Spice Blend and you have a delicious dish.

4 bone-in, skinless chicken thighs
8 slices of bacon

2 teaspoons Smoky Spice Blend
(recipe on page 232)

Preheat oven to 375°F.

Sprinkle the chicken thighs with 1 teaspoon of Smoky Spice Blend. Wrap each thigh in 2 strips of bacon. Sprinkle the chicken with the remaining Smoky Spice Blend, and bake for approximately 40 minutes or until the internal temperature of the chicken reaches 165°F.

NIGHTSHADE FREE?

Instead of the Smoky Spice Blend, try the Savory Spice Blend.

CHANGE IT UP

Try this recipe with pork tenderloin instead of chicken thighs. Simply follow the same instructions but bake the tenderloin until it reaches an internal temperature of 145°F (should be approximately 30-40 minutes).

NUTS
EGGS
NIGHTSHADES
FODMAPS

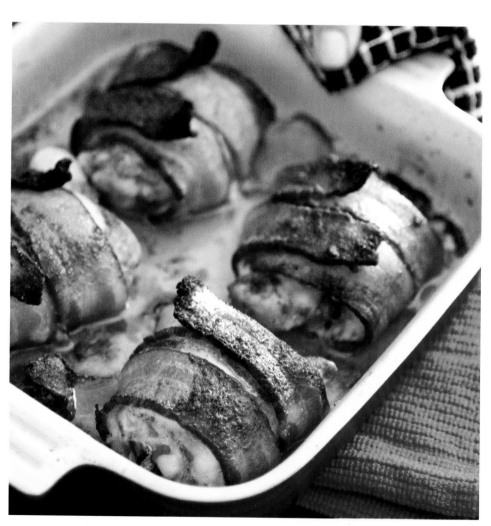

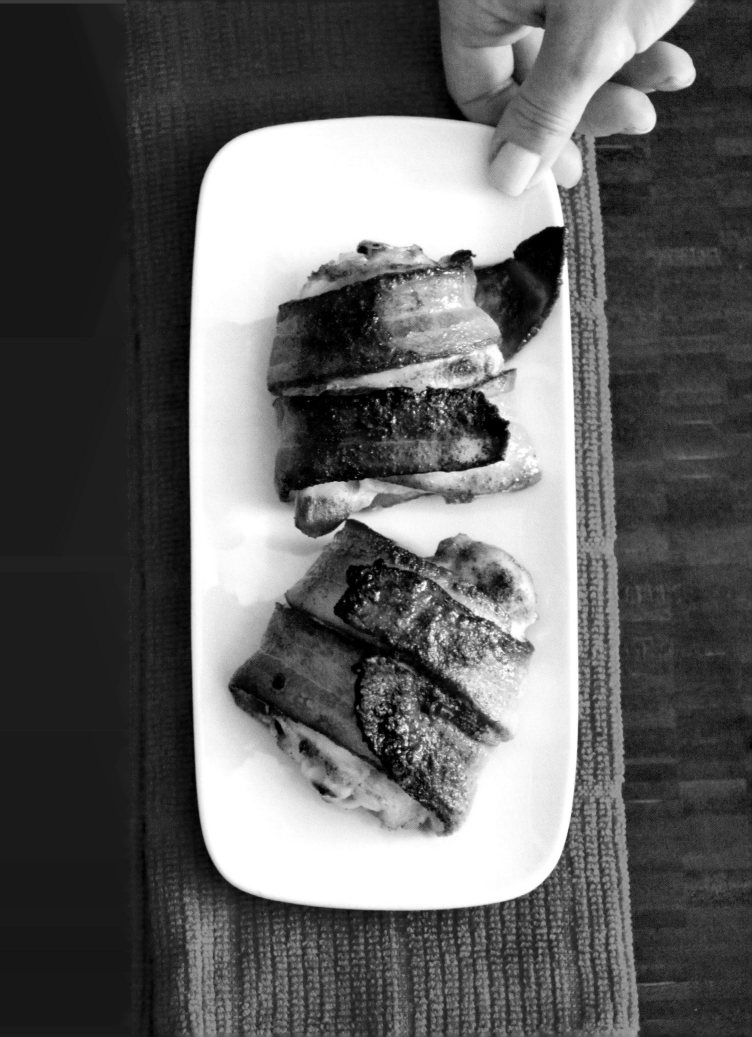

savory baked chicken legs

PREP TIME
5 minutes

COOKING TIME
45-60 minutes

YIELD
6 chicken legs (3-6 servings)

I love the ease and versatility of baked chicken. By using melted cooking fat and whatever spices you like, there are endless possibilities. To simplify things even further, I recommend that you choose one of the spice blend recipes to top the chicken legs.

6 chicken legs
1-2 tablespoons melted butter, ghee, bacon fat, or coconut oil

2 tablespoons of the spice blend of your choice
(recipes on pages 232-233)

NIGHTSHADE FREE?
Use only nightshade-free spice blends.

FODMAP FREE?
Use only FODMAP-free spice blends.

Preheat oven to 375˚F.

Place the chicken legs onto a baking sheet or into an oven-safe dish, and brush them with melted butter. Sprinkle the spice blend evenly over the chicken legs.

Bake for 45-60 minutes or until a thermometer reads 165˚F when inserted into the center of one of the chicken legs.

Pictured: Smoky Blend and Savory Blend.

CHANGE IT UP
Substitute bone-in, skin-on chicken breasts if you don't have chicken legs.

Serve with a simple green salad or with Roasted Rosemary Roots (recipe on page 350).

NUTS
EGGS
NIGHTSHADES
FODMAPS

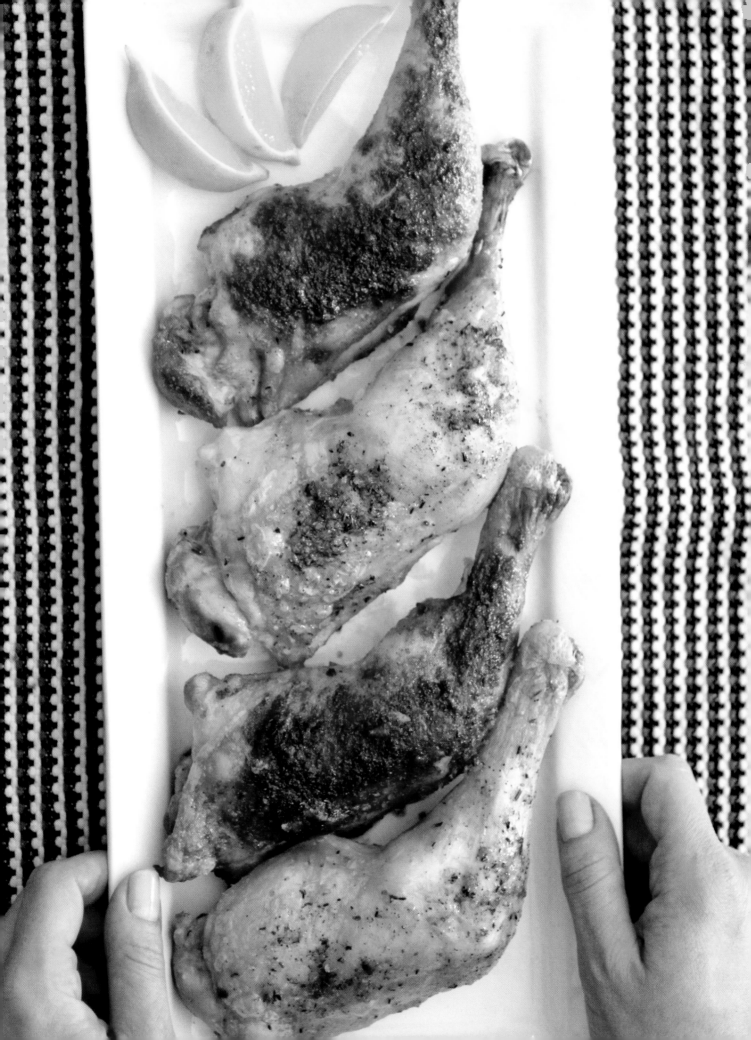

mustard glazed chicken thighs

PREP TIME
5 minutes

COOKING TIME
45 minutes

YIELD
12 chicken thighs
(4-6 servings)

SIDE NOTE
These are fantastic reheated in the oven or toaster-oven, and they make a delicious, mild breakfast as well.

Honey mustard is easily recreated without any sweetener when it's made with healthy fats like butter or coconut oil. Use whichever you like best, or try mixing the two.

1/4 cup melted butter
 or coconut oil
2 tablespoons gluten-free mustard
Black pepper to taste

1 teaspoon Sage Salt (recipe on page 230) or 1/2 teaspoon sea salt + 1/2 teaspoon dried sage
12 bone-in, skin-on chicken thighs

Preheat oven to 425°F.

In a small mixing bowl, combine the melted butter, mustard, black pepper, and Sage Salt. Place the chicken thighs on a baking sheet or oven-safe dish, and brush the mixture evenly over each one.

Bake for 45 minutes or until a thermometer reads 165°F when inserted into the center of one of the chicken thighs.

CHANGE IT UP
Use bone-in, skin-on chicken breasts if you don't have chicken thighs. Serve with Butternut Squash & Kumquats (recipe on page 360) or Mashed Faux-Tatoes (recipe on page 344).

NUTS

EGGS

NIGHTSHADES

FODMAPS

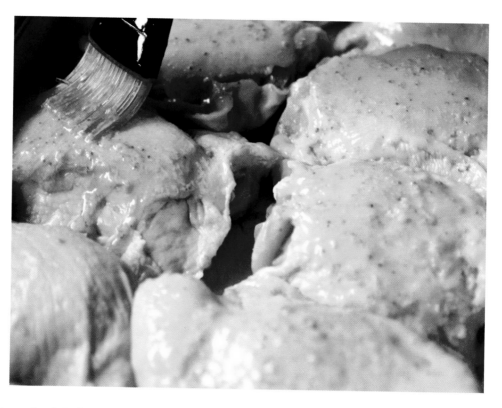

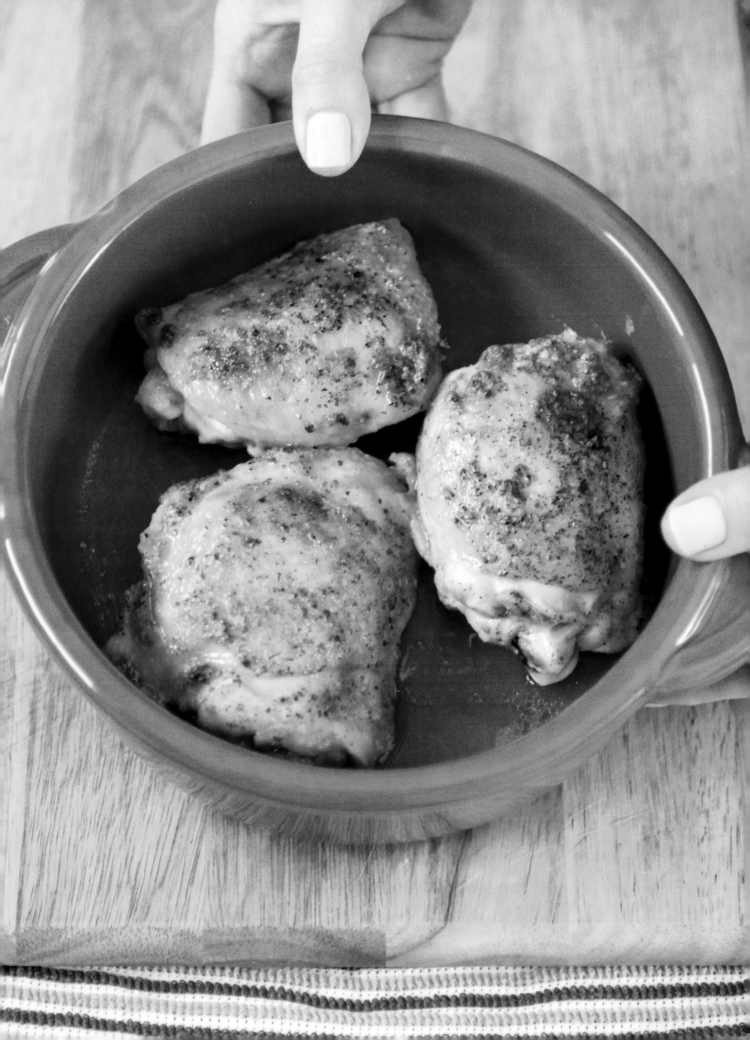

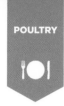

indian-spiced turkey burgers

PREP TIME
10 minutes

COOKING TIME
10 minutes

YIELD
Four burgers

Any of the spice blends are fantastic for kicking up a plain old burger. This version uses the Indian Spice Blend (recipe on page 233) and Red Roasted Garlic (recipe on page 370) garnish with cilantro. Pair it with a salad or roasted veggies for a super simple supper.

1 lb ground turkey
1 tablespoon Indian Spice Blend
   (recipe on page 233)

Sprigs of fresh cilantro for garnish

WRAP IT UP
Use a lettuce wrap or serve these burgers on a Portobello mushroom "bun" as-pictured. You can grill or bake the Portobellos at 350°F for about 10 minutes before using with these burgers.

FODMAP FREE?
Make your Indian Spice Blend without the onion powder.

In a large mixing bowl, combine turkey and Indian Spice blend until well integrated. Form the turkey into four 4-ounce patties, adding a thumb-print dimple in the center of each one to allow for even cooking.

Grill or skillet-cook the burgers for approximately 4 minutes per side over medium-high heat or until they are cooked through with no remaining pink and have reached an internal temperature of 165°F.

CHANGE IT UP
Substitute ground beef, bison, or lamb. Serve on a Sweet Potato Pancake bun (recipe on page 298) for a satisfying post-workout meal.

NUTS
EGGS
NIGHTSHADES
FODMAPS

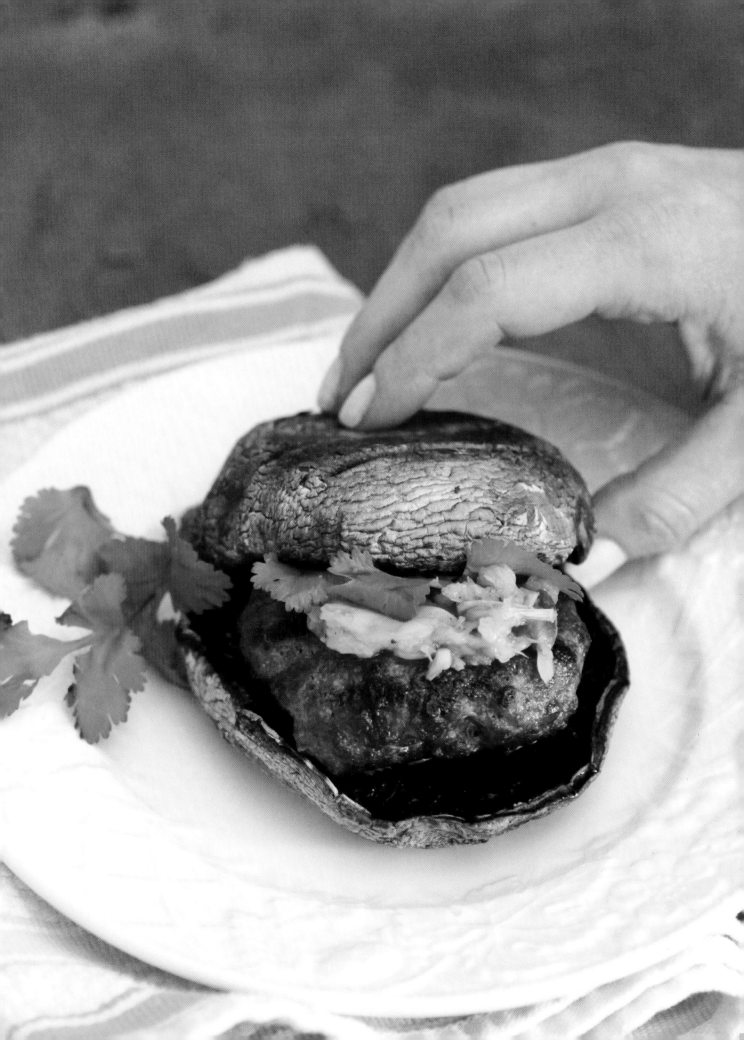

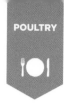
buffalo chicken lettuce wraps

PREP TIME
10 minutes

COOKING TIME
5-10 minutes

YIELD
2 large
or 4 small servings

Lettuce wraps are one of my favorite ways to take whatever random protein I have in the refrigerator and turn it into something delicious and handheld. The crunch and freshness of lettuce wrapped around this spicy chicken is a fun change of pace from Buffalo wings.

NIGHTSHADE FREE?
Toss the chicken in the spices with just garlic and onion powder, omitting the chipotle powder and tomatoes.

FODMAP FREE?
Omit the garlic, onion powder, avocado, and green onions; garnish with cilantro instead.

1 lb boneless, skinless chicken
   thighs
2 teaspoons chipotle powder
1/2 teaspoon garlic powder
1/2 teaspoon onion powder
Sea salt and black pepper to taste
2 tablespoons coconut oil

1 head of butter lettuce
   (or other variety)
1 avocado, sliced
1/2 cup cherry or grape tomatoes,
   halved
2 tablespoons chopped green
   onions

Slice the chicken thighs into 1/4-inch strips. Toss the chicken in a mixing bowl with the chipotle powder, garlic powder, onion powder, sea salt, and black pepper.

In a skillet over medium heat, melt the coconut oil, and then place the chicken thighs in the skillet. Cook for approximately 5-10 minutes, turning occasionally until the chicken is white all the way through.

Serve in lettuce cups, and top with sliced avocado, halved cherry or grape tomatoes, and chopped green onions.

CHANGE IT UP
Have a favorite hot sauce? Substitute 1 tablespoon in place of the chipotle powder, garlic powder, and onion powder.

NUTS
EGGS
NIGHTSHADES
FODMAPS

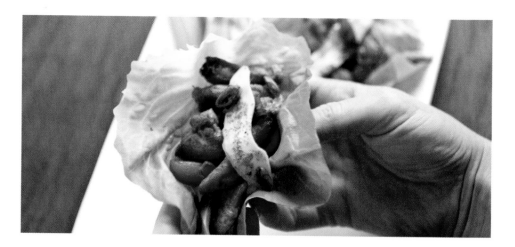

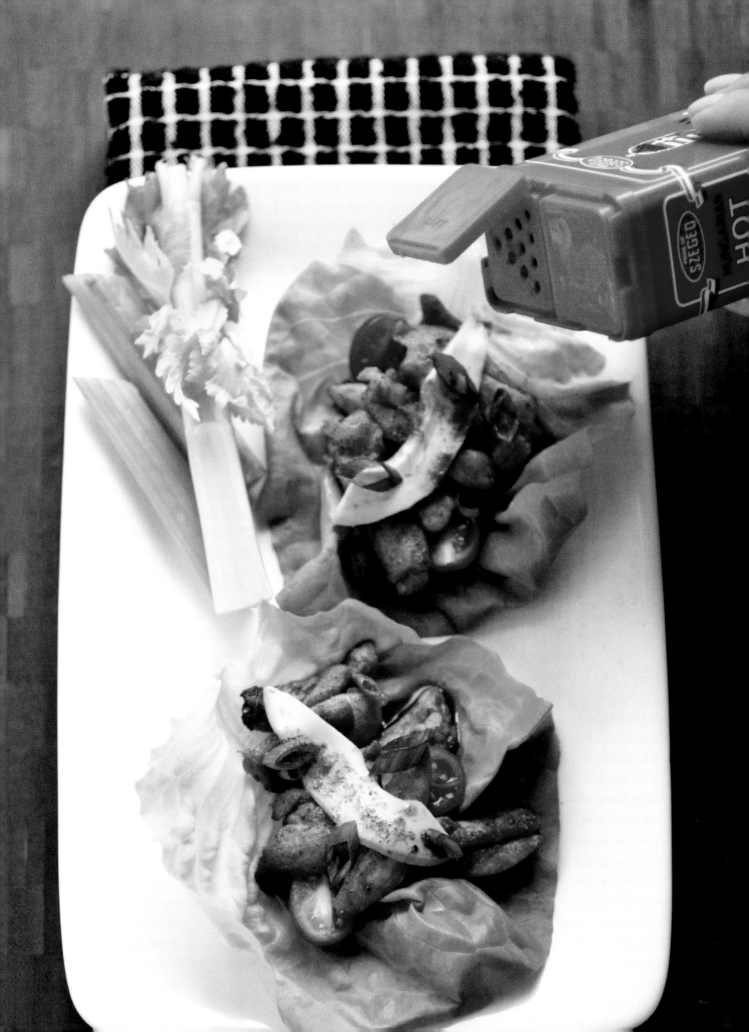

chinese 5-spice turkey lettuce cups

PREP TIME
45 minutes

COOKING TIME
15 minutes

YIELD
3-4 servings

NIGHTSHADE FREE?
*Leave the bell peppers
out of the toppings.*

FODMAP FREE?
*Leave the bell peppers
and red cabbage out of
the toppings.*

Asian flavors are tough to replace, but the deep, rich flavor that was once only found in soy sauce is brought out with a fermented coconut product called coconut aminos. You can find coconut aminos in most health food stores as well as from online retailers. As with soy sauce, a little bit goes a long way!

2 tablespoons coconut or palm oil
1 lb ground turkey
1 1/2 tablespoons Chinese 5-spice
Sea salt and black pepper to taste
2 tablespoons coconut aminos

SAUCE
2 teaspoon sesame tahini
    (or almond or sunbutter)
2 tablespoon coconut aminos
1 tablespoon cold-pressed
    sesame oil
1 teaspoon sesame seeds,
    for garnish

TOPPINGS
1 large carrot, shredded
(approximately 1/2 cup)
1/4 cup cilantro, chopped
1/2 cup bell peppers, assorted
    colors
1/2 cup chopped cucumber
1/4 cup red cabbage, shredded
1 lime, cut into wedges
1 tablespoon sesame seeds for
    garnish
1 head of butter or bibb lettuce

In a large skillet over medium heat, melt the coconut or palm oil. Add the ground turkey, Chinese 5-spice, salt, and pepper. With a wooden spoon or heat-resistant spatula, break the meat up in the pan and spread the spices around. Cook until browned.

To make the sauce, combine all ingredients except for the sesame seeds in a small mixing bowl.

Use as many or as few toppings as you like **and serve in cups of lettuce.**

NUTS
EGGS
NIGHTSHADES
FODMAPS

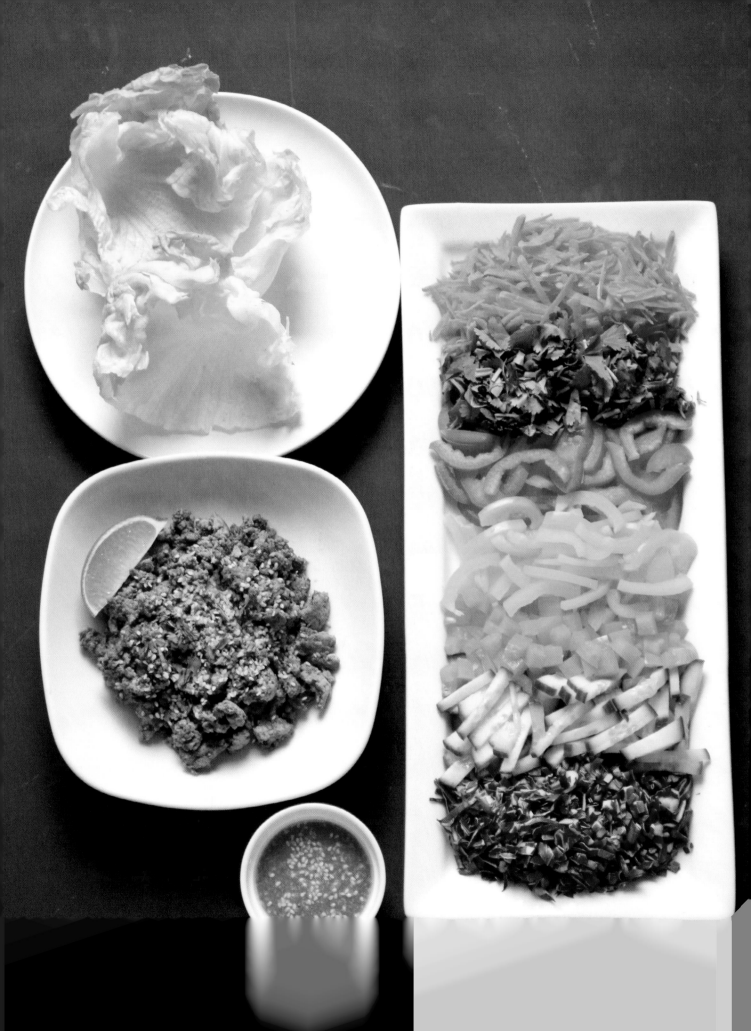

roasted duck with cherry sauce

PREP TIME
5 minutes

COOKING TIME
60-80 minutes

YIELD
2 duck legs (2 servings)

DUCK, DUCK...

Consider duck the next time you're planning on chicken. It takes a bit longer to cook, and special consideration needs to be made in order to render out the fat that comes with the skin. But it's a delicious alternative to chicken and turkey, and you end up with a lot of rendered duck fat for later use! Bonus!

FODMAP FREE?

Leave off the cherry sauce.

NUTS
EGGS
NIGHTSHADES
FODMAPS

Fruit and poultry are a fantastic combination any time of year. Try this recipe with figs or peaches. Use duck breast instead of legs if you prefer. If you'd like to sear the skin of the duck first, heat the skillet over medium-high heat, and then place the duck legs skin-side down in the pan for a few minutes before flipping them over to roast.

2 duck legs
1 teaspoon Herb Salt Blend with half rosemary and half sage (recipe on page 230) or use 1/4 teaspoon each of dried rosemary and sage with 1/2 teaspoon of coarse sea salt

CHERRY SAUCE

3/4 cup frozen or fresh cherries or 1/2 cup dried cherries that have been reconstituted in warm water for an hour
1 sprig of fresh rosemary

Preheat oven to 320°F.

Season the duck legs generously with the Rosemary & Sage Herb Salt Blend. Place the duck legs in an oven-safe skillet or roasting dish and put in the oven. Roast for 60-80 minutes until the skin is brown and the internal temperature of the duck legs reach 165°F.

While the duck cooks, simmer the cherries with the sprig of rosemary in a small sauce pan over low heat until the shape of the fruit begins to break down. Once the cherries have a soft consistency with liquid around them, remove the rosemary sprig, and then mash the fruit with a fork for a thicker texture (as pictured), or blend for a smoother texture. Set the sauce aside.

Top the roasted duck with the cherry sauce to serve. A lot of fat will remain. Strain and save this fat for cooking later. It's ideal for roasting potatoes or other root vegetables.

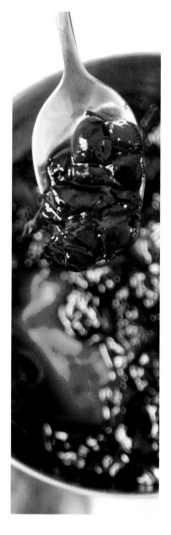

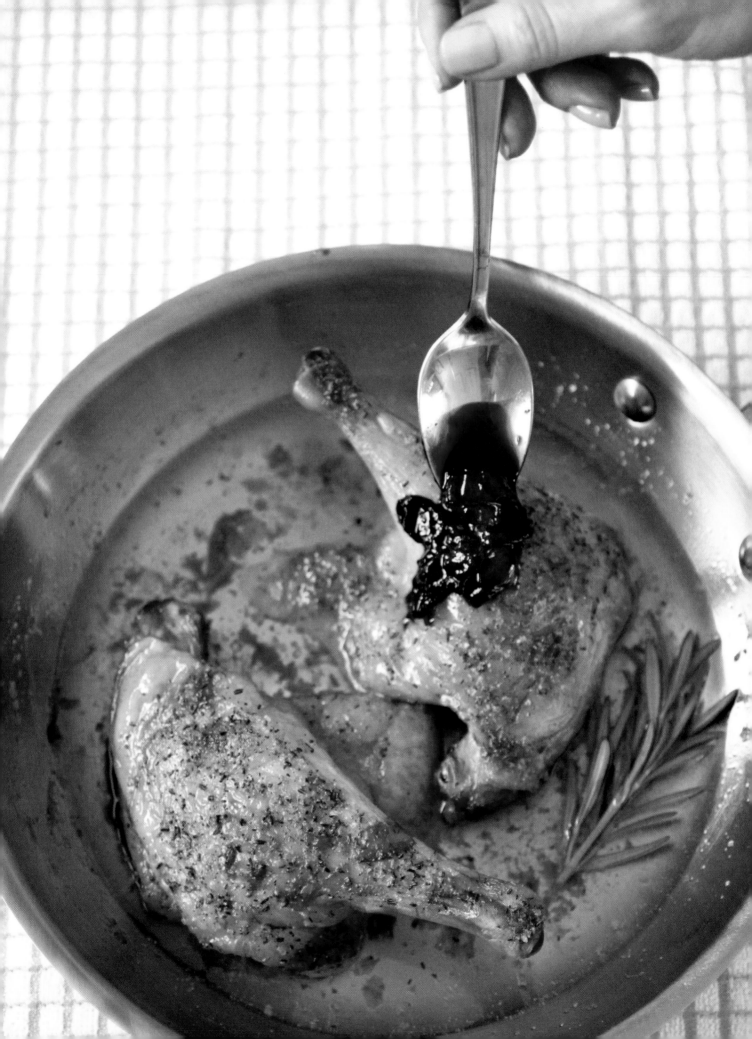

sage roasted turkey legs

PREP TIME
5 minutes

COOKING TIME
45-60 minutes

YIELD
2 turkey legs

Sage is a classic herb combination with turkey, and the smell will likely remind you of the holidays. This is an easy way to make use of the inexpensive cuts of turkey you often find at the grocery store.

2 large turkey legs
1 tablespoon melted butter or
coconut oil

1-2 teaspoons Herb Salt Blend
made with sage (recipe on page
230)
Black pepper to taste

Preheat oven to 375°F.

Brush the turkey legs with melted butter or coconut oil and season them generously with the Sage Salt Blend. Place the turkey legs in a shallow oven-safe roasting dish and cover with foil. Bake for 30 minutes.

Remove the foil and continue to bake until the internal temperature of the turkey reaches 165°F (another 15-30 minutes).

TURKEY TALK

High in tryptophan, selenium, vitamins B3 and B6, turkey is an excellent source of protein that is often overlooked outside of Thanksgiving. Keep an eye out for great deals on ground turkey, legs, or breast meat year-round. Opt for pasture-raised sources whenever possible (see page 31 for my Food Quality Guide). Fresh is always better than frozen.

CHANGE IT UP

Substitute chicken legs if you prefer. Pair the turkey with Cranberry Sauce (recipe on page 388) and Mashed Faux-Tatoes (recipe on page 344) for an anytime feast.

NUTS
EGGS
NIGHTSHADES
FODMAPS

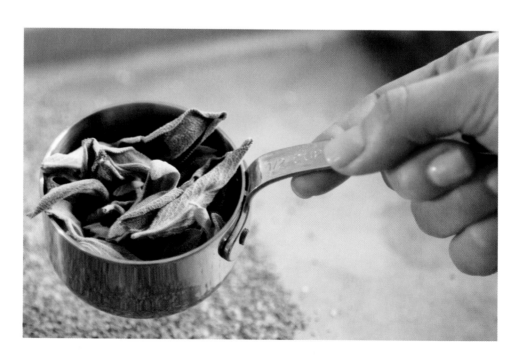

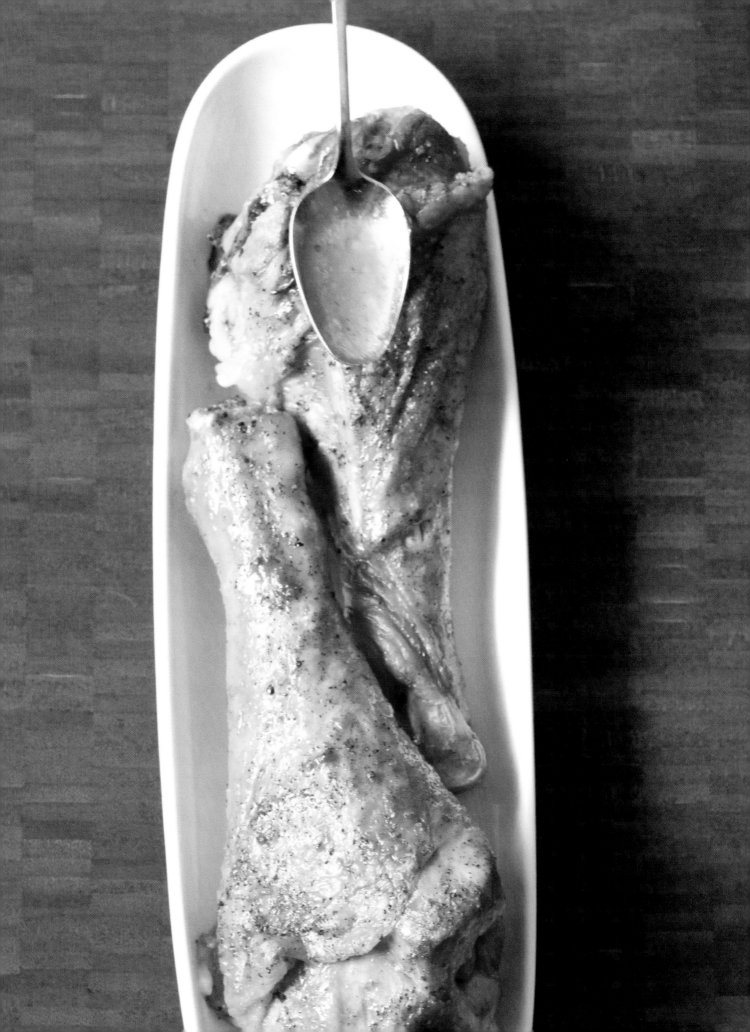

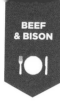
balsamic braised short ribs

PREP TIME
5 minutes

COOKING TIME
4-6 hours

YIELD
6-8 servings

There were a handful of favorite meals back in the day when I ran an organic meal delivery business, and braised balsamic BBQ beef was on the top of the list. I've updated this recipe to include dates as the sweetening element instead of brown sugar, and the result is a rich flavor that your family will love.

SIDE NOTE
This is also a fantastic dish to make for a pot-luck or Super Bowl party.

NIGHTSHADE FREE?
Replace the tomato sauce with beef Bone Broth (recipe on page 234).

FODMAP FREE?
Omit the garlic.

2 tablespoons Savory Spice Blend (recipe on page 233)
2-3 lbs of bone-in beef short ribs
1 tablespoon coconut oil
1 15-ounce can plain tomato sauce

1/2 cup balsamic vinegar
4 whole dried dates
6 cloves garlic, smashed

Rub the Savory Spice Blend into the short ribs.

Melt the coconut oil in a large skillet over medium-high heat, and sear the short ribs 1-2 minutes per side or until they are slightly browned.

Place the short ribs, tomato sauce, balsamic vinegar, dates, and garlic in a slow-cooker. Cover and cook on low for 4-6 hours or until the meat is tender enough to fall apart with a fork.

Shred the meat off of the bones and serve with Candied Carrots (recipe on page 340).

CHANGE IT UP
Don't have a slow-cooker? Use an enameled cast iron pot in an oven at 300˚F for 4-6 hours.

NUTS
EGGS
NIGHTSHADES
FODMAPS

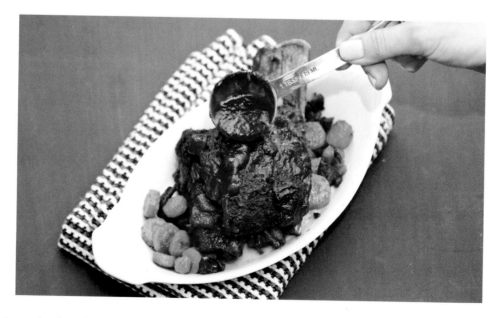

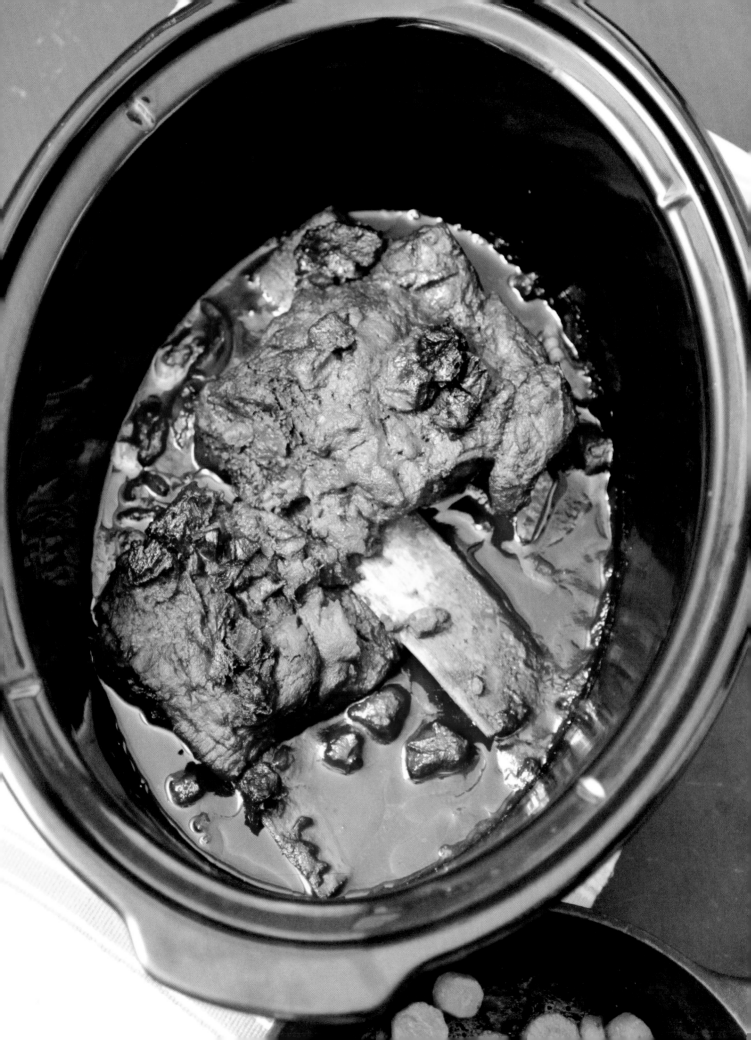

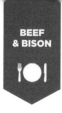
spaghetti squash bolognese

PREP TIME
15 minutes

COOKING TIME
60 minutes

YIELD
3-4 servings

CHANGE IT UP
You can also serve this sauce over zucchini noodles (see page 308).

A traditional meat sauce, Bolognese is usually made with heavy cream and a variety of meats. To keep this one dairy-free, I use coconut milk instead of cream.

1 spaghetti squash
Sea salt & black pepper to taste
2 tablespoons bacon fat
    or grass-fed butter
1 onion, finely diced
1 carrot, finely diced
1 stalk of celery, finely diced
1 clove of garlic, grated or
    finely diced

1/2 lb ground veal or beef
1/2 lb ground pork
4 slices bacon, chopped
1/2 cup full-fat coconut milk
3 ounces (1/2 small can) tomato
    paste
1/2 cup dry white wine (optional)
Sea salt and black pepper to taste

NUTS
EGGS
NIGHTSHADES
FODMAPS

Preheat oven to 375˚F.

Slice the spaghetti squash in half lengthwise so that two shallow halves remain. Scoop out the seeds and inner portion of the squash, and then sprinkle with sea salt and black pepper. Place both halves face down on a baking sheet. Roast for 35-45 minutes—until the flesh of the squash becomes translucent in color and the skin begins to soften and easily separate from the "noodles" that make up the inside.

Allow the squash to cool enough so that you can handle it, and then scoop the flesh out from the inside of the skin into a large serving bowl. Set aside until the sauce is finished.

While the squash bakes: In a large skillet over medium-high heat, melt the bacon fat or butter, and sauté the onions, carrots, and celery until they become translucent. Add the garlic and cook for an additional minute.

Add the ground veal, pork, and bacon, and cook until browned through. Once the meat is done, add the coconut milk, tomato paste, and white wine (optional), and simmer over medium-low heat for 20-30 minutes or until the sauce is well combined and any alcohol is cooked out (if you added it).

Add sea salt and black pepper to taste before removing the sauce from the heat.

Serve over the roasted spaghetti squash.

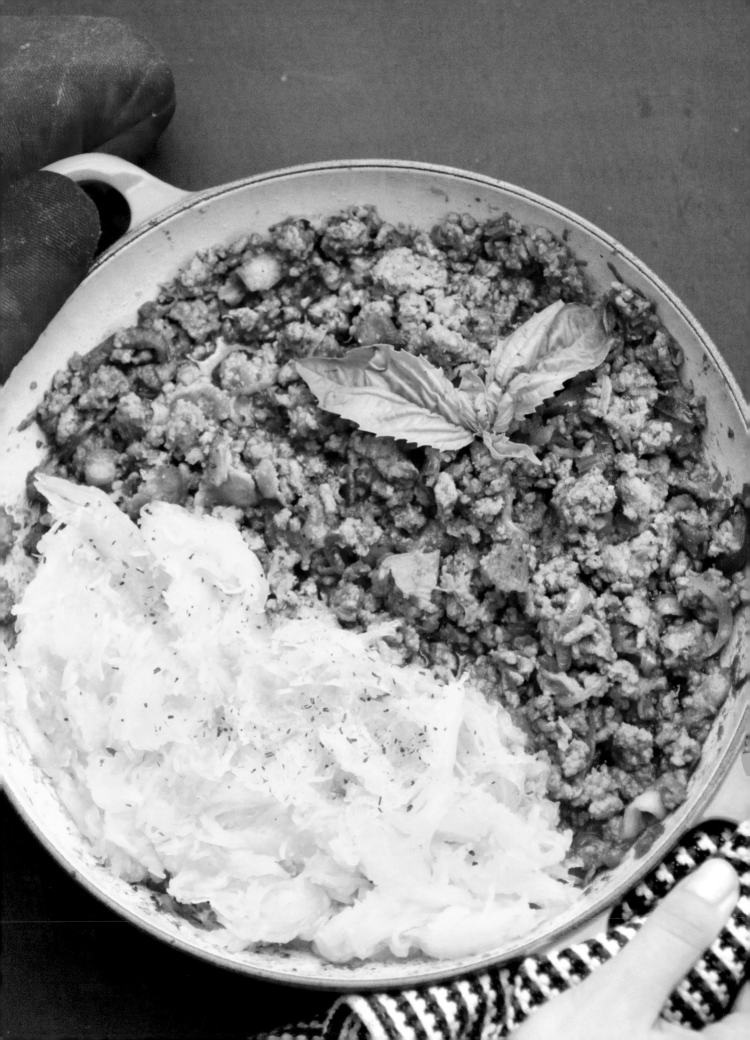

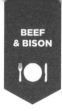

bison & butternut cocoa chili

PREP TIME
20 minutes

COOKING TIME
4-6 hours

YIELD
3-4 meal-sized servings

Before I went Paleo, my traditional chili recipe was a standard part of my cooking arsenal, but once I eliminated beans from my diet, chili was off the menu for a long time. That has changed with the creation of this fantastic recipe, which uses butternut squash and smoky flavors.

FODMAP FREE?
Leave out the garlic and onions. Add 3-4 chopped parsnips or carrots to make a bulkier dish.

3 cloves garlic, smashed
1 tablespoon smoked paprika
2 tablespoons chili powder
1 tablespoon chipotle powder
1 tablespoon cinnamon
1 tablespoon 100% cocoa powder
1 1/2 tablespoons sea salt
2 teaspoons black pepper

32 ounces diced tomatoes,
    canned—or 4 cups fresh, diced
1 lb bison stew meat
2 cups butternut squash, peeled
    and diced into 2-inch chunks
1 onion, diced into 2-inch pieces
1 bell pepper, diced into
    2-inch pieces

In a bowl, mix the garlic, smoked paprika, chili powder, chipotle powder, cinnamon, cocoa powder, sea salt, and black pepper with the tomatoes.

Place the bison, squash, onion, and bell pepper in the slow-cooker, and cover with the tomato mixture.

Cover and cook on low for 4 to 6 hours.

CHANGE IT UP
Don't have a slow-cooker? Use an enameled cast iron pot in an oven at 300°F for 4-6 hours.

This recipe can easily be made with ground beef or turkey instead of bison.

NUTS
EGGS
NIGHTSHADES
FODMAPS

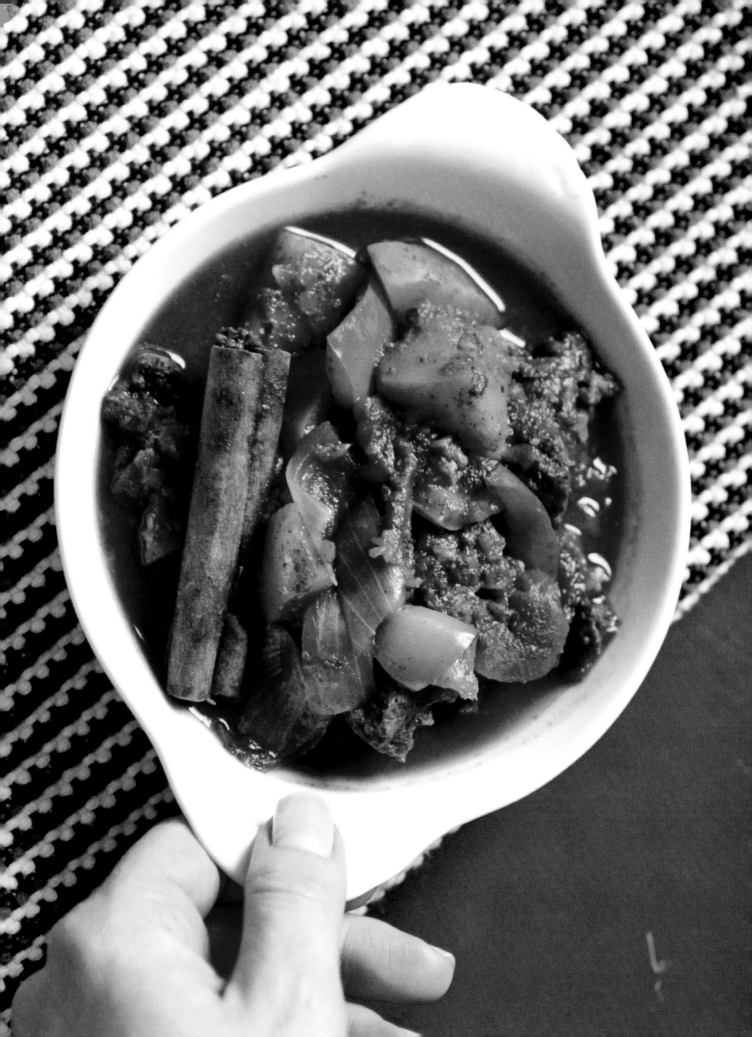

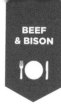
orange braised beef shanks

PREP TIME
10 minutes

COOKING TIME
4-6 hours

YIELD
6-8 servings

Beef shanks can be a confusing cut of meat, but they're often one of the most affordable, especially when you buy grass-fed. A slow-cooker or enameled cast iron Dutch oven pot do a good job of making this tougher cut of meat tender and delicious.

MAKE IT EASIER
Peel the sweet potato before dropping it into the slow-cooker.

FODMAP FREE?
Leave out the garlic.

2 teaspoons fennel seeds
1 teaspoon black peppercorns
32 ounces beef Bone Broth
    (recipe on page 234)
1 orange, sliced & juiced
1 teaspoon cumin
3 cloves garlic, smashed

6 beef shanks
    (approximately 3 lbs)
1 large sweet potato, cut into
    2-inch chunks

Place fennel seeds and peppercorns in a metal tea strainer ball or tie them up in a small piece of cheese-cloth. In the beef broth, mix the orange slices, orange juice, cumin, garlic, and the strainer that contains the seeds and peppercorns.

CHANGE IT UP
Don't have a slow-cooker? Use an enameled cast iron pot in an oven at 300˚F for 4-6 hours.

Place the beef shanks and sweet potato in the slow-cooker and add the spice ball (or bag) and broth mixture. Cover and cook on low for 4-6 hours or until the meat is tender enough to fall apart with a fork.

Shred the meat off of the bones, and peel the skin from the sweet potato before serving.

NUTS
EGGS
NIGHTSHADES
FODMAPS

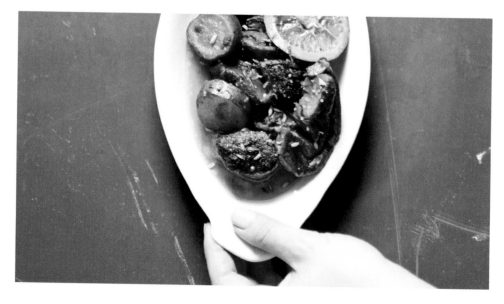

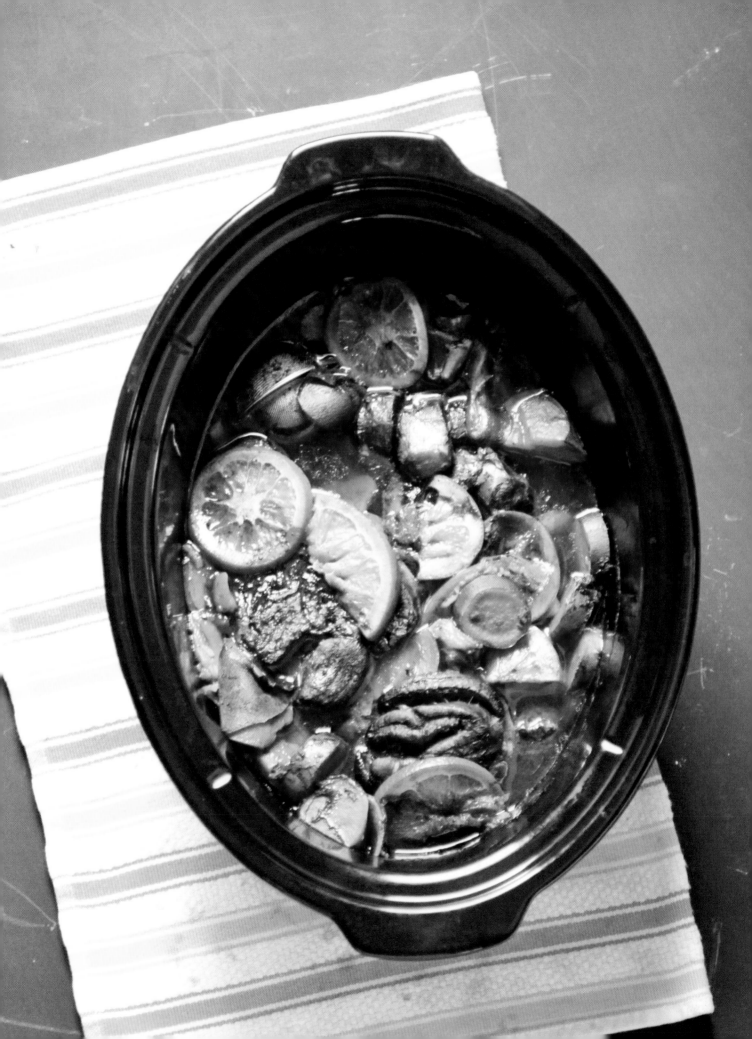

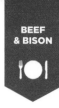
beef & mixed veggie stir-fry

PREP TIME
15 minutes

COOKING TIME
15 minutes

YIELD
2-4 servings

After a long week of cooking and using up almost all of the veggies you bought for the week, a stir-fry is the perfect answer to the "I don't feel like cooking" blues. Chop up whatever you have, add a few key ingredients like coconut aminos, water chestnuts, and sesame seeds, and you're all set.

CHOP, CHOP!
Learn how to chop veggies on pages 224-228.

NIGHTSHADE FREE?
Omit the bell peppers.

FODMAP FREE?
Use only vegetables from the Paleo foods list that are not marked as FODMAPs (page 29), and omit the garlic.

1 lb skirt steak
2 tablespoons coconut oil
1 cup red onion, julienned
1 cup broccoli, chopped
1 cup string beans, ends trimmed
1 cup bell peppers, julienned
(or use 4 cups total of whatever veggies you choose)
1 tablespoon sesame seeds, raw or toasted
2 tablespoons green onions/scallions, chopped
1/4 cup water chestnuts, sliced

STIR-FRY SAUCE
2 tablespoons coconut aminos
2 tablespoons warm water
2 cloves garlic, finely chopped or grated
1/4-1/2 teaspoon ginger, finely chopped or grated

NUTS
EGGS
NIGHTSHADES
FODMAPS

Spread the skirt steak across a large cutting board, and cut into sections that are approximately 4 inches long, cutting with the grain of the meat. Next, cut against the grain to slice each section into 1/4 inch strips.

CHANGE IT UP
Substitute chicken or pork for the beef.

Over medium-high heat, let the skillet get hot and melt the coconut oil. Place the steak in the skillet and allow it to brown on both sides, approximately 1-2 minutes per side. Remove the steak from the skillet and set aside.

Place the red onion, broccoli, string beans, and bell peppers (or whatever vegetables you decide to use) in the pan. Cook for about 5 minutes or until fork-tender.

While the vegetables cook, combine the sauce ingredients and mix well.

Add the meat back to the pan, followed by the sauce, and heat through for about 2 minutes.

Plate the stir-fry, and top with sesame seeds, green onions, and water chestnuts.

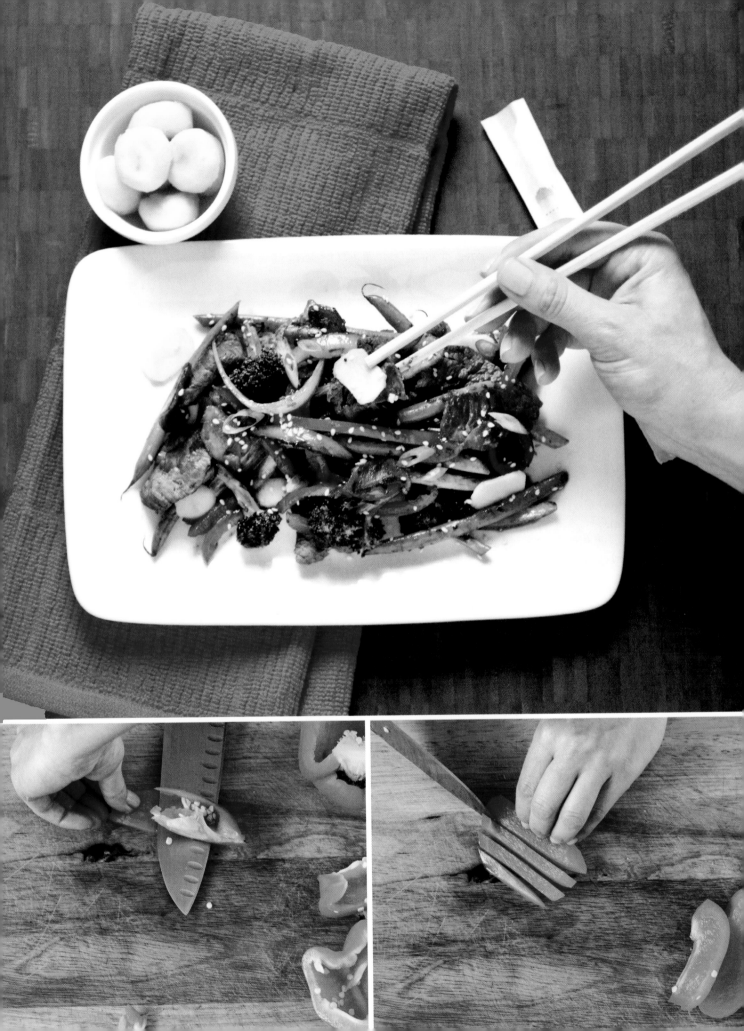

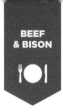
roasted marrow bones

PREP TIME
5 minutes

COOKING TIME
30 minutes

YIELD
3-4 servings

If you haven't made roasted marrow bones yet, stop what you're doing, find a local farmer who is pasture-raising cows on 100% grass, and get some bones. You won't believe how easy it is to enjoy this gourmet super-food at home. Your great grandmother would be proud. Use the bones to make broth (recipe on page 234) after you eat the marrow!

2 lbs beef marrow bones
Sea salt and black pepper to taste

Red Roasted Garlic
    (recipe on page 370) (optional)

SIDE NOTE

What's so great about bone marrow? It is rich in glycine and gelatin, both of which are fantastic for healing. Eating roasted marrow bones or drinking bone broth is extremely desirable when you're sick or as a way to prevent illness.

Preheat oven to 450°F.

Place the marrow bones in a shallow roasting pan and sprinkle with sea salt and black pepper. Roast for 30 minutes or until the bones and marrow are golden brown.

Serve and eat immediately with a spoon.

FODMAP FREE?

Make this without the roasted garlic-topper.

NUTS
EGGS
NIGHTSHADES
FODMAPS

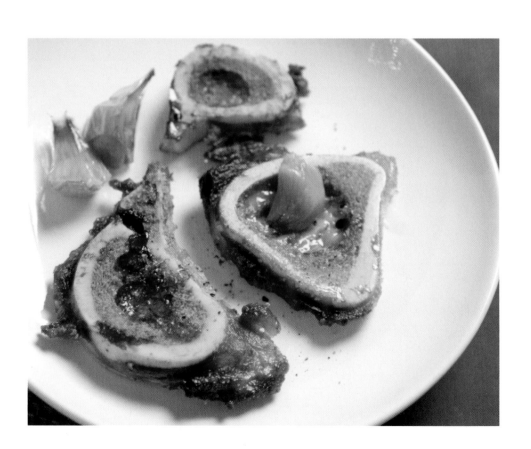

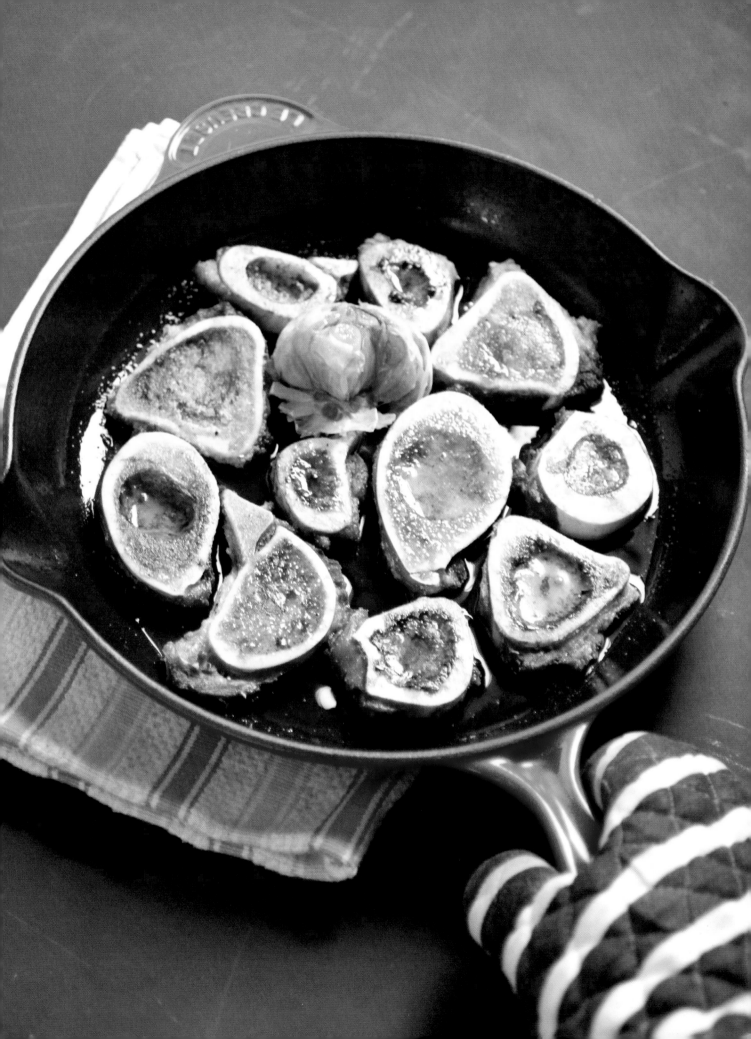

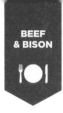

mom's stuffed cabbage rolls with tomato cranberry sauce

PREP TIME
30 minutes

COOKING TIME
45 minutes

YIELD
12-15 cabbage rolls
(serves 4-6 people)

SIDE NOTE
It's a good idea to make the Simple Cranberry Sauce ahead of time.

NIGHTSHADE FREE?
Replace the tomatoes with Bone Broth (recipe on page 234).

NUTS
EGGS
NIGHTSHADES
FODMAPS

This is a dish my mom has made for as long as I can remember. Her original recipe calls for canned, pre-made cranberry sauce, but this is a healthy alternative. Make a double batch and freeze them for later.

1 head Savoy cabbage, leaves carefully separated to remain intact
1 cup grated or shredded cauliflower
1 teaspoon butter or coconut oil
Sea salt and black pepper to taste
1 lb ground beef

1-2 cloves garlic, grated or finely diced
1/2 onion, finely diced
1 teaspoon dried rosemary
1 32-ounce can crushed or diced tomatoes
1 cup Simple Cranberry Sauce (recipe on page 388)

Preheat the oven to 350˚F.

Fill a large pot with 2 inches of water (use a steamer basket if you have one), and steam the whole cabbage leaves until they are soft. Set aside to cool.

While the cabbage is steaming, sauté the cauliflower in the butter in a large skillet over medium heat for just a few minutes until it is slightly softened. Add sea salt and black pepper to taste. Remove both the cabbage and cauliflower from the heat and set aside.

In a large mixing bowl, combine the ground beef, cooked cauliflower, garlic, onion, rosemary, and more sea salt and pepper until well incorporated.

Fill the end of one leaf of the cabbage at a time with approximately 1/4-1/3 cup of the mixture, and roll it like a burrito by rolling the bottom up, followed by the sides, and tucking the end underneath. Lay the cabbage rolls in a deep ovensafe dish with the tucked side down.

Combine the tomatoes and Simple Cranberry Sauce in the skillet that previously contained the cauliflower. Pour over the cabbage rolls.

Place the entire dish in the oven and cover with foil or a lid. Bake approximately 45 minutes or until the meat is cooked all the way through.

HELPFUL TIPS
Savoy cabbage is different from regular green cabbage, as it is softer and has curly edges. If you can't find it, regular green cabbage works fine.

You may need to steam the cabbage leaves in batches since they're very large. Allow time for this process.

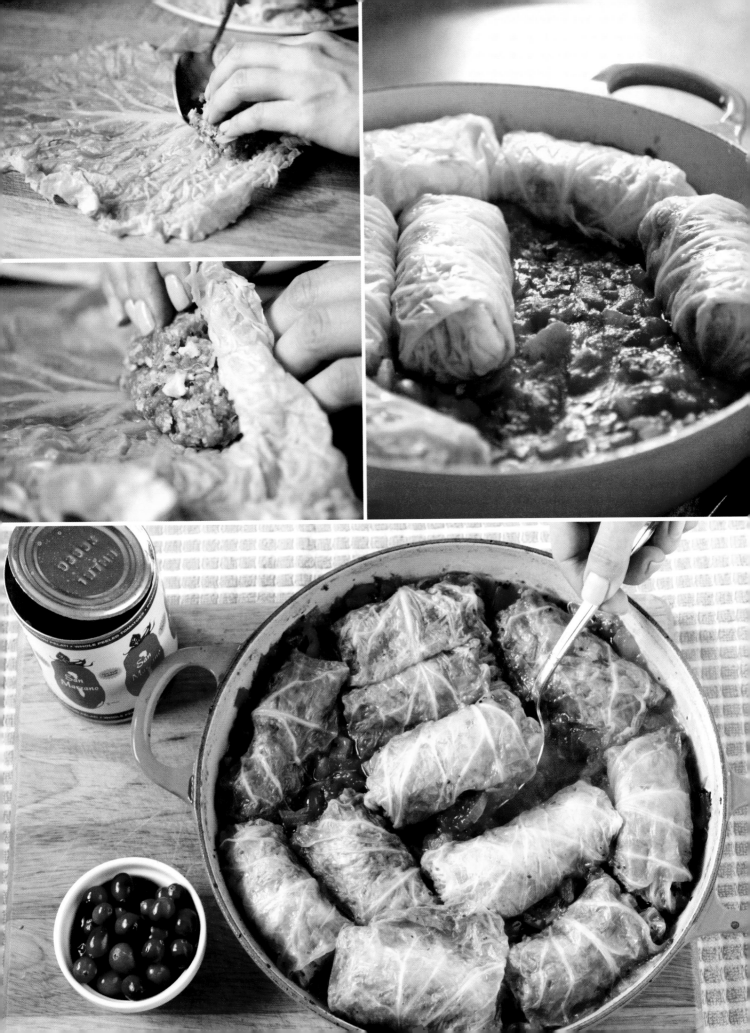

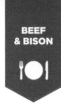
hayley's skirt steak tacos

PREP TIME
20 minutes

COOKING TIME
10-15 minutes

YIELD
3-4 meal-sized servings
or more if served as
an appetizer

NIGHTSHADE FREE?
*Omit the chili powder
and tomatoes, and top
with a Nightshade-Free
Salsa—either mango,
pineapple, or cucumber
(recipes on page 296).*

FODMAP FREE?
*Omit the garlic
and avocado.*

*Lettuce tacos are one of my favorite go-to weeknight meals. I wrap nearly any
kind of protein in lettuce, and top it with avocado. This recipe is named after
Hayley Mason, co-author of "Make it Paleo," who originated it.*

Juice and zest of one lime
1 clove garlic, grated or finely
   minced
1/2 teaspoon chili powder
1-1 1/2 lb skirt steak
Sea salt and black pepper to taste
1 head bib, butter, or Boston lettuce

TACO TOPPERS
2 dozen cherry tomatoes, halved
   (or one large tomato chopped
   into 1-inch pieces)
1 avocado, thinly sliced
1/4 cup chopped cilantro

Gently separate the leave of lettuce and rinse them off.
Set them aside to dry.

In a large mixing bowl, whisk together the lime juice,
zest, garlic, and chili powder. Place the skirt steak in
the bowl and massage the seasonings into it. Add sea
salt and black pepper to taste.

Grill for approximately 3 minutes per side. Set the
cooked steak aside to rest for 10 minutes, then slice against the grain into small
strips. You may want to divide the skirt steak into two or three sections before
slicing, as it is typically very long.

Serve the steak, tomatoes, cilantro, and avocado in your lettuce leaves.

CHANGE IT UP
*Top these simple steak
tacos with anything you
like, such as thinly sliced
red onions.*

*Add Five Kinds of Salsa
(recipe on page 296)*

NUTS

EGGS

NIGHTSHADES

FODMAPS

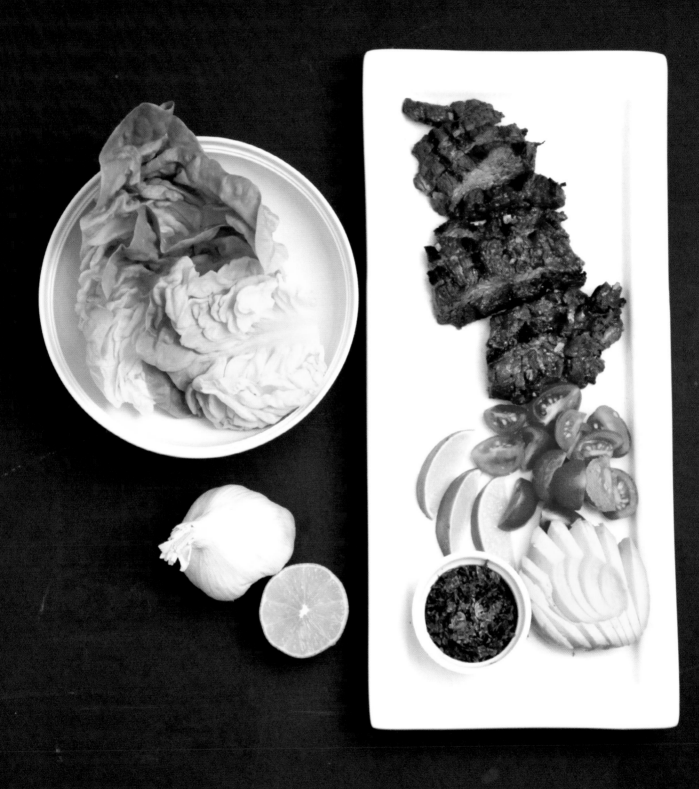

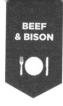

grilled garlic flank steak with peppers & onions

PREP TIME
20 minutes

COOKING TIME
10-15 minutes

YIELD
3-4 meal-sized servings

This is one of those go-to recipes for any weeknight or a cookout. Use leftover steak to top a salad or to pair with eggs for breakfast the next morning.

3 cloves garlic, grated or finely minced
1 1/2 - 2 lbs flank steak
Sea salt and black pepper to taste

1 tablespoon bacon fat, butter, ghee, or coconut oil
1 onion, diced into 1/2-inch pieces
1 bell pepper, diced into 1/2-inch pieces

NIGHTSHADE FREE?
Omit the pepper and serve over grilled squash and carrots.

FODMAP FREE?
Season only with sea salt and black pepper, and serve over grilled carrots instead of the peppers and onions.

Preheat an outdoor grill or indoor grill to medium-high heat. Massage the garlic into the steak, and season liberally with sea salt and black pepper.

Grill approximately 5 minutes per side, turning the steak one-quarter turn halfway through to achieve the grill marks. Set the cooked steak aside to rest.

In a large skillet over medium-high heat, melt the bacon fat and sauté the onion and peppers until soft and slightly browned on the edges.

Slice the steak on a slight angle against the grain. Serve the steak over the onion and pepper.

CHANGE IT UP
Serve this flank steak over any grilled or sautéed vegetables.

NUTS
EGGS
NIGHTSHADES
FODMAPS

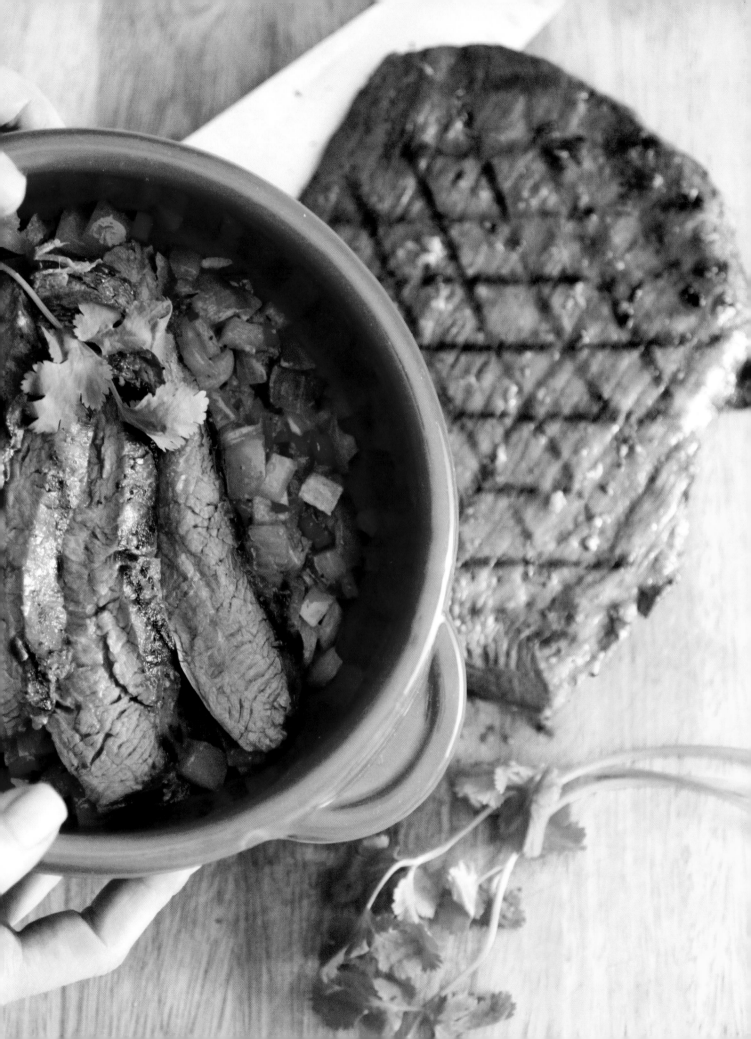

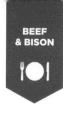
PREP TIME
30 minutes

COOKING TIME
10 minutes

YIELD
4 meal-sized salads

NIGHTSHADE FREE?
Omit the chili powder, tomatoes, and bell peppers. Use cucumber or fruit salsa instead, and add shredded carrots for color.

FODMAP FREE?
Omit the onion, garlic powder, and avocado.

NUTS

EGGS

NIGHTSHADES

FODMAPS

tangy taco salad

Ground beef gets kicked up to a whole new place when you make it into taco meat and pair it with some fun toppings.

1 lb ground beef
1 tablespoon chili powder
1 teaspoon onion powder
1 teaspoon garlic powder (or 2 cloves of fresh garlic, grated or finely chopped)
8 cups chopped romaine lettuce

1 cup sliced or chopped tomatoes
1/2 cup chopped bell peppers, any color
1 cup any kind of salsa (recipes on page 296)
1 avocado, sliced (or guacamole)
2 limes, halved

In a large skillet over medium-high heat, brown the meat, and add the spices (chili powder, onion powder, and garlic powder) when the meat is about halfway done.

While the meat is cooking, assemble the salad as you like with the lettuce, tomatoes, bell peppers, salsa, and avocado.

Top with the fully browned meat, and squeeze half a lime over each salad as dressing.

WRAP IT UP
You can also serve this as tacos with lettuce-leaf taco "shells."

Try substituting ground bison, turkey, or chicken in place of beef.

PREP TIME
30 minutes

COOKING TIME
-

YIELD
Approximately 8 servings

NIGHTSHADE FREE?
Use cucumber, pineapple, or mango for your salsa.

FODMAP FREE?
Use tomato or cucumber for your salsa.

NUTS

EGGS

NIGHTSHADES

FODMAPS

five kinds of salsa

Even if you don't eat tomatoes, there is no reason why you can't still enjoy salsa! Simply swap the traditional main ingredient with any of the other options in this recipe.

2 tablespoons fresh cilantro, finely chopped
1 shallot, minced
Juice of 1-2 limes (to taste)
1 tablespoon extra-virgin olive oil
Sea salt and black pepper to taste

2 cups of any one of the following, or a combination of two or more, diced:
Tomato
Mango
Cucumber
Bell pepper
Pineapple

In a medium-sized mixing bowl, combine the base ingredients: cilantro, shallots, lime juice, extra-virgin olive oil, sea salt, and black pepper to taste.

Add the main ingredient(s) and combine.

CHANGE IT UP
Here are some combination suggestions: tomato + cucumber; pineapple + mango; bell pepper + mango; pineapple + cucumber.

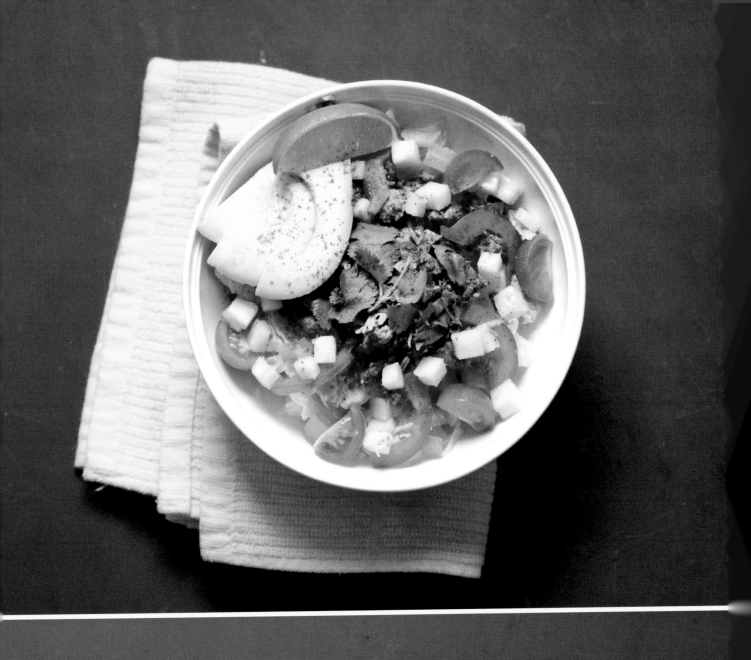

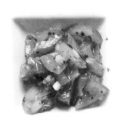 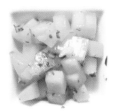 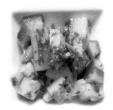 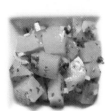 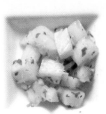

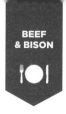

fiery jalapeño buffalo burgers

The sweetness of a Sweet Potato Pancake "bun" (recipe below) compliments the spiciness of this burger.

PREP TIME
15 minutes

COOKING TIME
10 minutes

YIELD
4 burgers

ON THE SIDE
Serve with a green salad or grilled vegetables to round out your plate.

NUTS

EGGS

NIGHTSHADES

FODMAPS

1 jalapeño pepper
1 teaspoon smoked paprika
1 teaspoon onion powder

Sea salt and black pepper to taste
1 lb ground bison

Place the jalapeño pepper over an open flame or on a grill until the skin is blackened all over. Remove from heat, and peel the skin off the pepper under cool running water. Chop the pepper, only including the white ribs and seeds if you like an extra spicy burger.

In a large mixing bowl, combine the meat, roasted pepper, and spices until well integrated. Form into four 4-ounce patties, adding a thumbprint dimple in the center to allow for even cooking.

Grill the burgers approximately 4-5 minutes per side or until they are done to your liking.

CHANGE IT UP
Use ground beef or lamb instead of bison. Top with bacon and Roasted Garlic Aioli (recipe on page 258) for some added depth of flavor.

sweet potato pancakes

Enjoy these pancakes for breakfast or use them as a bun for any burger! They can be made ahead of time and reheated to use within a few days. For a lower-carb option, make them with shredded carrots instead of sweet potatoes.

PREP TIME
15 minutes

COOKING TIME
20 minutes

YIELD
4-5 large pancakes

EGG FREE?
Omit the eggs and coconut flour then sauté the ingredients in a pan instead to create a delicious hash.

NUTS

EGGS

NIGHTSHADES

FODMAPS

3 eggs
2 teaspoons coconut flour
1/2 teaspoon cinnamon
1/4 teaspoon ground ginger
1/4 teaspoon sea salt

2 cups shredded sweet potatoes
(using a food processor with a shredding disc is ideal, or shred them by hand)
Coconut oil for pan frying
(amount will vary)

In a medium-sized mixing bowl, beat the eggs with the coconut flour, cinnamon, ground ginger, and sea salt. Mix in the shredded sweet potatoes until well combined.

Add about 1/8 inch of coconut oil to a large skillet over medium-low heat. Spoon the mixture into the skillet in "cakes" that are 4-6 inches in diameter, and cook approximately 2-3 minutes per side until they hold together, flipping once as you would a regular pancake.

CHANGE IT UP
Replace the cinnamon and ginger with 1/4 teaspoon of rosemary.

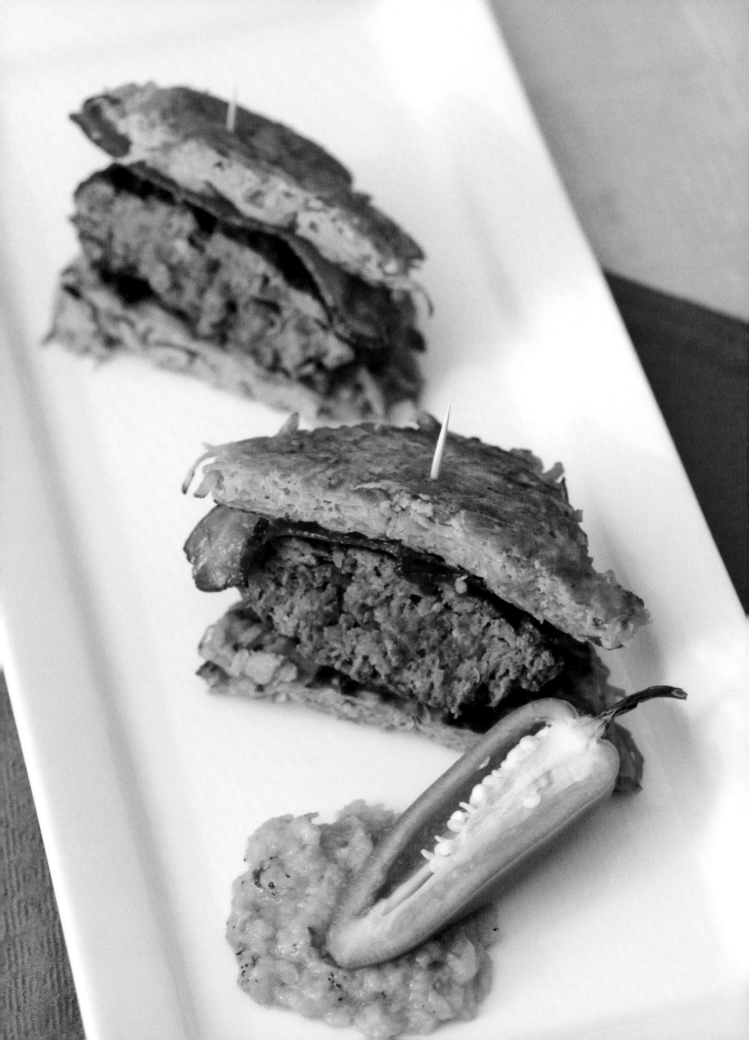

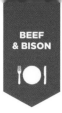
italian style stuffed peppers

PREP TIME
20 minutes

COOKING TIME
25-35 minutes

YIELD
3-4 meal-sized servings

NIGHTSHADE FREE?
Stuff squash instead of peppers, and omit the tomatoes.

FODMAP FREE?
Omit the onions and garlic and stuff the mixture into squash instead of peppers.

NUTS
EGGS
NIGHTSHADES
FODMAPS

One of the easiest ways to make ground meat into a special meal is by stuffing it into an elegant "package." Use any colored bell peppers, or even another type of vegetable, like a summer or winter squash, to make this all-in-one meal.

2 bell peppers, halved and cleaned
1 tablespoon bacon grease or coconut oil
1/2 large onion, diced
Sea salt and black pepper to taste
4 cloves garlic, pressed or chopped

1/2 cup diced tomatoes, fresh or canned
1 lb ground beef, bison, turkey, or chicken
6 fresh basil leaves, finely chopped
Extra basil leaves for garnish

Preheat oven to 375˚F.

Place the bell pepper halves in a roasting dish face down for 10-15 minutes. (You can skip this step if you want to keep the peppers more firm/raw.)

While the bell peppers are cooking, heat the bacon grease or coconut oil in a large skillet over medium-high heat. Sauté the onions, adding sea salt and black pepper to taste, until they're translucent and slightly browned on the edges. Add the tomatoes and garlic to the onions, and simmer for about two minutes.

Add the meat and cook until fully done. Taste the mixture, and adjust seasoning to your liking (more sea salt, more black pepper, etc.). Mix in the chopped basil.

Remove the peppers from the oven - they should be just a bit softened - and flip them over. Spoon the stuffing mixture into each one. You can go ahead and eat them at this point, or put them back in the oven for 15-20 minutes to allow the flavors of the bell pepper and the meat mixture to blend together more.

You can refrigerate or freeze and reheat later.

CHANGE IT UP
Add 2 cups of finely chopped baby spinach to the meat.

COOKING TIP
It's best not to use acidic ingredients (like tomatoes or vinegars) in cast iron cookware since the acid will interact with the iron. This is a good time to use an enameled cast-iron or stainless steel skillet.

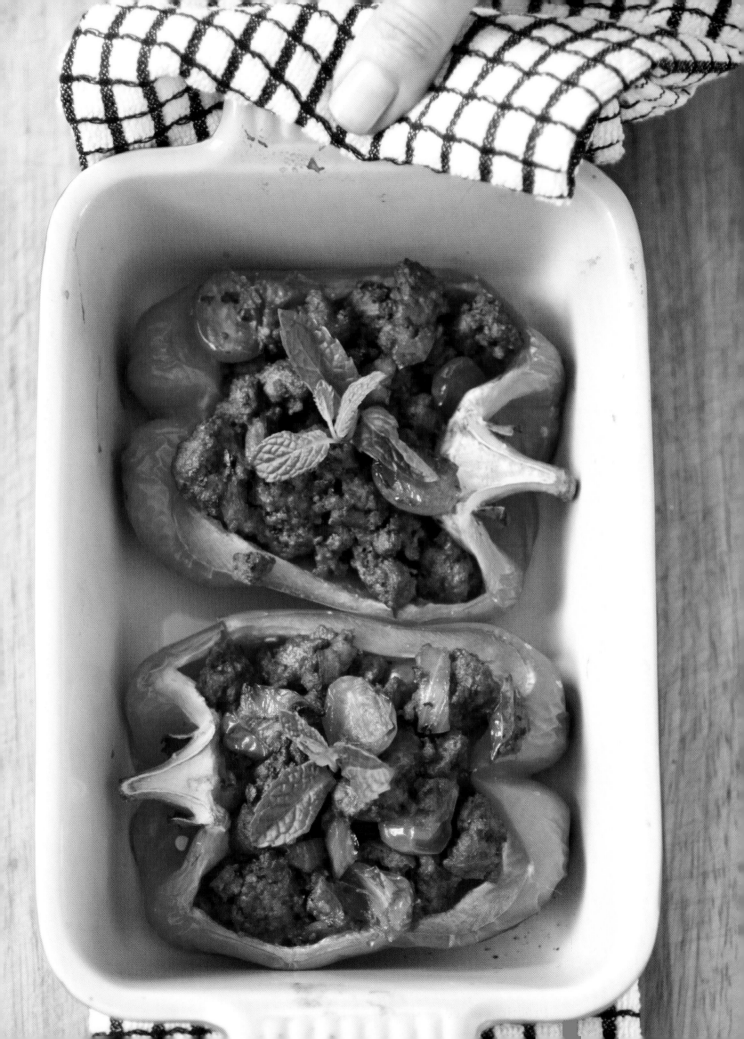

red palm & coriander tuna over daikon noodle salad

PREP TIME
25 minutes

COOKING TIME
10 minutes

YIELD
3-4 servings

Grilled tuna is a fantastic treat, especially in the summertime. The cold daikon noodle salad is a fresh and tasty way to compliment the grilled fish. If you don't have an outdoor grill, a grill pan will do the trick!

1 tablespoon red palm oil, melted
1 lb wild tuna steaks
1/2 teaspoon Lemon Salt (recipe on page 230) or use 1/4 teaspoon salt and the zest of half a lemon
1/4 teaspoon coriander
Black pepper to taste
1/2 of a lemon
1 tablespoon extra-virgin olive oil

DAIKON NOODLE SALAD
2-3 daikon radishes
1 large carrot
1 tablespoon fresh cilantro, chopped
Juice of 1/2 lemon
1 tablespoon extra-virgin olive oil or cold-pressed sesame oil
Sea salt and black pepper to taste

CHANGE IT UP

Don't like or can't find daikon radish? You can make the noodles for the salad out of zucchini or yellow squash—or use all carrots.

GET THE TOOLS

You can find a julienne peeler easily online as well as in most kitchen gadget shops locally.

Find red palm oil online at Tropical Traditions or in a local, organic grocery store or food co-op.

NUTS
EGGS
NIGHTSHADES
FODMAPS

Brush the red palm oil over each side of the tuna. Combine the lemon salt, coriander, and black pepper in a small bowl, and sprinkle the mixture evenly over both sides of the tuna.

Grill the tuna for 3 minutes on each side or until done to your liking. If you are enjoying wild, sashimi-grade tuna, you can leave it nearly rare. If you are eating a wild but lower grade tuna, cook until it is just pink in the center.

For the Daikon Noodle Salad: Rinse and peel the outer skin of the daikon radishes with a standard vegetable peeler. Using a julienne peeler (or continue with the standard peeler if you don't have a julienne peeler), continue to "peel" the radishes into noodle-shaped pieces. Repeat this process with the carrot.

In a large mixing bowl, toss the julienned radishes and carrots with the chopped cilantro, lemon juice, oil, salt, and pepper. Serve immediately to retain the crunch, as the daikon will become soggy if it sits too long before serving.

Plate the tuna over the Daikon Noodle Salad and finish with a squeeze of lemon; drizzle the extra-virgin olive oil over the tuna before serving.

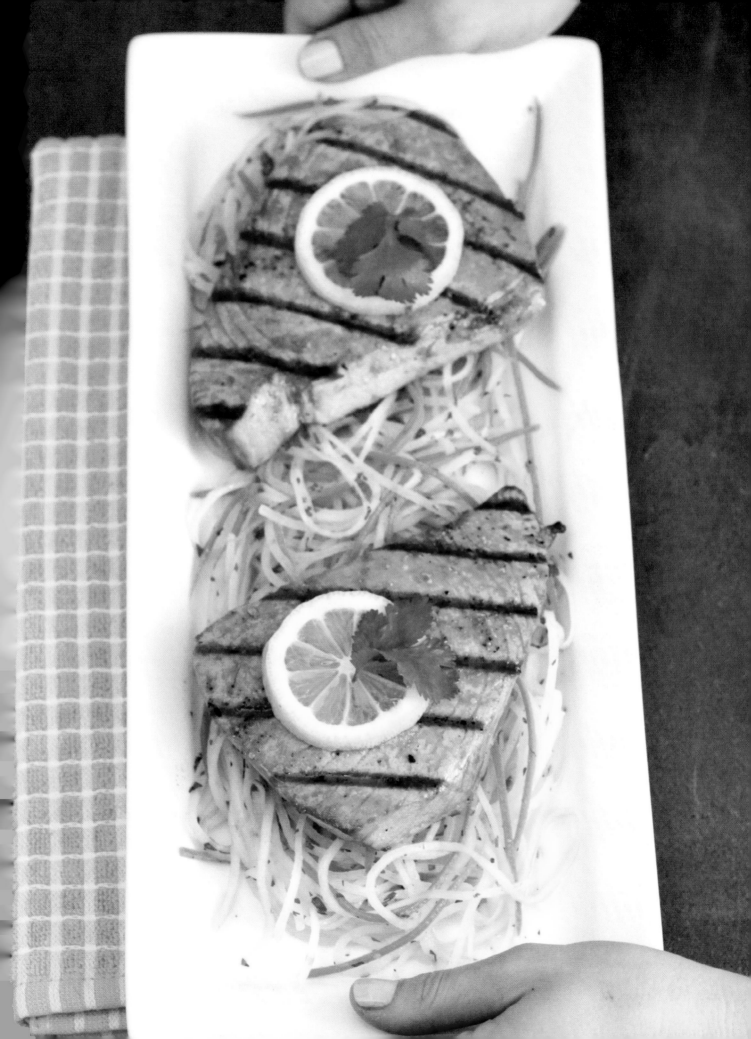

asian orange
pan-seared scallops

PREP TIME
5 minutes

COOKING TIME
20 minutes

YIELD
2 large or
3-4 small servings

Scallops are very simple to cook, but they require your undivided attention as over-cooking them will yield a rubbery result. This recipe is ideal to use with fresh scallops; it is not recommended for previously frozen scallops because they tend to give off a lot of water and are difficult to sear.

CHANGE IT UP
This sauce would work very nicely with any other type of seafood that you like or with chicken or pork.

Try it with bone-in pork chops for a gourmet weeknight treat!

FODMAP FREE?
Leave out the garlic powder.

1 lb large wild scallops
Sea salt and black pepper to taste
Garlic powder (a few pinches)
2 tablespoons butter, ghee,
   or coconut oil
Zest of 1 orange

DEGLAZING LIQUID
2 tablespoons coconut aminos
2 tablespoons freshly squeezed
   orange juice (about 1 orange)
1 tablespoon warm water
1 tablespoon butter or coconut oil

NUTS
EGGS
NIGHTSHADES
FODMAPS

Lay the scallops on a paper or cloth towel and pat them on each side to remove excess moisture. Sprinkle both sides lightly with sea salt, black pepper, and a few pinches of garlic powder.

Melt the butter, ghee, or coconut oil in a stainless steel skillet or a well-seasoned cast iron pan over medium-high heat, and place the scallops into the hot pan, allowing at least 1 inch of room between them. Allow the scallops to sear for approximately 2-3 minutes before turning to sear the other side or until the scallops are white all the way through and no longer translucent. Cooking time will vary with the thickness of the scallops.

While the scallops are cooking, combine the deglazing liquid ingredients in a bowl.

After removing the scallops from the pan, turn the heat to high and pour in the deglazing liquid.

Deglazing is the process of pouring liquid into a very hot pan that has flavor-filled bits seared into the bottom of it. Use a whisk to remove the seared bits from the pan to flavor the sauce.

Reduce the remaining liquid over high heat for 2-3 minutes.

Remove the scallops from the pan to serve, and spoon about 1/2 teaspoon of the sauce over each scallop, garnishing with orange zest.

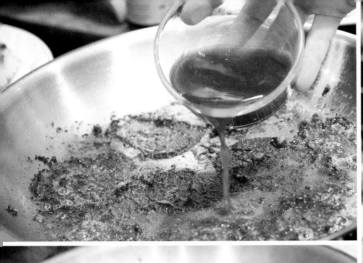

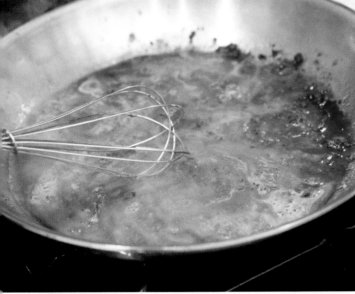

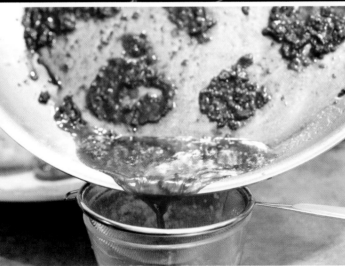

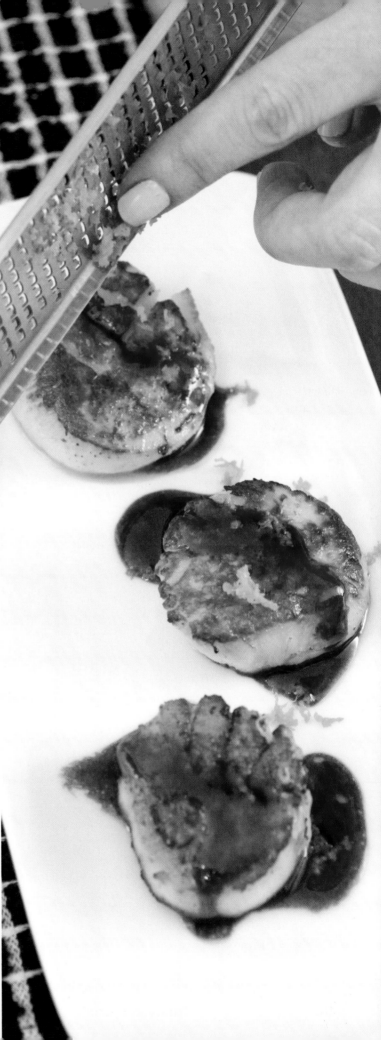

HOW TO DEGLAZE A PAN:

Pour your liquid of choice into a very hot pan that has flavor-filled bits seared into the bottom of it. Follow the liquid with a whisk to remove the bits from the pan and help flavor the sauce. Then allow the remaining liquid to simmer over high heat for just a few minutes before straining the sauce to serve.

lemon rosemary broiled salmon

PREP TIME
5 minutes

COOKING TIME
15 minutes

YIELD
3-4 servings

Homemade Rosemary Salt (recipe on page 230) has been a go-to in my kitchen for a long time. This recipe was a happy-accident since I never would have thought to pair rosemary with fish, but I tried it—and it was delicious!

2 tablespoons butter, ghee,
    or coconut oil
1 lb wild salmon,
    either whole or in portions

1 lemon
1 teaspoon Rosemary Salt
    (recipe on page 230)

SIDE NOTE

If you don't have a broiler or if your oven doesn't have a broil setting, you can bake the salmon at 350˚F for about 10-15 minutes.

These seasonings also work beautifully with chicken.

Preheat oven to a low broil setting.

Place thinly sliced pats of butter in a baking dish, or spread ghee or coconut oil over the bottom of the dish. Place the salmon in the dish and sprinkle with the Rosemary Salt. Add more thin pats of butter on top of the salmon, and top with slices of lemon.

Broil on low for approximately 10-12 minutes or until the salmon is cooked to your liking.

NUTS

EGGS

NIGHTSHADES

FODMAPS

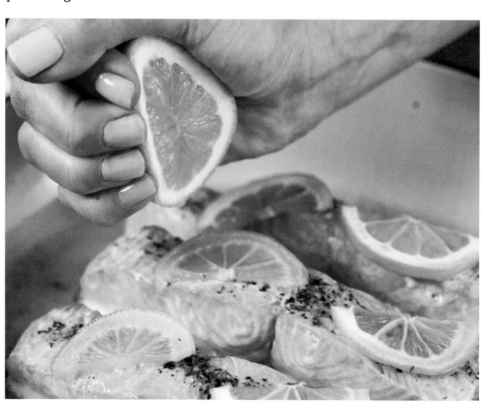

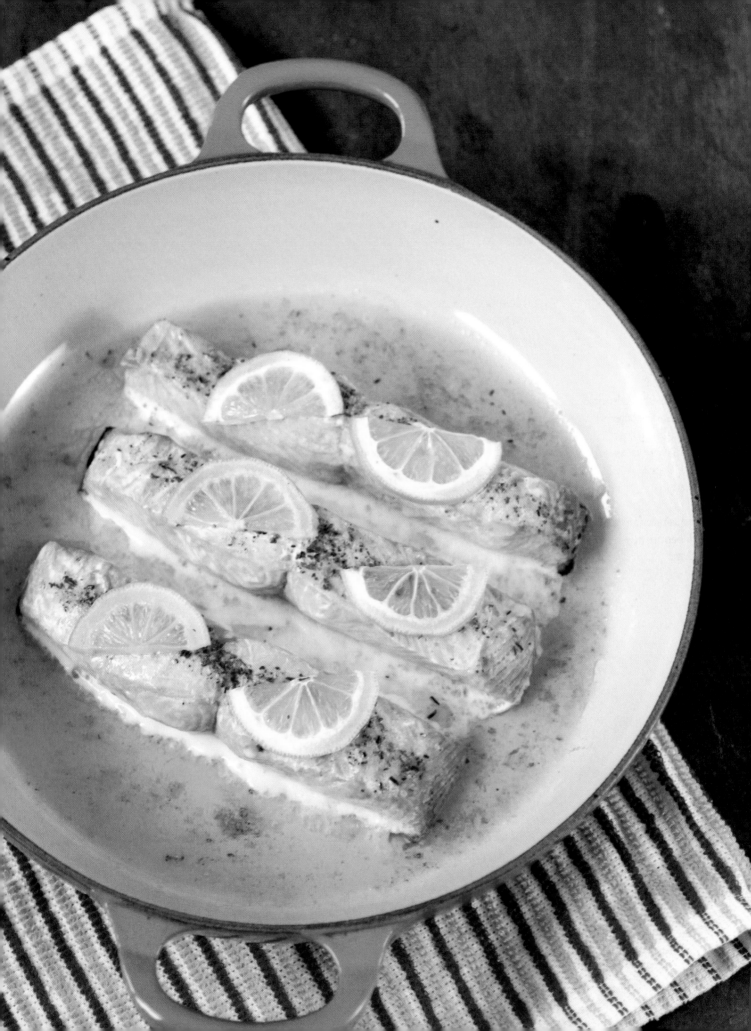

pesto shrimp & squash fettuccine

PREP TIME
30 minutes

COOKING TIME
25 minutes

YIELD
2 meal-sized portions or
4 side dish-sized servings

If you miss pasta, zucchini noodles are a fantastic replacement. They're more flavorful, nutrient-dense, and can carry a sauce just like other noodles. Use a julienne or regular vegetable peeler to make them, depending upon the shape of noodles you want.

2 dozen large shrimp
4 zucchini or yellow squash
Sea salt and black pepper to taste

PESTO
1/2 cup macadamia nuts
1 bunch cilantro, rinsed
1 clove garlic
1/2 cup extra-virgin olive oil or
    macadamia nut oil
Sea salt and black pepper to taste

SIDE NOTE

If you have precooked shrimp to use, be sure they're warm before tossing with the sauce and noodles.

For instructions on deveining shrimp, see page 312.

FODMAP FREE?

Omit the garlic

NUT FREE?

Try substituting shredded coconut instead, or simply leave the nuts out of the pesto.

NUTS

EGGS

NIGHTSHADES

FODMAPS

Make the pesto first. Combine the macadamia nuts, cilantro, garlic, extra-virgin olive oil, sea salt, and black pepper in a food processor, and blend until smooth.

Peel and devein the shrimp (see page 312 for details) before they are cooked, pulling the tail off first, then the rest of the shell. (Doing this before cooking allows you to serve the dish warm, as deveining after cooking would require you let the shrimp cool first.)

Place a steamer basket in a large sauce pot, and boil about an inch of water. While the water is heating, run a julienne or regular vegetable peeler along each of the squash until you reach the center, seedy part. Steam the squash for about 3-5 minutes. Set the steamed squash "noodles" aside.

Steam the shrimp for approximately 3 minutes or until they're pink all the way through.

Place the steamed squash into a mixing bowl with the pesto and toss until well combined.

Top the noodles with the shrimp, and serve warm.

CHANGE IT UP

Use a julienne peeler to make spaghetti-shaped noodles versus fettuccine shapes.

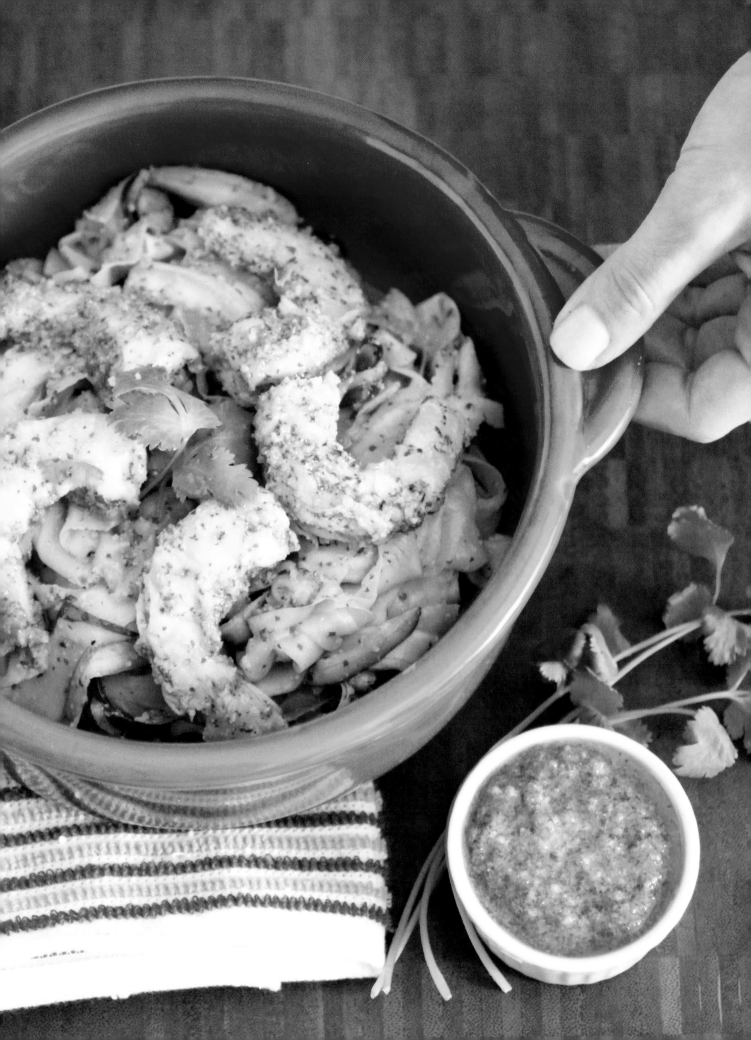

quick & easy salmon cakes

PREP TIME
10 minutes

COOKING TIME
20 minutes

YIELD
4 patties

If you're looking to dress-up the wild canned salmon you've been buying, this is the recipe for you! It's quick and easy, and it can be made mostly from the ingredients you tend to have on-hand.

FODMAP FREE?
Leave out the shallots, garlic, and green onions—season with extra fresh herbs.

Do not use the coconut flour or coconut oil.

2 6-ounce cans of wild salmon, drained
2 eggs, beaten
3 tablespoons minced shallots
1-2 cloves garlic, minced or grated
2 tablespoons green onions (scallions), minced

1 teaspoon Savory Spice Blend (recipe on page 233)
2 teaspoons gluten-free mustard (optional)
1-2 teaspoons coconut flour (optional)
1/4 cup coconut oil or butter

Combine the salmon, eggs, shallots, garlic, green onions, Savory Spice Blend, and mustard (optional) in a small mixing bowl. If the consistency is runny, sift the coconut flour over the mixture, and combine well.

CHANGE IT UP
Change the seasonings for a new taste experience—try the Curry Spice Blend instead of Savory.

In a large pan over medium heat, melt enough coconut oil to create a layer about 1/4-inch thick. Form the salmon mixture into 4 equally sized patties, and place them in the pan, all at once or 2 at a time. Allow the patties to brown on one side before flipping, and cook all the way through.

Serve warm or cold as leftovers.

NUTS
EGGS
NIGHTSHADES
FODMAPS

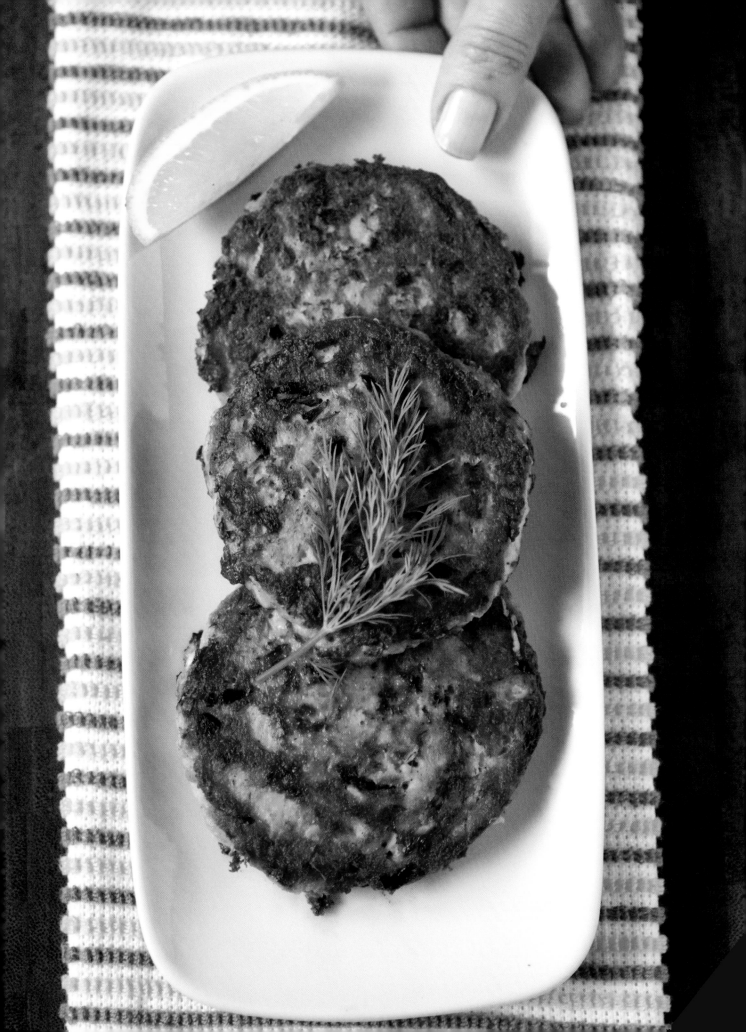

tomatillo shrimp cocktail

PREP TIME
40 minutes

COOKING TIME
5 minutes

YIELD
Approximately 1 cup of cocktail sauce. Servings of shrimp will vary by size/weight: 4-6 shrimp per person work well as an appetizer; 10-12 shrimp work well as an entree.

Shrimp cocktail is a classic favorite amongst my friends, and it makes an appearance at every party we throw. Enjoy this variation on the classic sauce that's typically made with red tomatoes.

- 2+ lbs wild jumbo or colossal shrimp
- 2 cups tomatillos, outer skin peeled and fruit quartered
- 1 teaspoon jalapeño pepper, minced
- 1/2 teaspoon garlic, minced or grated

- 1-2 teaspoon fresh horseradish, minced or grated (to taste, using more will yield a spicier sauce)
- 1 tablespoon apple cider vinegar or distilled vinegar
- 1 tablespoon extra-virgin olive oil

HOT, HOT, HOT

For a less spicy version, leave out the jalapeño and adjust the amount of horseradish.

NIGHTSHADE FREE?

Make the cocktail sauce from mangoes, peaches, or pineapple instead of tomatillos.

Peel, devein, and then steam the shrimp for approximately 2-3 minutes if fresh, 3-5 minutes if frozen. Note: You can either devein fresh shrimp before or after cooking. If they are frozen, you will need to cook them first. Set the cooked shrimp aside and allow them to chill before serving.

Combine the tomatillos, jalapeño, garlic, horseradish, vinegar, and extra-virgin olive oil in a food processor, and pulse until smooth.

Serve chilled.

CHANGE IT UP

If you can't find tomatillos, you can use regular red tomatoes.

Also, try tossing the shrimp in the sauce and eating over a salad.

NUTS

EGGS

NIGHTSHADES

FODMAPS

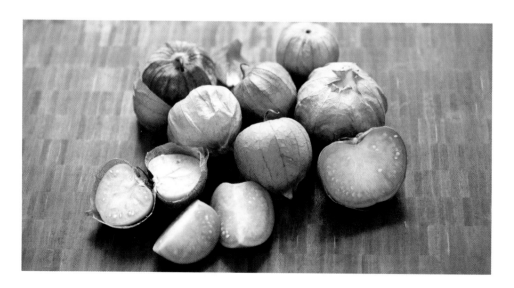

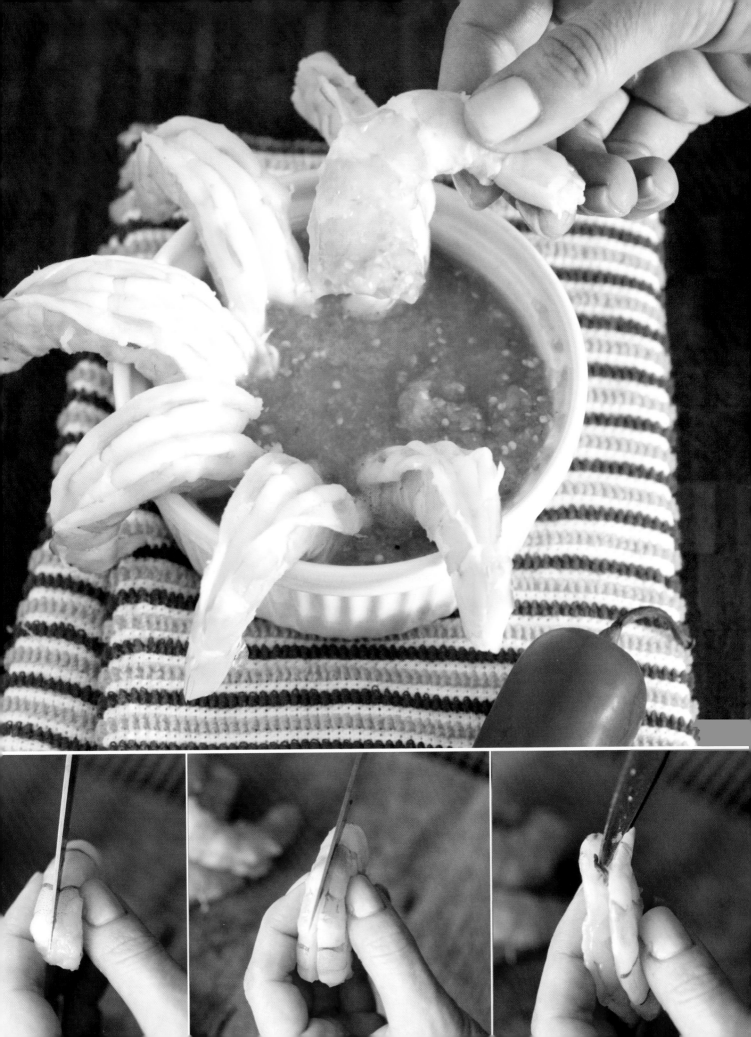

citrus macadamia nut sole

PREP TIME
10 minutes

COOKING TIME
15 minutes

YIELD
3-4 servings

Growing up, my mom used to make nut-topped fish nearly every week. Her recipe would change from time to time, but the basics always included butter and some kind of light or white fish. Try this with flounder or halibut if you prefer.

1/4 cup macadamia nuts, chopped
Zest of one orange
1 lb lemon sole, or other white fish

Sea salt and black pepper to taste
2 tablespoons butter or coconut oil

CHANGE IT UP
Use another type of nut if you prefer, and try it with lemon or lime zest instead of orange.

Preheat oven on a low broil setting.

In a small mixing bowl, combine the macadamia nuts and orange zest. Set aside.

Place the lemon sole on a baking sheet, season with sea salt and black pepper to taste, then top evenly with the butter or coconut oil and nut/zest topping.

Place the fish in the broiler and cook approximately 10 minutes or until opaque white all the way through.

NUTS
EGGS
NIGHTSHADES
FODMAPS

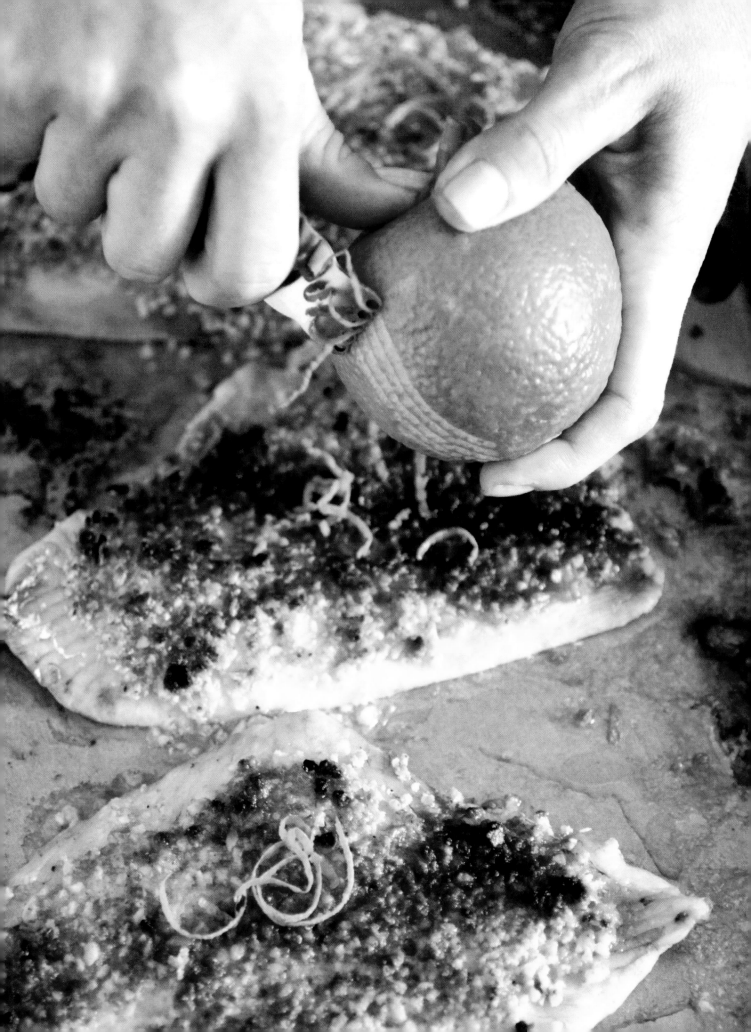

nori salmon handroll

PREP TIME
5 minutes

COOKING TIME
-

YIELD
1 snack-sized hand roll

For a super-fast snack or lunch option, roll your favorite fish or even leftover chicken or turkey into a seaweed paper and off you go!

1 toasted nori (seaweed) sheet
1/4 avocado, mashed or sliced
2 ounces wild smoked salmon (lox)
2 slices cucumber

1 green onion (scallion), finely chopped
1 very thin slice of lemon (optional)

CHANGE IT UP
Use wild canned salmon if you don't have or don't care for smoked.

Place the nori paper on a cutting board, and layer the avocado, smoked salmon, cucumber, green onion, and lemon on top of it.

Wrap the paper around the ingredients, and enjoy.

NUTS
EGGS
NIGHTSHADES
FODMAPS

---

simple shrimp ceviche

PREP TIME
40 minutes

COOKING TIME
-

YIELD
4 cups

This recipe is always a hit at parties, and it is fantastic for an outdoor barbecue. For the best flavor, prepare the ceviche a couple of hours ahead and let it marinate in the citrus. Add 1 ripe, diced avocado right before serving.

1 lb cooked, peeled, and deveined wild shrimp (cooled)
1/4 red bell pepper, finely diced
1/4 orange or yellow bell pepper, finely diced
1/2 jalapeño pepper, finely diced (seeds and white ribs removed)
1/4 cup diced raw jicama

1/4 cup diced cucumber (skin-on)
1 tablespoon shallot, finely diced
2 tablespoons cilantro, chopped
2 tablespoons extra-virgin olive oil
Juice of 1 lime
Juice of 1 lemon
2 cups of sliced cucumber, for dipping

NIGHTSHADE FREE?
Omit the bell peppers.

Chop the cooked, cooled shrimp into 1/4-1/2-inch pieces. Combine red bell pepper, orange/yellow bell pepper, jalapeño, jicama, cucumber, shallot, cilantro, olive oil, lime juice, and lemon juice in a large mixing bowl.

Chill the mixture in the refrigerator for 30 minutes before serving with cucumber slices.

NUTS
EGGS
NIGHTSHADES
FODMAPS

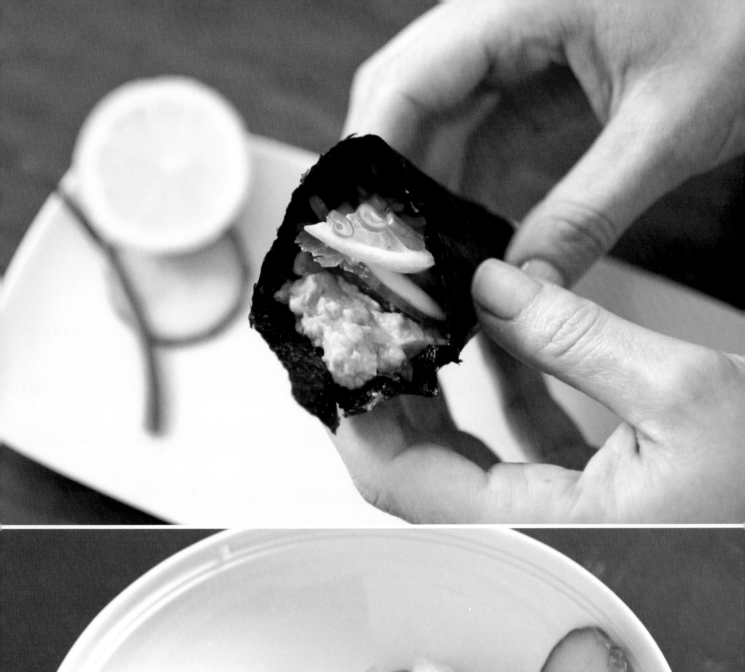
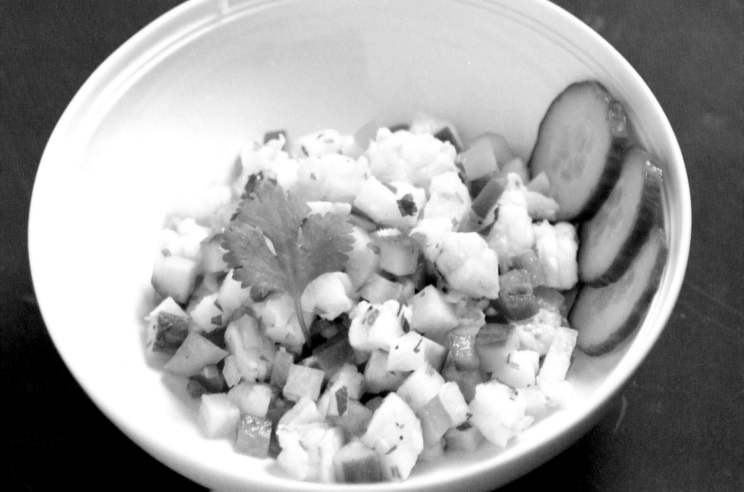

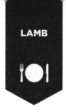

lemony lamb dolmas (stuffed grape leaves)

PREP TIME
40 minutes

COOKING TIME
50 minutes

YIELD
20-24 dolmas
(serves 4 as an entrée)

FODMAP FREE?
Omit the onions and cauliflower.

This dish works great with the following recipes: Taramasalata on page 386, Roasted Garlic Tahini Sauce on page 386, Avo-ziki on page 322, and Olive Tapenade on page 326.

1 tablespoon coconut oil
1 small onion, finely diced
1 lb ground lamb
1 teaspoon nutmeg
1/2 teaspoon cinnamon
1 teaspoon cumin
1 teaspoon dried oregano
2 tablespoons dried currants or
    raisins
1 cup cauliflower, shredded
    or grated

Juice of 1 lime
Sea salt and black pepper to taste
20 grape leaves
    (approximately 16-ounce jar)
1 lemon
1/4 cup water
2-3 bay leaves
2 tablespoons raw sliced almonds

NUTS
EGGS
NIGHTSHADES
FODMAPS

Preheat oven to 350°F.

In a large skillet over medium heat, melt the coconut oil and sauté the onion until clear. Add the ground lamb, nutmeg, cinnamon, cumin, dried oregano, and dried currants or raisins, and cook until the lamb is still just slightly pink inside.

Add the shredded cauliflower, and combine with the meat mixture, cooking an additional 2-3 minutes. Squeeze the lime juice over the meat mixture, and stir. Set the meat and cauliflower mixture aside to cool slightly before rolling in the grape leaves.

Gently separate and unroll the grape leaves, as they are somewhat delicate. Spoon a small amount of the lamb mixture into the center of the end of the leaf (pictured), and roll the bottom of the leaf up. Then, fold the sides over and continue to roll until the end is tucked underneath.

Lay the dolmas in an oven-safe dish with the finished end side down. Slice the lemon thinly, and then squeeze juice over the tray. Pour the water over the tray, and top with bay leaves and sliced almonds.

Cover with foil, and bake for 30-45 minutes until the leaves turn a darker shade and the water evaporates. Remove the bay leaves before eating.

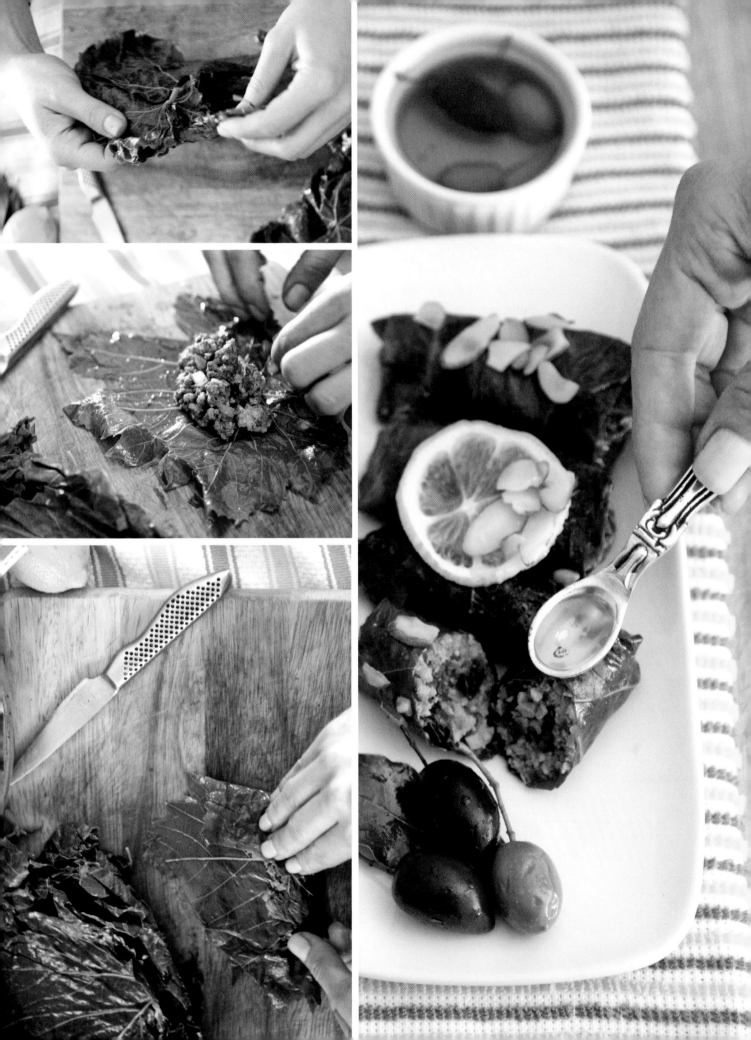

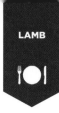
mediterranean lamb roast

PREP TIME
10 minutes

COOKING TIME
6-8 hours

YIELD
6-8 servings

When your days are busy and filled with activity, slow-cooker recipes make life really easy. Set up this lamb roast in the morning and come home to an amazingly flavorful roast after work!

4 lbs lamb roast
2 onions, cut into quarters
4 large carrots, chopped into
    1-inch pieces
6-8 cloves of garlic, smashed

1/4 cup Kalamata olives
1/4 cup brine/liquid from olives
32-ounce can whole peeled plum
    tomatoes

SIDE NOTE
I like Kalamata olives for this recipe, but you could also use green olives if you have them on-hand.

Place all ingredients in a slow-cooker, and cook on low for a minimum of 6 hours or overnight.

If you don't have a slow-cooker, use an enameled cast iron Dutch oven, and braise the ingredients at 275˚F for six hours or overnight at 200˚F.

Serve alone or over Mashed Faux-Tatoes (recipe on page 344).

NIGHTSHADE FREE?
Leave out the tomatoes and use 24 ounces of Bone Broth on page 234 instead as your braising liquid.

NUTS
EGGS
NIGHTSHADES
FODMAPS

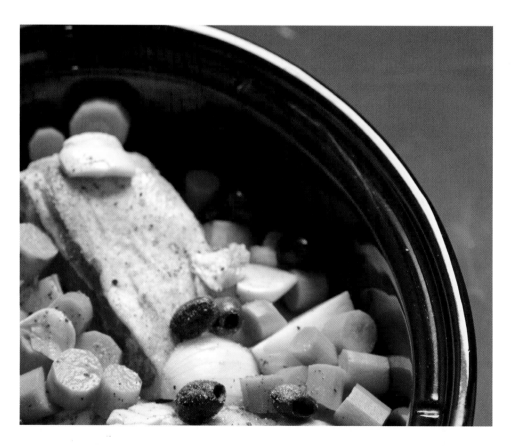

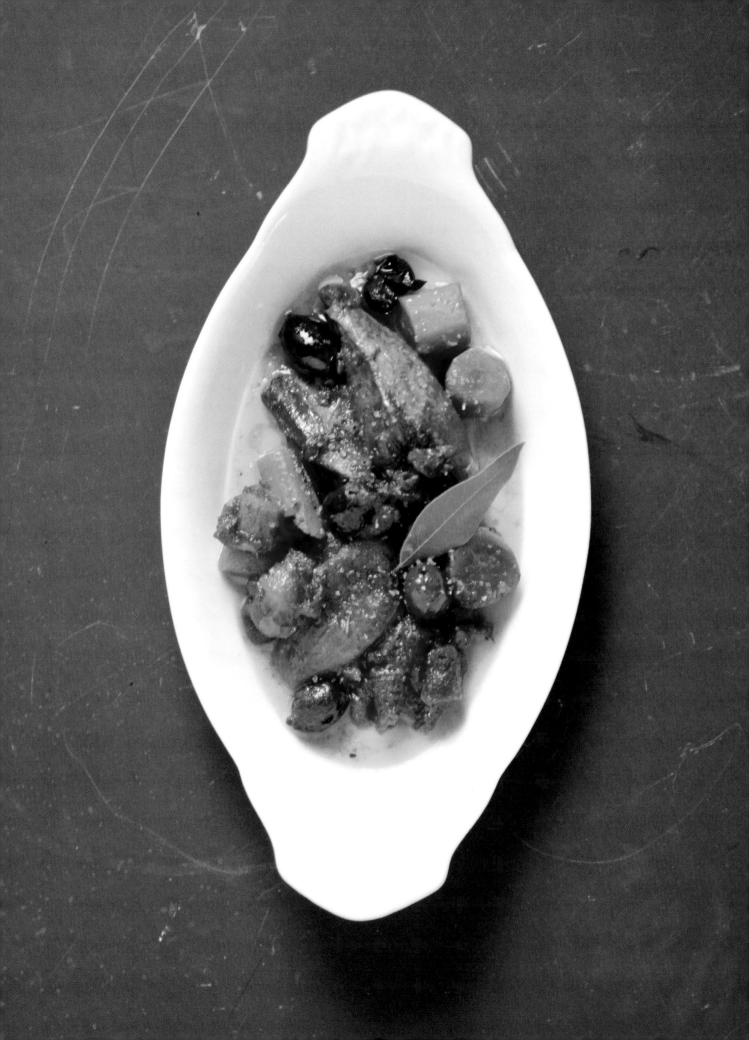

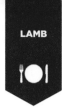
lamb lettuce boats
with avo-ziki sauce

PREP TIME
20 minutes

COOKING TIME
10 minutes

YIELD
2-3 entrée-sized portions

I've been known to wrap pretty much anything in lettuce—and lamb is no exception! This combination is fresh and tasty and has bold flavors. It's an unexpected and fun way to present lamb to your family.

SIDE NOTE

These are fantastic with the Olive Tapenade on page 326 as well! (pictured)

NIGHTSHADE FREE?

Leave off the tomatoes.

FODMAP FREE?

Leave off the Avo-Ziki Sauce.

1 lb lamb stew meat
Sea salt and black pepper to taste
1/2 teaspoon dried or fresh oregano
1 tablespoon coconut oil, melted
4-6 large romaine lettuce leaves, cleaned
1 cup cherry tomatoes, halved (or regular tomato, diced)
1/2 cucumber, finely diced
1 lemon, cut in half

AVO-ZIKI SAUCE
1 ripe avocado
1/4 cup grated cucumber
1 small clove garlic, grated
Juice of 1 lemon
2 tablespoons extra-virgin olive oil
Sea salt and black pepper to taste
1 teaspoon fresh dill, finely chopped

In a small mixing bowl, season the lamb with sea salt, black pepper, and oregano. In a skillet over medium-high heat, melt the coconut oil, and then place the lamb pieces in the pan. Cook the lamb approximately 2-3 minutes or until it is browned on one side, and flip to brown the other side for another 2 minutes or so.

Once the meat is cooked, chop it into 1/2-inch pieces.

Place the romaine lettuce leaves onto serving plates and top with the chopped lamb, cherry tomatoes, and cucumber. Squeeze lemon over each lettuce boat, then top with the Avo-Ziki Sauce.

For the Avo-Ziki: Combine all ingredients in a small food processor or with a hand blender.

NUTS

EGGS

NIGHTSHADES

FODMAPS

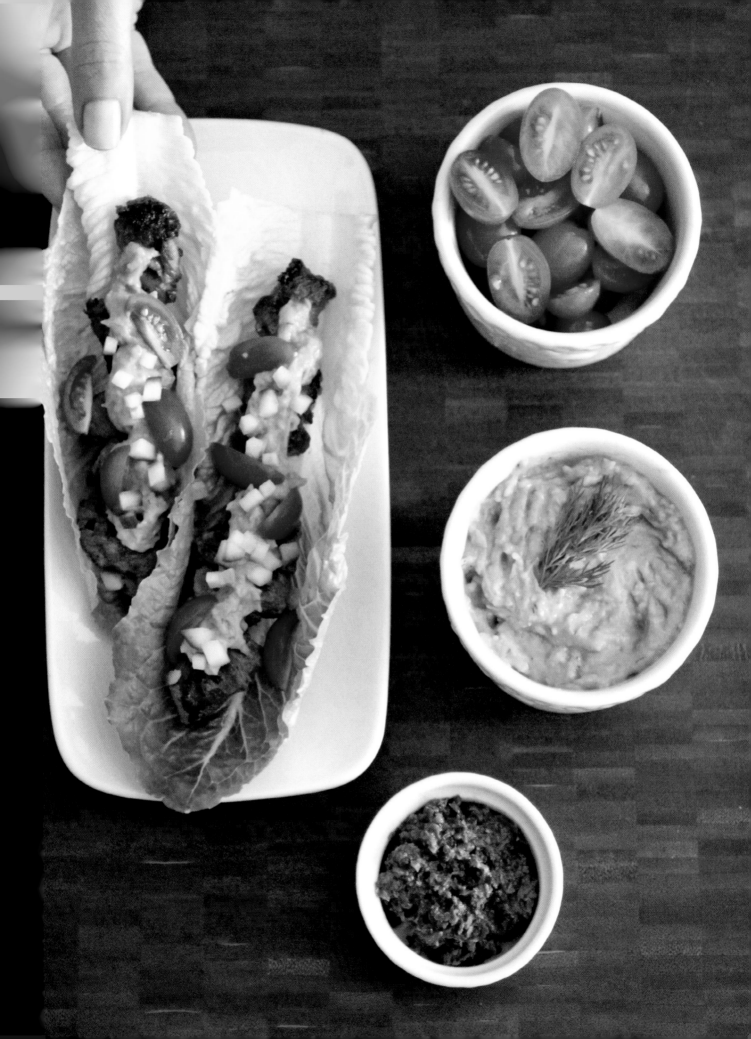

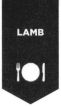

spiced lamb meatballs with balsamic-fig compote

PREP TIME
20 minutes

COOKING TIME
30 minutes

YIELD
16 mini meatballs + sauce

These spiced meatballs are delicious with a dipping sauce, but if pairing them with a fruit sauce isn't your thing, have no fear! They're also fantastic with Roasted Garlic Tahini Sauce (recipe on page 386) or Olive Tapenade (recipe on page 326).

1 lb ground lamb
1 teaspoon cumin
1/4 teaspoon allspice
1/4 teaspoon cinnamon
1 teaspoon onion powder
Sea salt and black pepper to taste

BALSAMIC-FIG COMPOTE
1/2 cup water
1/2 cup balsamic vinegar
4 dried figs, sliced
1 sprig fresh rosemary

SIDE NOTE

This recipe is a simple way to take dried fruit to a whole other level. You can use fresh figs if you have, which requires less water and less cooking time. I love the sweet and tangy combination of the figs and the vinegar.

FODMAP FREE?

Omit the onion powder and enjoy these meatballs with olive tapenade instead of the fig compote.

Preheat oven to 375˚F.

In a mixing bowl, combine the lamb and spices with your hands. Form into approximately 16 small meatballs (1 1/2 inch diameter, 1 ounce each), and place in a large baking dish. Bake for 25 minutes.

While the meatballs bake: in a small saucepan, combine water, balsamic vinegar, figs, and rosemary. Simmer until the texture becomes thick. Add more vinegar if it tastes too sweet, and reduce the sauce further if it tastes too tart.

Serve the meatballs warm from the oven with the compote.

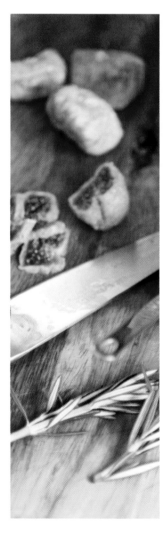

NUTS
EGGS
NIGHTSHADES
FODMAPS

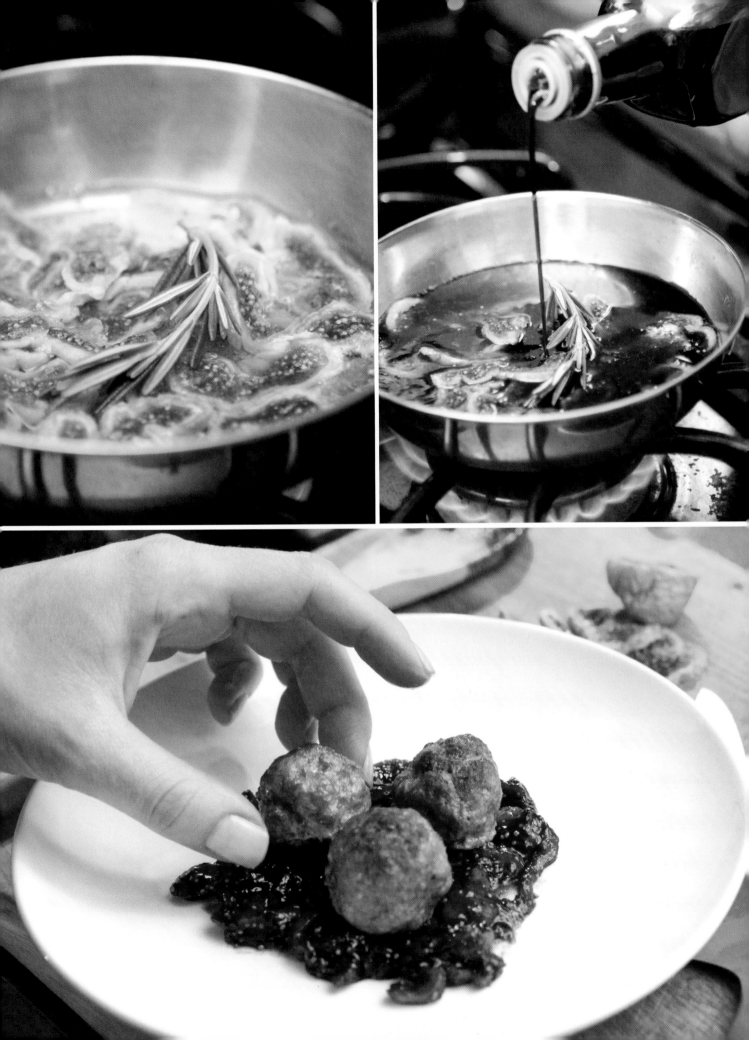

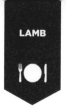
greek-style lamb kabobs

Kabobs are an easy way to make a fantastic presentation out of an inexpensive cut (like stew meat). It's a perfect alternative to tired cookout burgers.

PREP TIME
30 minutes

COOKING TIME
15 minutes

YIELD
2-4 meal-sized portions

CHANGE IT UP
Use cilantro instead of oregano for a quick change of flavor profile!

NUTS
EGGS
NIGHTSHADES
FODMAPS

1 lb lamb stew meat, cubed
1 bell pepper, cut into 1-inch pieces
2 zucchini, cut into 1-inch pieces
1 red onion, cut into 1-inch pieces
Juice of 2 lemons or limes

1/2 teaspoon dried oregano
1/2 teaspoon sea salt
1/4-1/2 teaspoon black pepper to taste
1/4 cup extra-virgin olive oil

Preheat an outdoor or indoor grill to medium-high heat.

Arrange the cubes of lamb on heat-safe skewers, alternating with the bell peppers, zucchini, and onions (or other vegetables).

In a small mixing bowl, combine the lemon or lime juice with the oregano, sea salt, and black pepper. Brush the citrus mixture over the skewers and allow them to marinate for 10 minutes.

Place the skewers onto the grill or grill pan and cook for approximately 3-4 minutes per side or until done to your liking. Drizzle the skewers with the extra-virgin olive oil just prior to serving.

---

lamb chops with olive tapenade

Lamb and olives are a perfect combination. Enjoy these simple chops with the salty and delicious olive spread.

PREP TIME
10 minutes

COOKING TIME
5-10 minutes

YIELD
4 servings

CHANGE IT UP
Enjoy these with a green salad or Sautéed Spinach (recipe on page 366).

NUTS
EGGS
NIGHTSHADES
FODMAPS

2 tablespoons bacon fat
   or coconut oil
2 lbs lamb chops
1 tablespoon Greek Spice Blend
   (recipe on page 233)

OLIVE TAPENADE
1/2 cup Kalamata olives, pitted
1/2 teaspoon dried oregano
2 tablespoons extra-virgin olive oil
1 tablespoon capers
1/2 teaspoon anchovy paste
Juice of 1/2 lemon

Preheat oven to 400°F.

In an oven-safe pan over medium heat, melt the bacon fat. While the pan heats, sprinkle both sides of the lamb chops with the Greek Spice Blend. Sear the lamb chops for 2 minutes on each side, and place the entire pan in the hot oven for 2 minutes. Remove the lamb chops from the oven

To make the tapenade: Combine all ingredients in a food processor or hand blender. Top each lamb chop with a dollop of the tapenade.

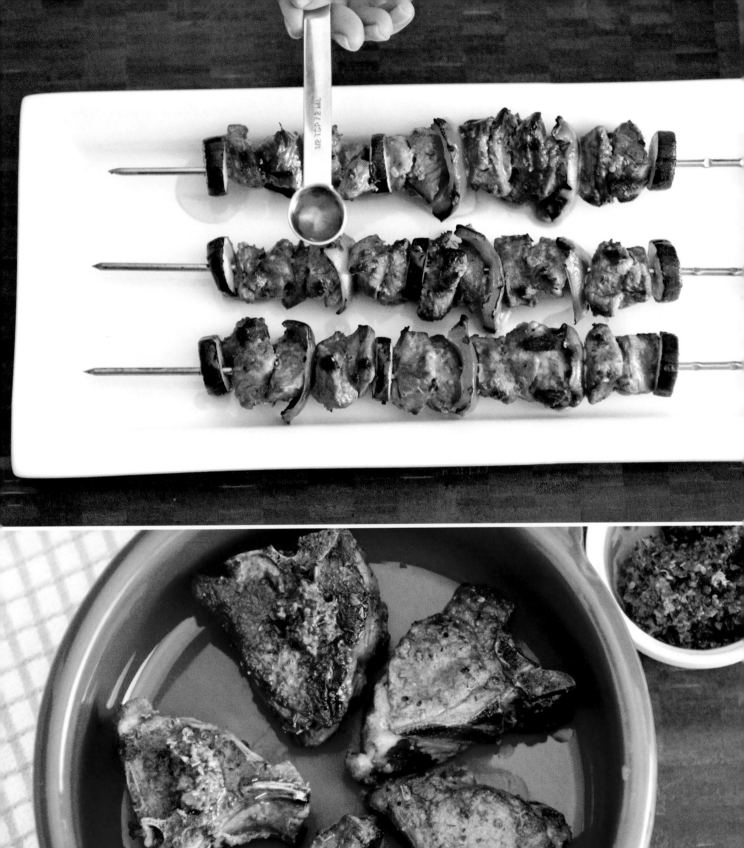
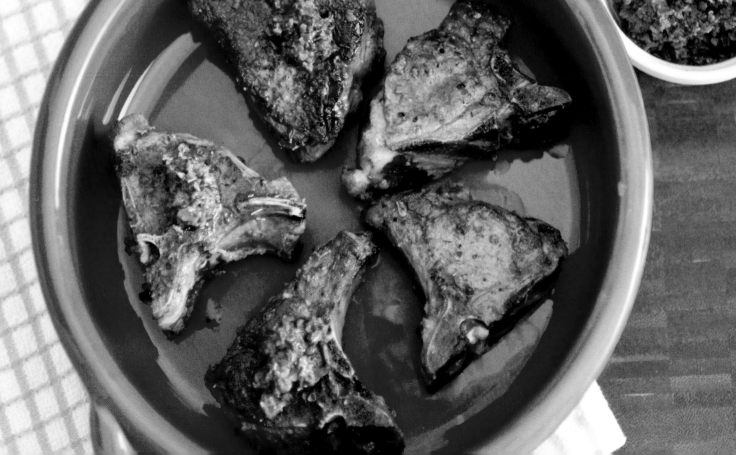

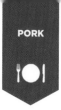
cumin spiced pork tenderloin with root vegetables

PREP TIME
20 minutes

COOKING TIME
45 minutes

YIELD
4-6 entree-sized portions

SIDE NOTE
This dish pairs nicely with Roasted Brussels with Fennel (recipe on page 350).

FODMAP FREE?
Omit the onion and garlic, and substitute carrots for the parsnips.

NUTS
EGGS
NIGHTSHADES
FODMAPS

A cooking class I took while living in San Francisco called "Food of Spain" inspired this dish. The combination of the cumin and garlic complement the pork nicely. Served over roasted root vegetables, this dish is simple enough for a weeknight meal, but creates an elegant enough presentation to serve to dinner guests.

1 tablespoon cumin
1 tablespoon coriander
1 tablespoon granulated garlic or garlic powder
1 teaspoon sea salt
Black pepper to taste
2 pork tenderloins
2 tablespoon bacon fat (or other cooking fat)

2 onions, chopped into large slices
4 parsnips, peeled and chopped
2 cloves fresh garlic, smashed
1 large orange, peeled and segmented
Seeds of 1 pomegranate (approximately 1/4 cup) (optional)

Preheat oven to 375˚F.

In a small mixing bowl, combine the cumin, coriander, granulated garlic, sea salt, and black pepper.

Using paper towels, pat the pork tenderloins dry, and apply the spice blend to the meat generously to create a crust. Heat a large skillet over medium-high heat, and melt the bacon fat. Place the pork tenderloins in the skillet, and sear on all sides for approximately 2 minutes per side.

Place the onions, parsnips, garlic, orange segments, and pomegranate seeds in a large roasting dish, topped by the seared pork tenderloins. Roast for 30-40 minutes or until the internal temperature of the pork tenderloins reaches 145˚F. If you need to continue to roast the vegetables until they are soft, simply remove the pork and set it aside on a cutting board to rest while the vegetables finish roasting for another 10-15 minutes.

Slice the tenderloin on the bias (diagonally) and serve over the vegetables.

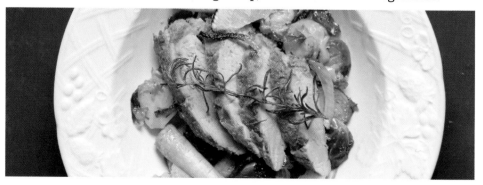

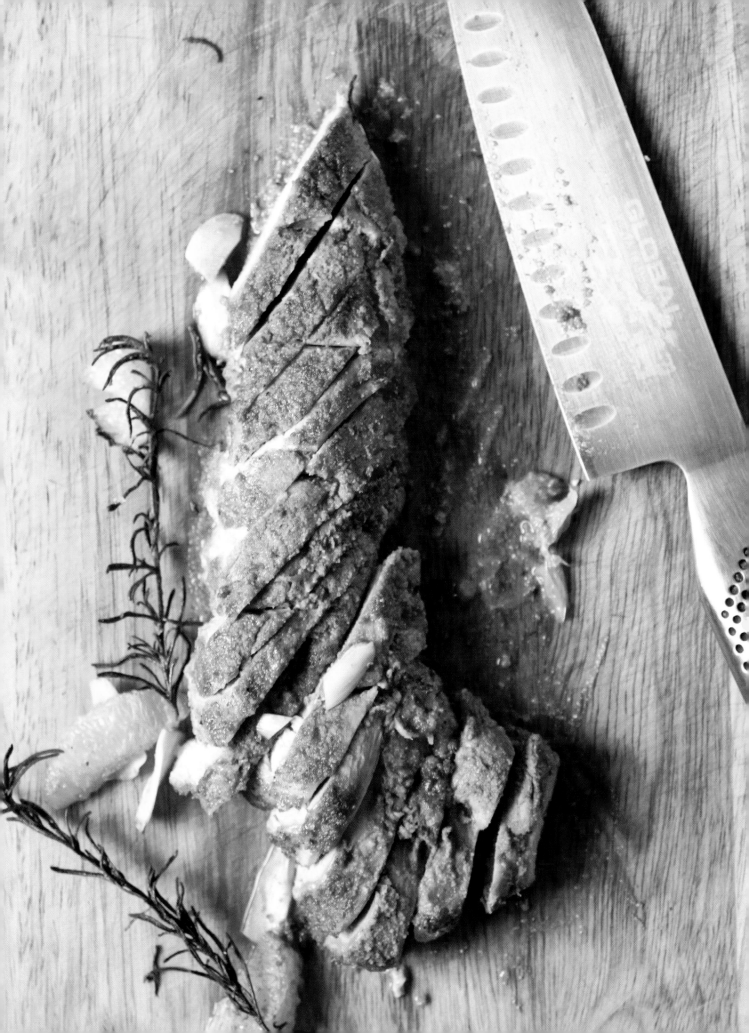

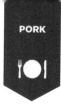

chorizo meatballs

PREP TIME
10 minutes

COOKING TIME
20-25 minutes

YIELD
1 dozen meatballs

This recipe is simple if you make the Chorizo Spice Blend (recipe on page 232) ahead of time and keep it on-hand for a quick weeknight dinner. These are also great as an appetizer at a party or as a meal served over Mashed Faux-Tatoes (recipe on page 344).

1 lb ground pork
2 tablespoons Chorizo Spice Blend

1 tablespoon apple cider vinegar

CHANGE IT UP
Substitute beef or a combination of ground pork and chicken. Double or triple the recipe and make extras for leftovers or to freeze for later use.

Preheat oven to 425°F.

In a medium-sized mixing bowl, mix the ground pork, spices, and apple cider vinegar with your hands until well combined and the spice mixture looks evenly dispersed.

Form the meat into a dozen 1-ounce meatballs, and then place in an oven-safe baking dish or on a baking sheet. Bake for 20-25 minutes.

NUTS
EGGS
NIGHTSHADES
FODMAPS

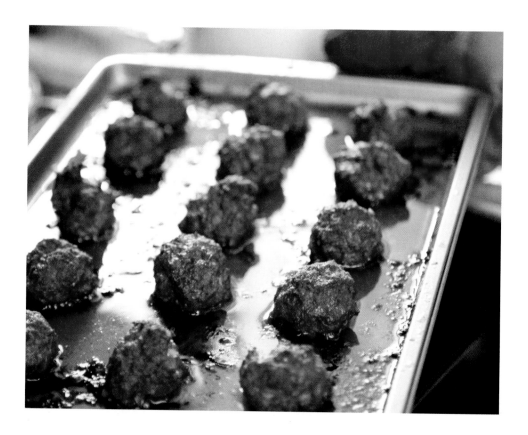

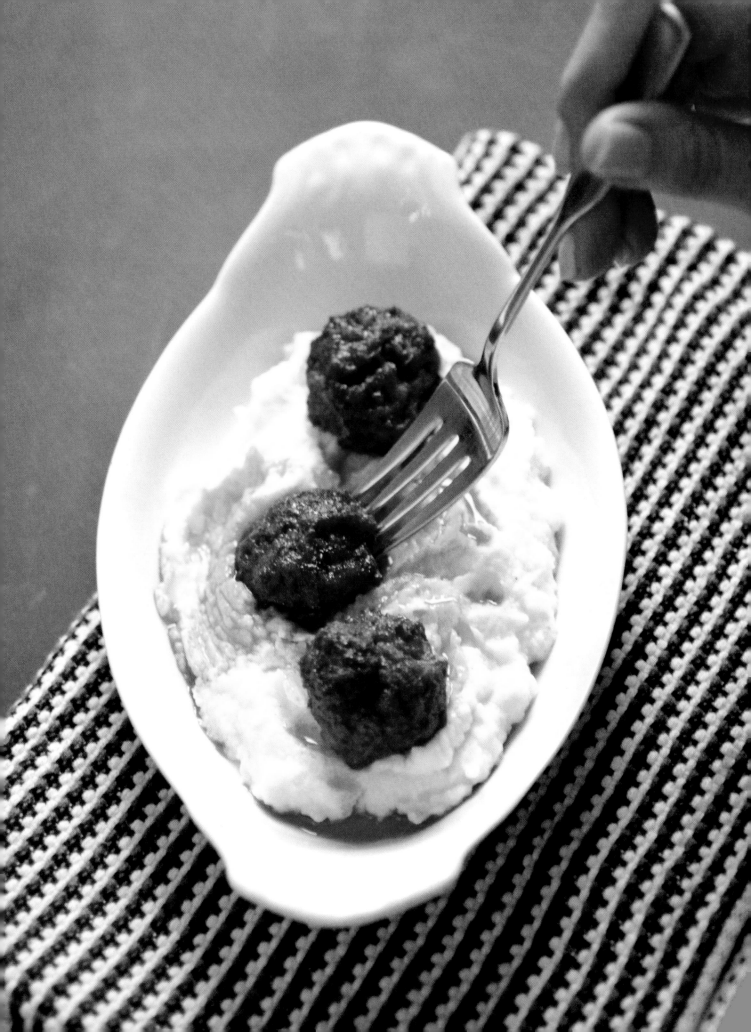

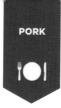
grandma barbara's stuffed mushrooms

PREP TIME
20 minutes

COOKING TIME
30 minutes

YIELD
3-4 entree-sized portions /
12 mushrooms

CHANGE IT UP
*Substitute ground turkey
for the pork. Stuff 4 large
Portobello caps instead
of 12 baby mushrooms.*

NIGHTSHADE FREE?
*Leave out the bell
peppers.*

NUTS
EGGS
NIGHTSHADES
FODMAPS

*My grandma used to make a big spread of appetizers every holiday, and I always
requested her stuffed mushrooms. The original recipe calls for breadcrumbs, so
this is an adaptation, but don't worry—the tops of these get crispy even without
the grains.*

1 dozen baby Portobello
    mushroom caps, cleaned
1 tablespoon bacon fat
    (or other cooking fat)
1/4 cup bell pepper, minced
1/4 cup yellow onion, minced

1 lb ground pork sausage (use
    ground pork plus Italian Sau-
    sage blend, recipe on page 233)
2 cups spinach, finely chopped or
    processed
1 clove garlic, grated

Preheat oven to 450°F.

Place the mushrooms on a baking sheet with the "cup" side facing down, and
bake for 10 minutes or just enough to allow some of the moisture to release
from the mushrooms. Do this before or while you prepare the filling mixture.

In a large skillet over medium heat, melt the bacon fat, and place the bell peppers and yellow onions in the pan, sautéing until the onions are clear and soft.
Add the sausage to the pan, and cook it until little or no pink meat remains
(approximately 5 minutes), stirring occasionally to break up any large chunks of
meat.

Add the spinach and garlic, and combine together in the pan. Spoon the mixture into each of the mushroom caps, and place them back onto the baking
sheet.

Bake for approximately 20 minutes or until golden brown on top.

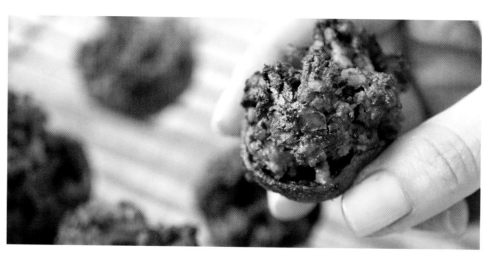

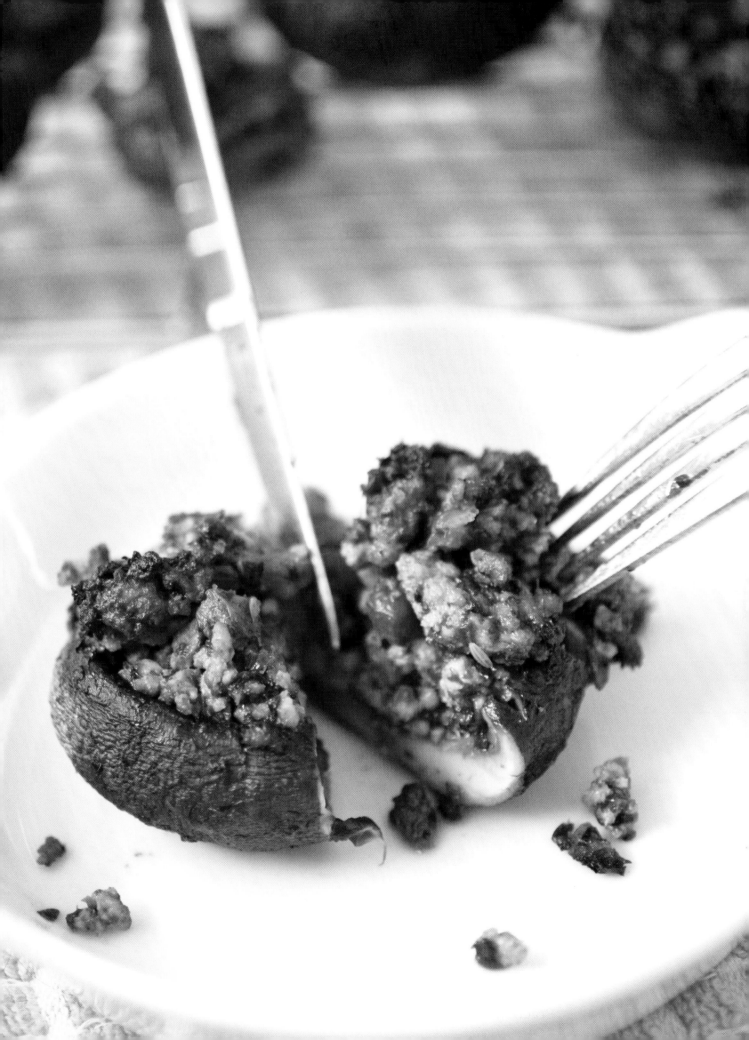

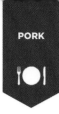

thanksgiving stuffing meatballs

PREP TIME
20 minutes

COOKING TIME
25-30 minutes

YIELD
24, 1 ounce meatballs

SIDE NOTE
Make these into patties instead of meatballs to freeze and save for future breakfasts that are quick and easy!

NUTS
EGGS
NIGHTSHADES
FODMAPS

If you've ever wished you could eat something that tastes like Thanksgiving any time of the year without cooking a whole feast, here's your chance! These tiny pork meatballs pack all the flavor of the season and are perfect with the Simple Cranberry Sauce (recipe on page 388) for dipping.

2 lb ground pork
2 tablespoons Italian Sausage
    Spice Blend (recipe on page 233)
2 teaspoons butter, bacon fat, or
    coconut oil
1/4 cup onion, finely chopped

1/4 cup celery, finely chopped
1/4 cup carrot, grated or shredded
1/4 cup chestnuts, finely chopped
    (use walnuts or pecans if
    chestnuts are not available)

Preheat oven to 425°F.

In a medium-sized mixing bowl, combine the pork and Italian Sausage Spice Blend until the spices are well incorporated evenly throughout the meat.

In a large skillet over medium heat, melt the butter, bacon fat, or coconut oil. Place the onions, celery, and carrots in the pan, and sauté until the onions and celery appear translucent. Add the chestnuts, and continue to cook for another 2 minutes.

Set the onion, celery, carrot, and chestnut mixture aside to cool until you can touch it comfortably. Then, combine the mixture with the meat, and form the pork into 24 meatballs.

Place the meatballs in an oven-safe dish or on a baking sheet, and bake approximately 25-30 minutes or until cooked all the way through.

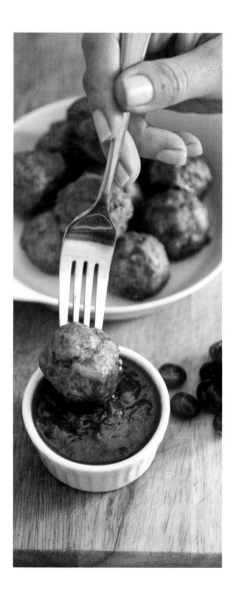

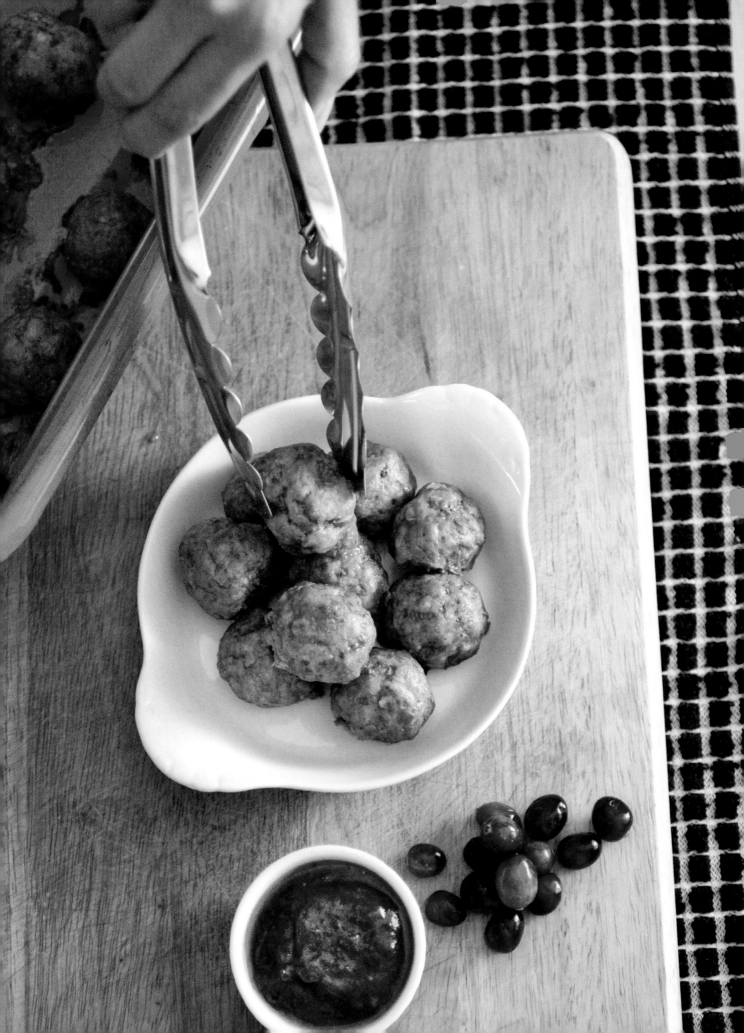

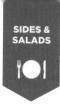
broc-cauli chowder with bacon

PREP TIME
30 minutes

COOKING TIME
30 minutes

YIELD
Approximately 8 servings

CHANGE IT UP
You can make the soup with just broccoli or just cauliflower.

If you're looking for an easy way to eat your veggies, this chowder is it! In every bowl of this creamy side dish, you get a heaping helping of both broccoli and cauliflower.

4 cups broccoli, chopped and steamed
2 cups chicken or beef broth (recipe on page 234)
4 cups cauliflower, chopped and steamed

4-6 cloves of roasted garlic (optional, recipe on page 370)
Sea salt & black pepper to taste
4 slices of bacon, baked and chopped (recipe on page 236)

Using a blender, liquefy the broccoli with half of the broth until smooth. Repeat the process with the cauliflower and the remaining broth. Add the roasted garlic to either of the batches before blending again.

Combine the soup purees in a large pot over medium heat. Add sea salt and black pepper to taste. Simmer for 10 minutes, stirring to combine the two purees. Add more stock, 1/4 cup at a time, if the soup is too thick.

Garnish with baked, chopped bacon.

NUTS

EGGS

NIGHTSHADES

FODMAPS

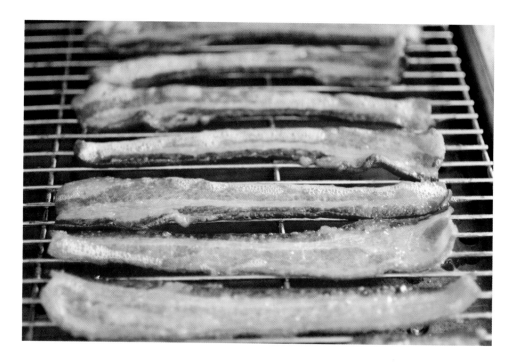

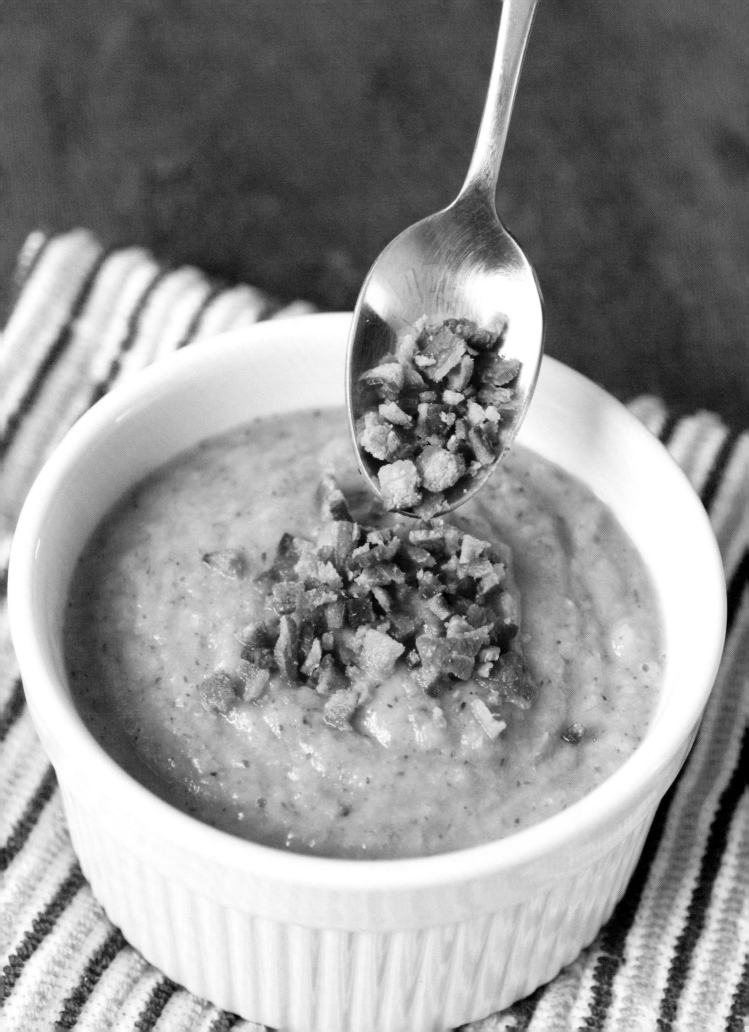

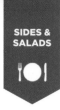
asparagus with lemon & olives

PREP TIME
5 minutes

COOKING TIME
10-15 minutes

YIELD
4 servings

Simply grilling, roasting, or steaming asparagus yields a delicious result, but topping asparagus with some citrus and olives takes it to a new level. Enjoy this as a side to the salmon recipe on page 306 or with any simply-grilled meat.

1 lb asparagus
1 tablespoon butter or
    coconut oil, melted
1/2 teaspoon garlic powder
Sea salt and black pepper

1 lemon
1 tablespoon extra-virgin olive oil
1/4 cup Kalamata olives,
    pitted & halved

CHANGE IT UP
This recipe also works with green olives and orange zest.

Preheat oven to 375 ° F.

Chop the ends off of the asparagus, and rinse under water. Place the asparagus on a baking sheet, and toss with the melted butter or coconut oil. Sprinkle with garlic powder, sea salt, and black pepper to taste. Roast for approximately 10-15 minutes - less time for very thin asparagus, more time for very thick asparagus.

While the asparagus is roasting, use a microplane grater to remove the zest from the lemon, and set the zest aside.

When the asparagus is bright green and fork tender, remove it from the oven, drizzle with extra-virgin olive oil, and top with the lemon zest and halved olives.

NUTS
EGGS
NIGHTSHADES
FODMAPS

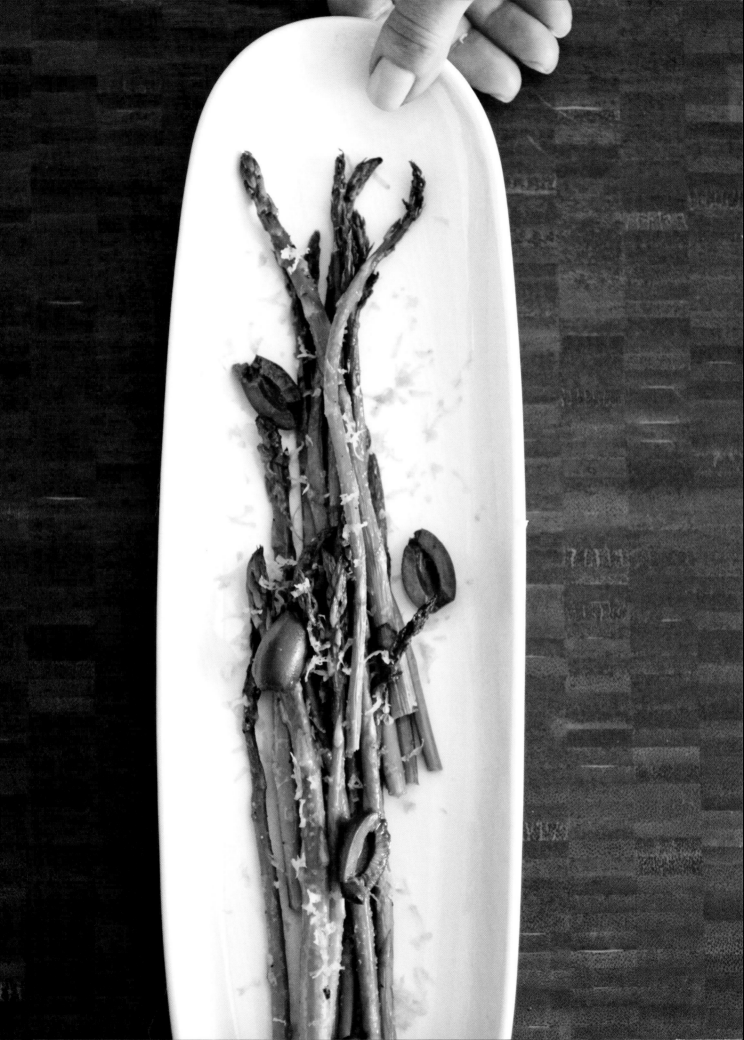

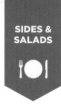
candied carrots

PREP TIME
10 minutes

COOKING TIME
20-30 minutes

YIELD
4 servings

Serve these with Balsamic Braised Short Ribs (recipe on page 278).

8 large carrots, peeled and chopped into 1/2-inch pieces

4 dates, pitted and chopped

2 tablespoons melted butter or coconut oil

Sea salt to taste

SIDE NOTE

These carrots are a treat—not a recipe to make every week.

NUTS

EGGS

NIGHTSHADES

FODMAPS

Preheat oven to 375˚F.

Place the carrots and dates into an oven-safe dish, and top with the melted butter or coconut oil. Toss to coat, and sprinkle with sea salt to taste.

Bake for approximately 20-30 minutes or until the carrots are fork-tender.

cilantro cauli-rice

PREP TIME
20 minutes

COOKING TIME
5 minutes

YIELD
4 servings

This rice-replacement pairs well with any Mexican dish and is especially delicious under the Grilled Garlic Flank Steak with Peppers & Onions (recipe on page 294).

1 head of cauliflower

1 tablespoon coconut oil or butter

Sea salt and black pepper to taste

1/4 cup fresh cilantro, finely chopped

CHANGE IT UP

Instead of cilantro, use any fresh herb you like: try basil or chives!

NUTS

EGGS

NIGHTSHADES

FODMAPS

Remove the outer leaves and stem from the cauliflower, and chop it into large chunks. Shred the cauliflower using a box grater or food processor.

In a large skillet over medium heat, melt the coconut oil, and place the shredded cauliflower into the skillet. Add sea salt and black pepper to taste. Sauté for about 5 minutes or until the cauliflower begins to become translucent, stirring gently to ensure it cooks through.

Place the cooked cauliflower into a serving bowl, and toss with the chopped cilantro before serving.

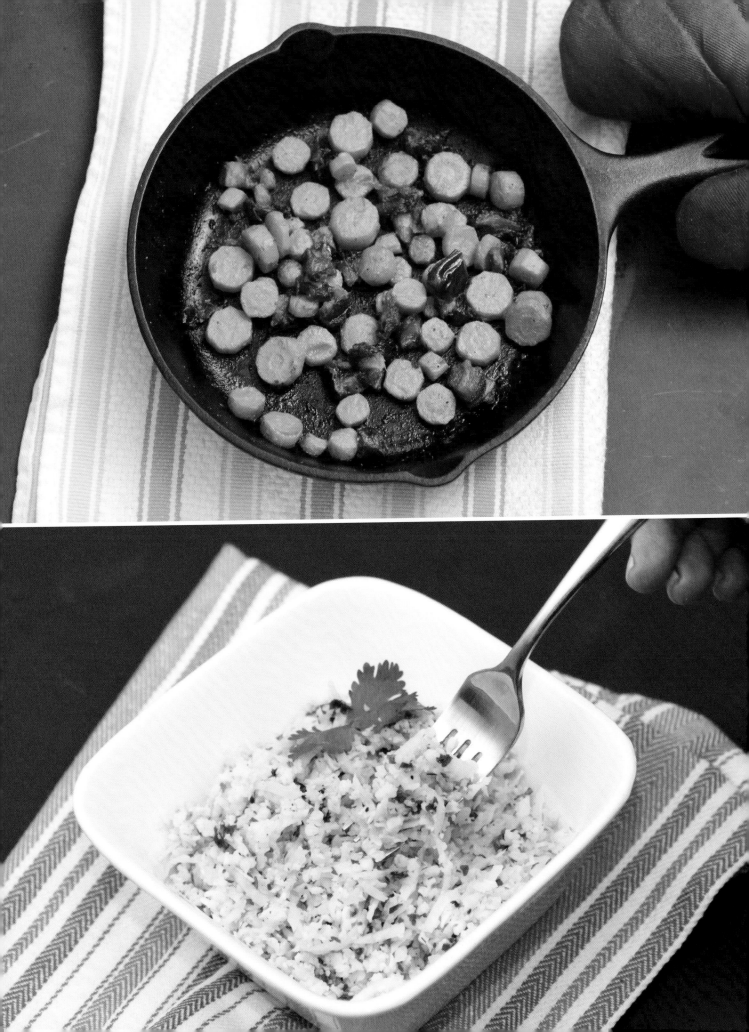

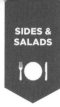

grilled squash & pineapple

PREP TIME
15 minutes

COOKING TIME
45 minutes

YIELD
8 servings

Grilling foods that are sweet usually yields a delicious result—and these two beautiful, carb-rich foods are no exception.

1 whole butternut squash
1/2 of a pineapple, skinned and
    sliced into 1 inch pieces
1/4 cup melted butter, ghee,
    or coconut oil

1-2 tablespoons Smoky Spice Blend
    (recipe page 232)
Sea salt to taste
1/4 cup shredded coconut for
    garnish

SIDE NOTE
If you don't have an outdoor grill, you can use a grill pan indoors to get the same effect.

Preheat oven to 375°F.

Remove the skin from the butternut squash with a vegetable peeler, then slice it in half lengthwise and remove the seeds. Slice into 1 inch pieces and roast for 30 minutes or until fork-tender.

Brush the roasted butternut squash and pineapple slices with the melted butter or coconut oil, season with spice blend and sea salt, then place onto a grill over medium heat.

Grill the butternut squash and pineapple for approximately 3-5 minutes per side, or until grill marks appear.

Garnish with shredded coconut and serve warm.

CHANGE IT UP
Grill any kind of fruit that you can slice into thick pieces: apples, pears, peaches, or even whole figs!

NUTS
EGGS
NIGHTSHADES
FODMAPS

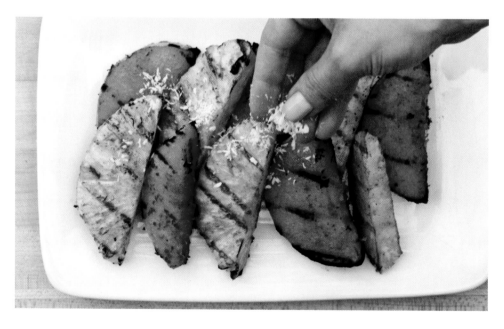

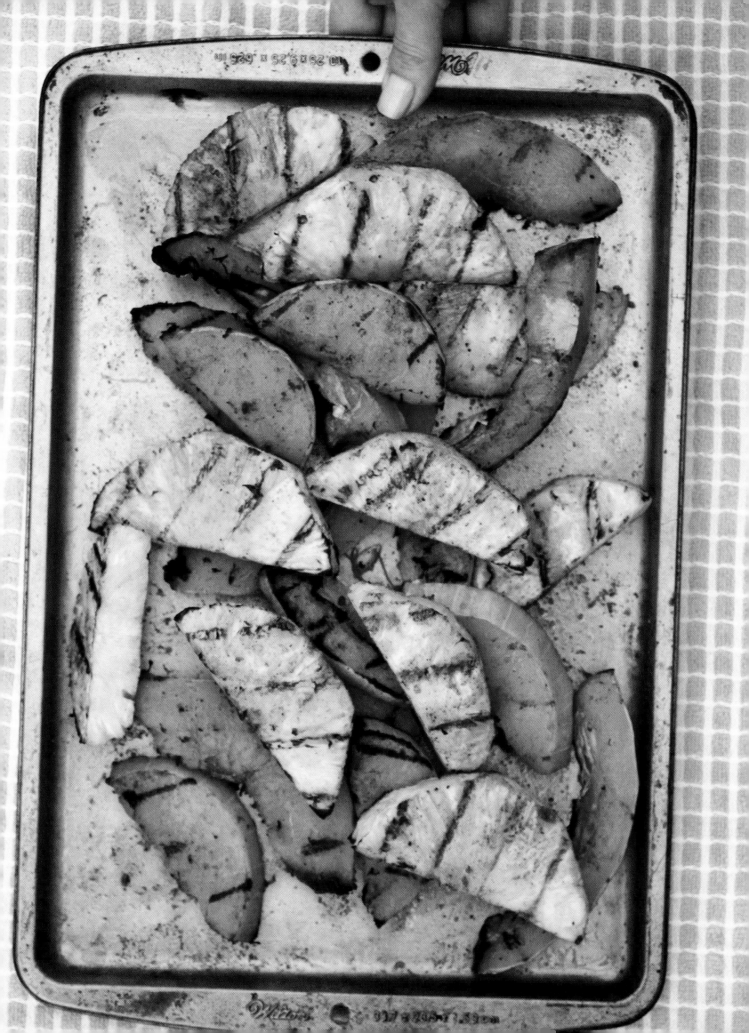

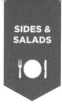
mashed faux-tatoes

PREP TIME
10 minutes

COOKING TIME
20 minutes

YIELD
4-6 servings

This is the most amazing alternative to mashed potatoes you can make. My entire family was fooled when I served these up for Thanksgiving dinner a few years ago, and there were no leftovers!

1 head of cauliflower (about 4 cups)
4 tablespoons butter or coconut oil

1/2 teaspoon Herb Salt Blend
   (recipe on page 230)
Black pepper to taste

SIDE NOTE
If you can't eat butter, try adding roasted garlic for more depth of flavor.

Chop the cauliflower into roughly 2-3-inch pieces.

Steam the cauliflower until it is fork-tender, and place it in a food processor. Add the butter, Herb Salt Blend, and black pepper.

Purée until smooth and creamy.

CHANGE IT UP
If you don't have a food processor, mash the cauliflower by hand with a potato masher. Try serving it with Mini Chorizo Meatballs (recipe on page 330).

NUTS

EGGS

NIGHTSHADES

FODMAPS

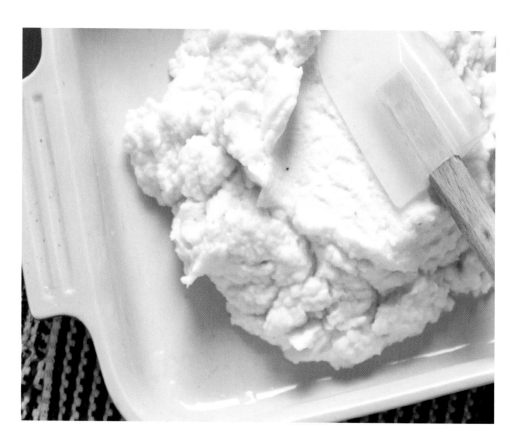

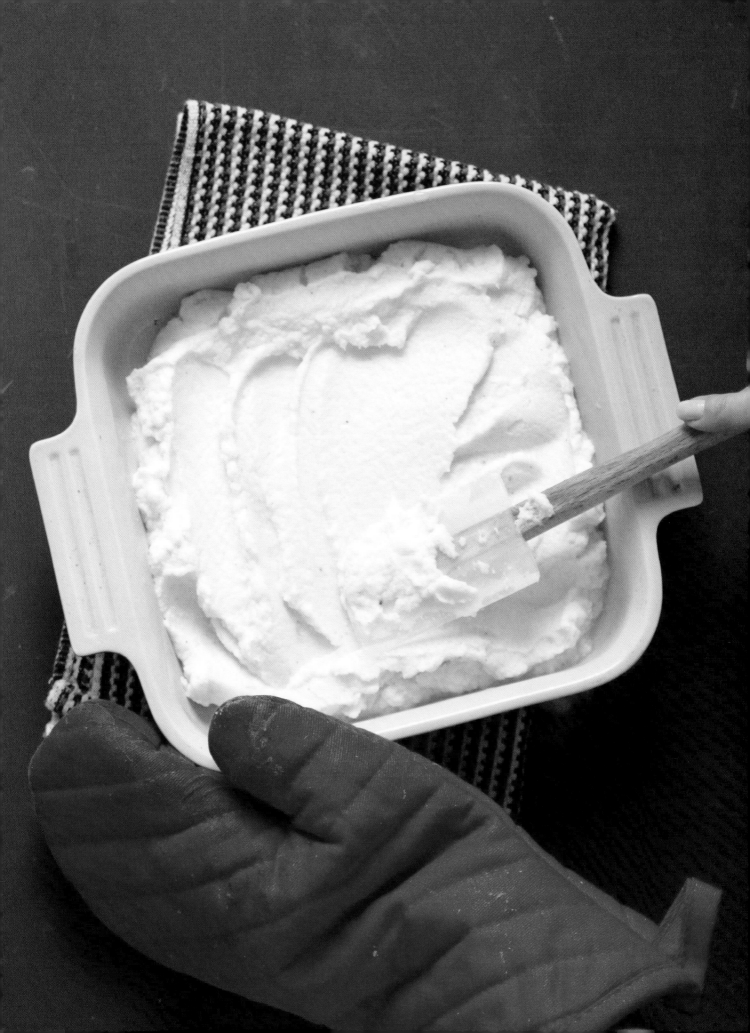

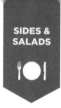
lemon roasted romanesco

PREP TIME
10 minutes

COOKING TIME
20-25 minutes

YIELD
3-4 servings

CHANGE IT UP
Can't find romanesco in your grocery store or farmers market? No problem! Substitute cauliflower or broccoli instead.

Romanesco can be a novelty, but whenever I see it, I pick it up for its unique look and color. Keep your cooking interesting by trying as many different kinds of vegetables as you can.

8 small or 2 large heads of romanesco (small heads are pictured, but it's often available in a larger size, almost as big as you'd find standard cauliflower)

2 tablespoon butter, bacon fat, or coconut oil
Sea salt and black pepper to taste
1/2 lemon, very thinly sliced

Preheat oven to 375°F.

Remove the outer leaves of the romanesco, chop it into 2-inch pieces, and place it in the center of a baking sheet. Pour the melted butter, bacon fat, or coconut oil over the romanesco, and toss gently with your hands to coat the pieces evenly. Sprinkle with sea salt and black pepper, and top with the lemon slices.

Roast for approximately 20-25 minutes or until the edges are golden brown and the romanesco is fork-tender.

NUTS

EGGS

NIGHTSHADES

FODMAPS

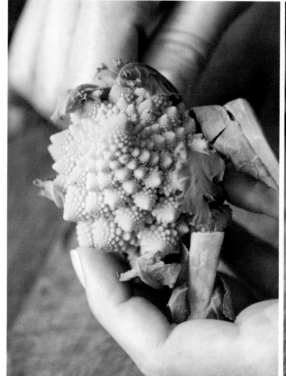
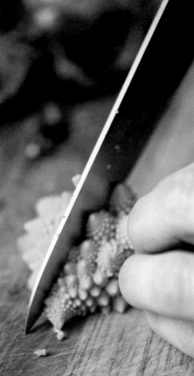

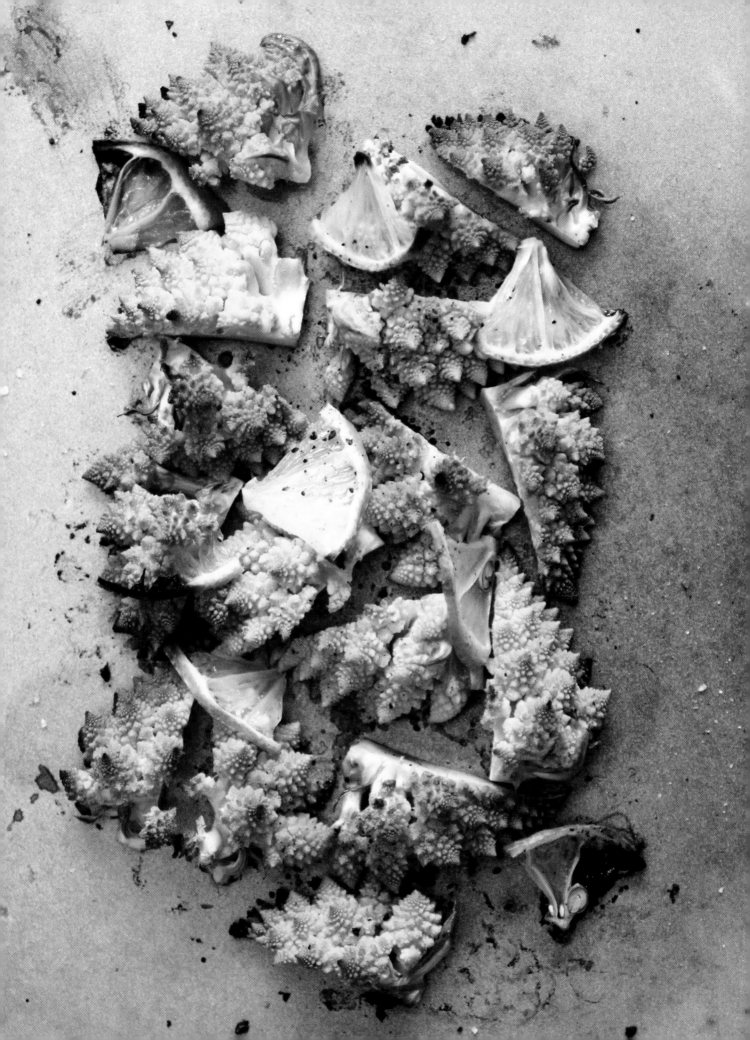

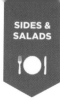
butternut sage soup

PREP TIME
30 minutes

COOKING TIME
45 minutes

YIELD
4-6 servings

FODMAP FREE?
Omit the onion, garlic, and coconut milk.

NUTS
EGGS
NIGHTSHADES
FODMAPS

This soup is so rich and creamy you won't miss the dairy!

1 butternut squash
4 tablespoons bacon fat,
    coconut oil, or ghee, divided
1 yellow onion, diced
4 cloves of garlic, peeled and
    smashed
1 teaspoon Sage Salt Blend (recipe
    on page 230) or a few pinches
    each of dried sage and sea salt

Black pepper to taste
16 ounces Bone Broth, chicken is
    ideal (recipe on page 234)
2 tablespoons coconut milk
    (optional)
Juice of 1 orange
2 tablespoons water
    (more or less as needed)
8-12 fresh sage leaves

Preheat the oven to 400°F.

Peel and chop the butternut squash. Toss the squash in 1 tablespoon of the bacon fat in a roasting dish and bake for about 40 minutes or until fork-tender.

While the squash roasts, use a large pot to sauté the onions in the rest of the bacon fat until the onions begin to brown on the edges. Add the garlic to the skillet, followed by the Sage Salt Blend and pepper. Cook for approximately 2 minutes to take the edge off of the raw garlic. Add broth, coconut milk, and water.

Add the roasted squash, and stir together. Finally, add the orange juice just before turning off the heat.

After the soup has cooled a bit, pour it into a blender, and blend until smooth. Be careful not to fill the blender to the top because the steam will expand the liquid.

Once the soup is in bowls, use a small frying pan or cast iron skillet to fry the sage in 1-2 tablespoons of butter or ghee until it looks bubbly and is crispy to the touch.

Garnish each bowl with a couple of sage leaves.

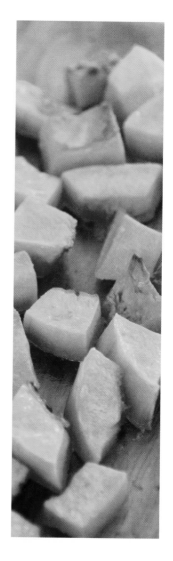

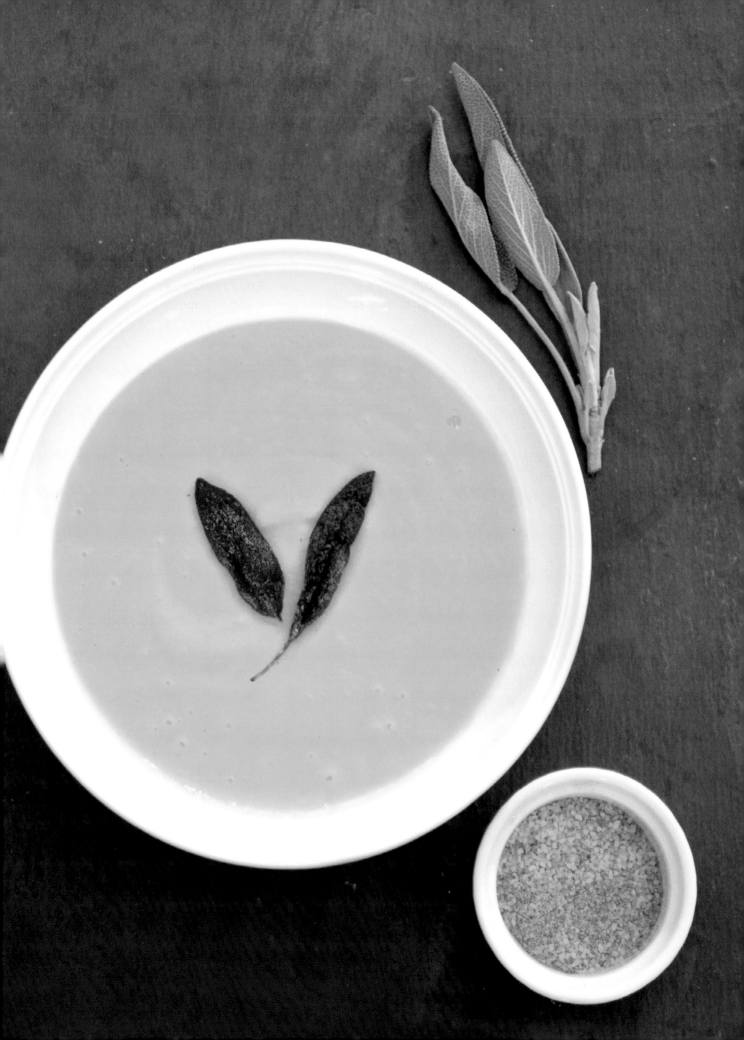

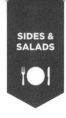
PREP TIME
10 minutes

COOKING TIME
20 minutes

YIELD
4 servings

CHANGE IT UP
If fennel is not in season, use shallots instead.

NUTS
EGGS
NIGHTSHADES
FODMAPS

brussels sprouts with fennel

The easiest way to make Brussels sprouts is also the best: simply roasted with bacon fat, sea salt, and pepper. It doesn't take more than that to make these tiny cabbage-head-looking vegetables taste fantastic.

4 cups Brussels sprouts
1/2 cup fennel, thinly sliced
    (about 1 bulb)
2 tablespoons melted bacon fat,
    butter, or coconut oil

2 tablespoons chopped fennel
    fronds (the tops that look
    like dill)
Sea salt and black pepper to taste

Preheat oven to 375°F.

Slice the Brussels sprouts into 1/8-inch pieces, removing the ends and outer-most leaves. Place the sliced Brussels sprouts onto a large baking sheet, and top with the fennel fronds.

Toss all of the vegetables with the melted bacon fat, butter, or coconut oil, and top with sea salt and black pepper.

Roast for 20 minutes.

PREP TIME
15 minutes

COOKING TIME
30-40 minutes

YIELD
4 servings

FODMAP FREE?
Substitute carrots for the sunchokes, and omit the garlic.

NUTS
EGGS
NIGHTSHADES
FODMAPS

roasted rosemary roots

This recipe calls for sunchokes and parsnips, but this simple roasting method and flavor combination is perfect for any root vegetable. Try it with carrots or sweet potatoes, or combine one white and one orange-colored vegetable for a more colorful presentation.

8 sunchokes, rinsed
4 parsnips, peeled
3 tablespoons melted butter, ghee,
    or coconut oil

1 teaspoon fresh rosemary,
    finely chopped
1 clove garlic, grated or finely
    chopped (optional)

Preheat oven to 425°F.

Chop the sunchokes and parsnips into roughly 1/4-inch sticks that are 2-3 inches long.

CHANGE IT UP
Use any other savory herb you like instead of rosemary; try sage, parsley or thyme.

Toss the chopped vegetables with the melted butter, ghee, or coconut oil and rosemary. If you are using garlic, add it while tossing the vegetables together.

Spread the vegetables on a baking sheet, and roast for 30-40 minutes or until fork-tender and golden brown on the edges.

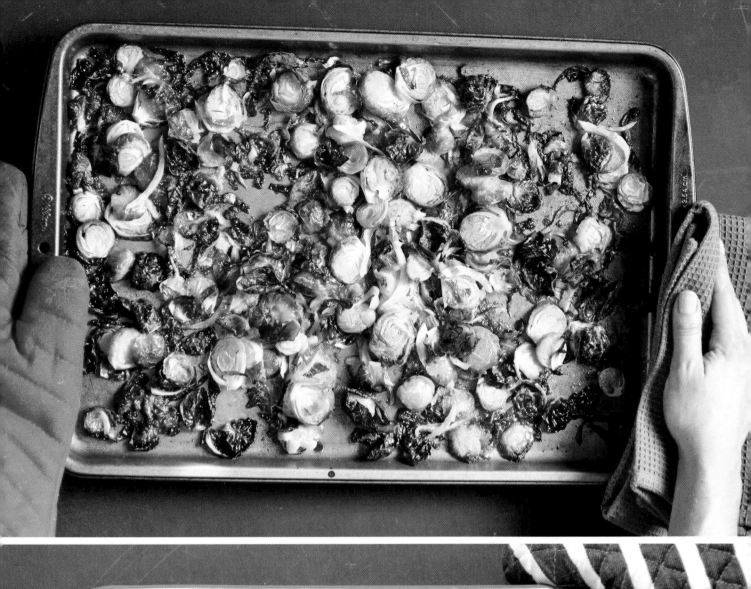
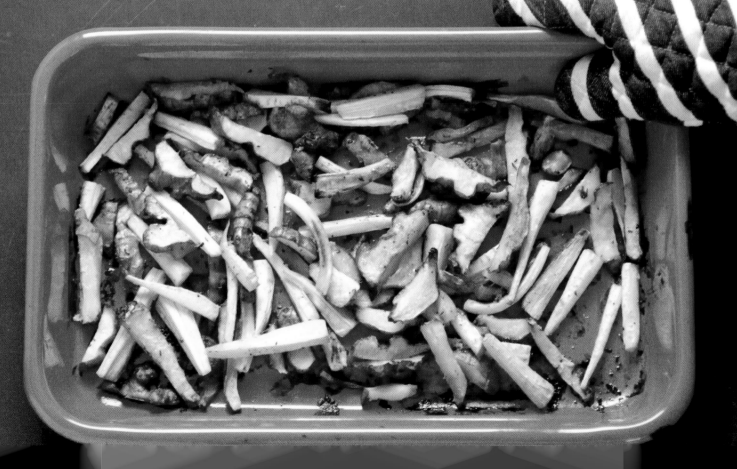

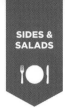
sautéed red cabbage with onions and apples

PREP TIME
15 minutes

COOKING TIME
20-30 minutes

YIELD
4 servings

This sweet and savory dish is great when paired with any type of roasted or grilled meat, and it also works well as a side dish to eggs in the morning.

1 large yellow onion, thinly sliced
1 tablespoon bacon fat or coconut oil
1/2 head of red cabbage, thinly sliced
2-4 tablespoons unfiltered apple cider vinegar

1 tablespoon Rosemary Salt Blend (recipe on page 230)
1 green apple, sliced into matchstick-sized pieces

SIDE NOTE
Though I often recommend cooking in cast iron skillets, I don't recommend cooking this dish in cast iron since it includes vinegar, which is very acidic and may react to the cast iron.

In a large enameled pot or pan, sauté the onion in the fat or oil. When it is mostly translucent, add the cabbage and cook until it begins to soften.

Add the vinegar and Rosemary Salt blend, and allow the cabbage and onion mixture to cook until everything is softened / fork-tender.

Add the apples, and cook them until soft. Add more vinegar or some water if the mixture becomes too dry.

CHANGE IT UP
Instead of using plain bacon fat, chop and render 2-3 slices of bacon for the cooking fat, and add the cooked bacon meat back to the mixture when plating.

For a slightly sweeter version, add about 2 tablespoons to 1/4 cup of chopped, dried cranberries (find a no-sugar-added brand or dry some yourself).

NUTS
EGGS
NIGHTSHADES
FODMAPS

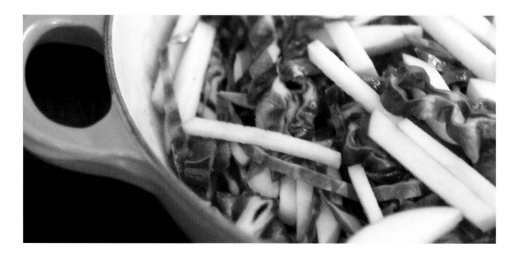

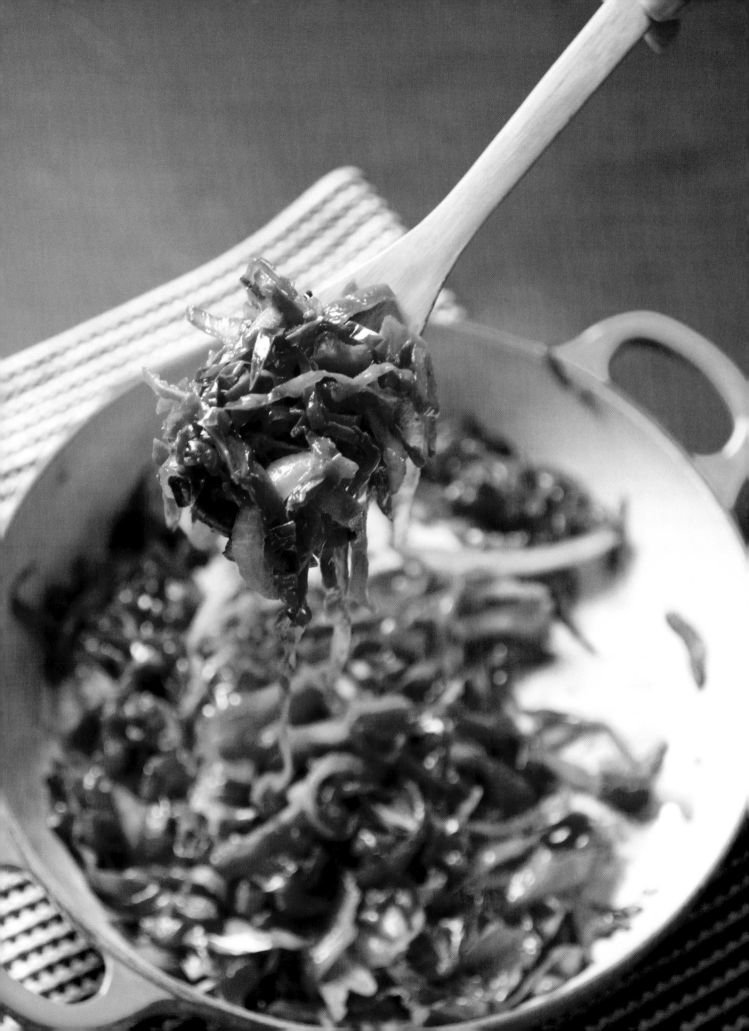

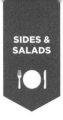
roasted figs with rosemary

PREP TIME
15 minutes

COOKING TIME
10-15 minutes

YIELD
4 servings

SIDE NOTE
This simple fig recipe can be made as-is, of course, or you can wrap each bite of fig with some prosciutto to serve it as a snack or appetizer.

Fresh figs are only in season for a couple of months each year—typically late summer into early fall in most parts of the U.S. They have an entirely different taste and texture from dried figs, which are great used in sauces, as in the Balsamic-Fig Compote on page 234.

12 whole, fresh figs
2 teaspoons fresh rosemary, finely
   minced

2 tablespoons extra-virgin olive oil
Coarse sea salt

Preheat oven to 425˚F.

Slice off the tip of the figs, and cut them into quarters. Place the fig quarters onto a baking sheet. Sprinkle the finely minced rosemary over the figs, and roast for 10-15 minutes or until the edges of the figs are slightly browned.

Remove the figs from the oven, and drizzle with extra-virgin olive oil and sea salt before serving.

NUTS
EGGS
NIGHTSHADES
FODMAPS

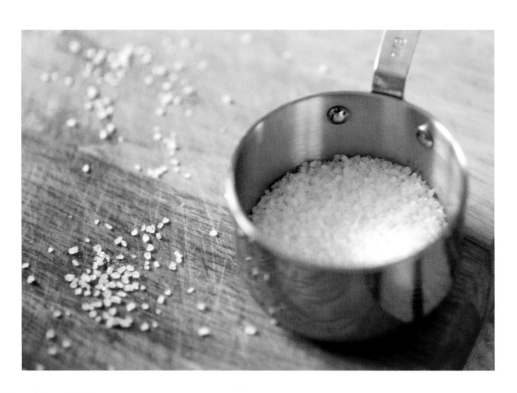

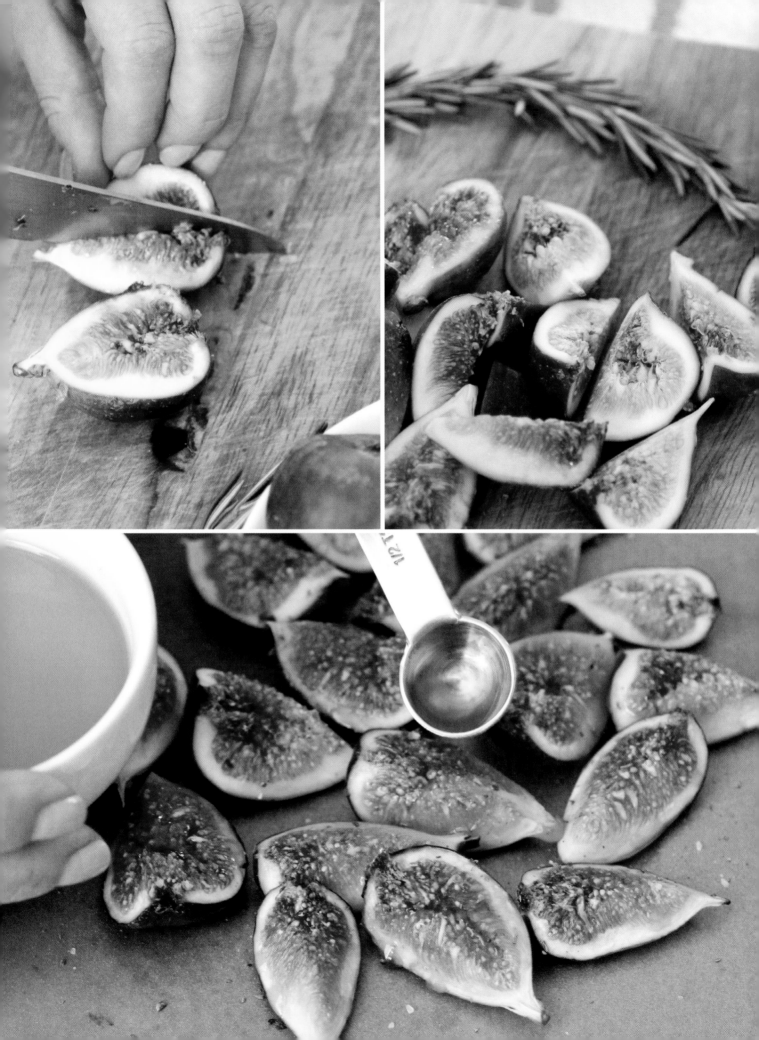

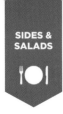
simple baked kale chips

PREP TIME
10 minutes

COOKING TIME
20 minutes

YIELD
4 servings

Kids especially enjoy these chips! This is a quick way to make use of a lot of kale, and you'll find yourself making this recipe often, as it goes faster than you'd expect!

2 bunches of curly kale
   (or other variety)
1 tablespoon melted coconut oil

1/2 teaspoon garlic powder
   (optional)
Sea salt and black pepper to taste

SIDE NOTE
Keep a close eye on the kale as it bakes—it can burn quite quickly if you're not paying attention!

FODMAP FREE?
Leave out the garlic powder; use other spices you like instead.

Preheat oven to 350°F.

Rinse the kale leaves under cold water, and pat them dry with a towel. Pull the leaves from the stalk by holding tightly onto the end and running your hand up the sides of the stem. You can also just cut the stem out.

Roughly chop the kale into large pieces, and place them in a large mixing bowl. Top the kale with the melted coconut oil, and massage the oil gently into the pieces of kale, spreading it evenly over all of the leaves.

Arrange the kale in a single layer onto two baking sheets, and sprinkle them with garlic powder, sea salt, and black pepper to taste.

Bake for 10-15 minutes or until the kale becomes crispy.

CHANGE IT UP
Add any seasonings you like! This recipe is especially good with a few pinches of cayenne pepper or onion powder instead of garlic powder.

NUTS

EGGS

NIGHTSHADES

FODMAPS

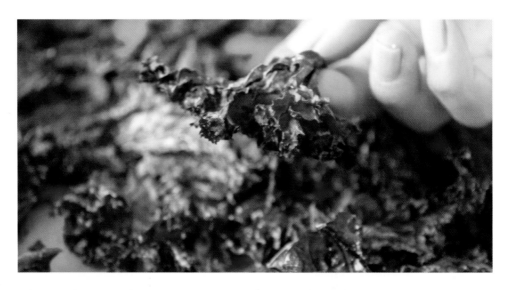

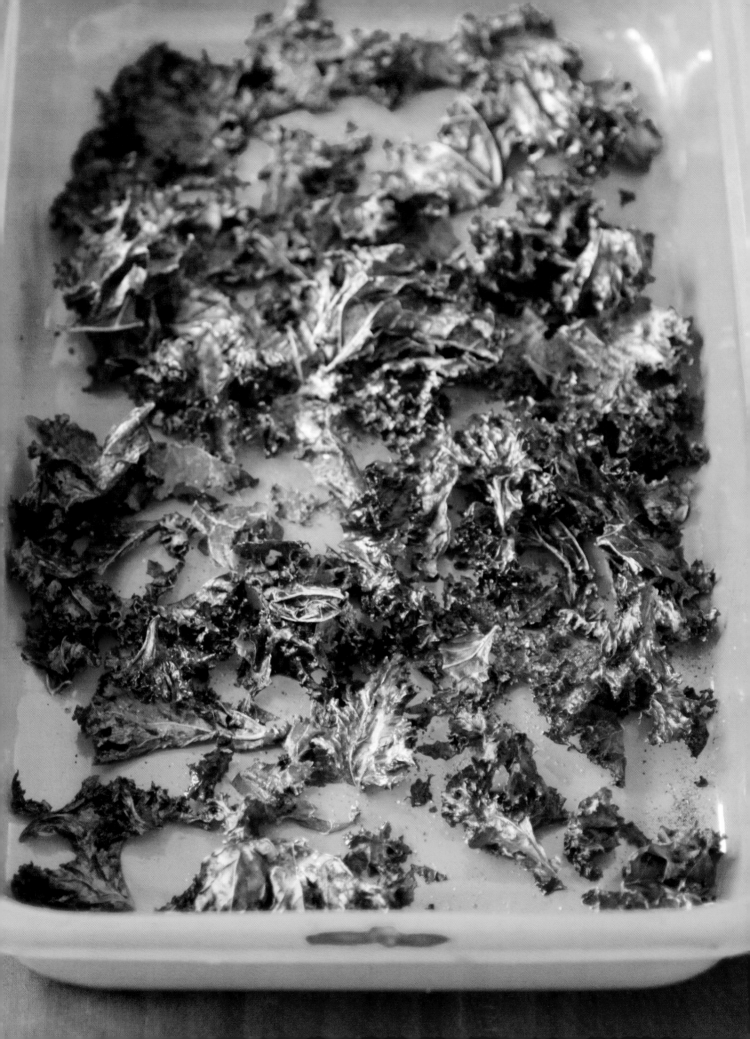

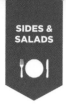
acorn squash with cinnamon & coconut butter

Roasting winter squash is a soul-warming experience. The aroma that comes from the oven as the food roasts and nears doneness is amazing. This dish is almost a dessert, but without any added sweeteners.

PREP TIME
5 minutes

COOKING TIME
35-45 minutes

YIELD
4 servings

CHANGE IT UP
Try this with sweet potatoes, yams, or any kind of winter squash.

NUTS
EGGS
NIGHTSHADES
FODMAPS

1 acorn squash
1/4 tablespoon coconut butter or coconut manna (coconut cream concentrate)
Few pinches of cinnamon

Pinch of sea salt
2 tablespoons raisins or currants (optional)
2 tablespoons sliced almonds or chopped walnuts (optional)

Preheat oven to 375˚F.

Slice the squash down the middle lengthwise, and place it face down in an oven-safe baking dish. Bake for approximately 35-45 minutes or until fork-tender and the edges begin to brown.

When the squash is cooked, remove it from the oven. While it's still warm, fill the center sections with even amounts of the coconut butter. Dust with cinnamon and a pinch of sea salt. Top the squash with any other ingredients you like, such as raisins, currants, almonds, walnuts, or other nuts. Serve warm.

---

green beans with shallots

While it has "bean" in its name, the green bean is mostly pod, not bean, so they're a perfectly healthy green vegetable to enjoy.

PREP TIME
5 minutes

COOKING TIME
15 minutes

YIELD
4 servings

FODMAP FREE?
Leave out the shallots and season with lemon zest instead!

NUTS
EGGS
NIGHTSHADES
FODMAPS

1 lb fresh green beans
2 tablespoons butter or coconut oil, divided

2 shallots, sliced
Sea salt and black pepper to taste

Steam the green beans in a basket over about 1-inch of boiling water for approximately 8 minutes or until they become a brighter shade of green.

While the green beans are steaming, melt 1 tablespoon of the butter or coconut oil in a medium-sized skillet over medium heat. Place the shallots in the skillet, and sauté until they are translucent and the edges are golden brown. Add sea salt and black pepper to taste.

Remove the green beans from the steamer basket, and place them in a serving bowl. Top with the remaining 1 tablespoon of cooking fat, and toss to combine.

Place the cooked shallots on top of the green beans, and serve.

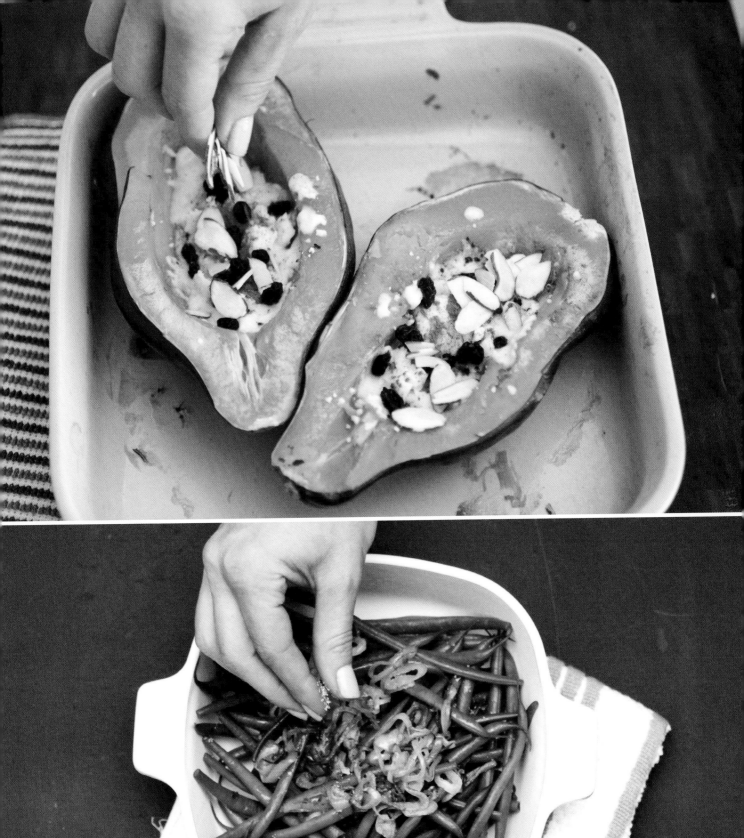

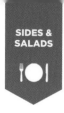
butternut squash & kumquats

PREP TIME
10 minutes

COOKING TIME
40 minutes

YIELD
6 servings

Looking for a way to use those cute, little, not-quite-oranges citrus fruits you've seen at the grocery store or farmers market? Well, here's something I whipped up to make use of kumquats. The bitter, citrus-y bite of the kumquats pairs nicely with the sweetness of the butternut squash.

1 butternut squash
1/2 cup kumquats, sliced
1 small shallot, finely sliced

2 tablespoons coconut oil, butter, or ghee, melted
Sea salt and black pepper to taste

SIDE NOTE
Kumquats are quite bitter, so pairing them with a sweet, starchy vegetable works nicely!

FODMAP FREE?
Leave out the shallots.

Preheat oven to 400˚F.

Peel and chop the butternut squash, and place it in a roasting dish with the kumquats, shallots, and melted coconut oil, butter, or ghee.

Toss the ingredients to combine, and sprinkle with sea salt and black pepper to taste.

Bake for approximately 40 minutes or until the squash is fork-tender and the edges are browned.

CHANGE IT UP
This dish can also be made with sweet potatoes, yams, delicata squash, or kabocha squash.

NUTS
EGGS
NIGHTSHADES
FODMAPS

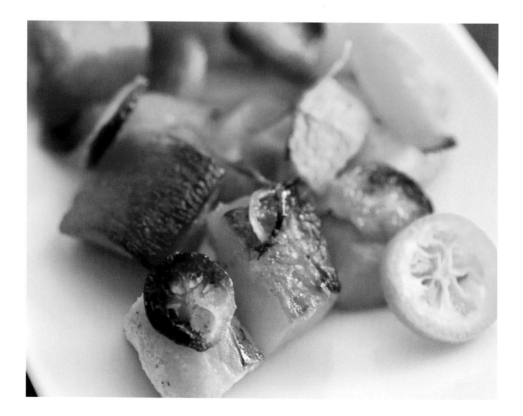

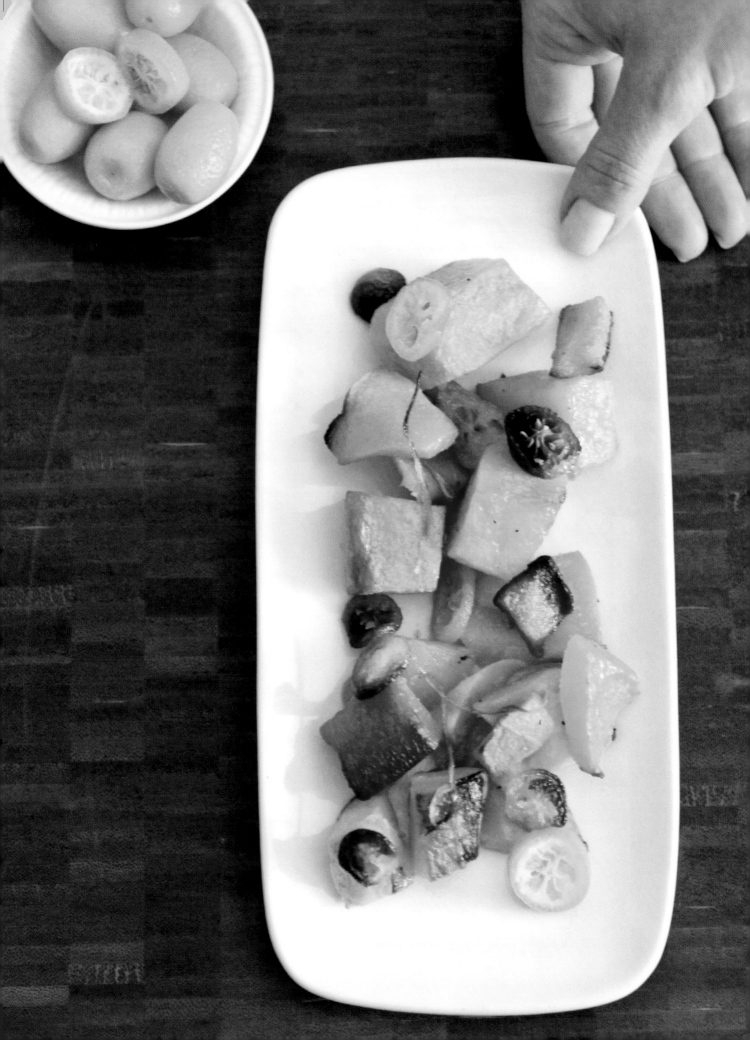

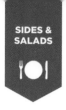
sweet & savory potatoes

Sweet potatoes can be roasted and enjoyed simply with salt and black pepper, but to kick them up, use a few different spices. The result is a whole new taste experience!

PREP TIME
15 minutes

COOKING TIME
30 minutes

YIELD
2 servings

FODMAP FREE?

Omit the onion & garlic powder, and add 1/2 teaspoon dried rosemary.

NUTS

EGGS

NIGHTSHADES

FODMAPS

2 large sweet potatoes
(to yield 2 cups chopped)
1 teaspoon duck or bacon fat,
melted, or coconut oil

1/4 teaspoon onion powder
1/4 teaspoon garlic powder
1/2 teaspoon cinnamon
Sea salt and black pepper to taste

Preheat oven to 375°F.

Peel the sweet potatoes, and chop them into 1-inch pieces. In a medium-sized mixing bowl, toss the sweet potato pieces with the duck fat, bacon fat, or coconut oil, coating coat them evenly.

In a small mixing bowl, combine the onion powder, garlic powder, cinnamon, sea salt, and black pepper. Add the spice blend to the sweet potatoes, and toss again to spread the spices evenly.

Place the potatoes evenly on a baking sheet, and bake for approximately 30 minutes or until the potatoes are fork-tender.

baked beets with fennel

Beets are amazingly nutrient-dense and are recommended in nearly every meal plan in this book! Save some of these for a salad topping the next day.

PREP TIME
15 minutes

COOKING TIME
30-40 minutes

YIELD
2-3 servings

FODMAP FREE?

Bake carrots or parsnips with fennel instead of beets.

NUTS

EGGS

NIGHTSHADES

FODMAPS

2 large beets
1 bulb of fennel
1/2 orange (optional)

2 tablespoons coconut oil or butter
Sea salt and black pepper to taste

Preheat oven to 375°F.

Peel the beets with a vegetable peeler, and chop them into 1-inch cubes. Chop the tops (fronds) off the fennel bulb, and slice the bulb into 1/4-inch strips. Slice the orange into 1/2-inch pieces, or use segments if you prefer.

Top the beets, fennel, and oranges with the melted coconut oil or butter, and toss to combine. Spread evenly in an oven-safe dish, and bake for 30-40 minutes or until the beets are fork-tender.

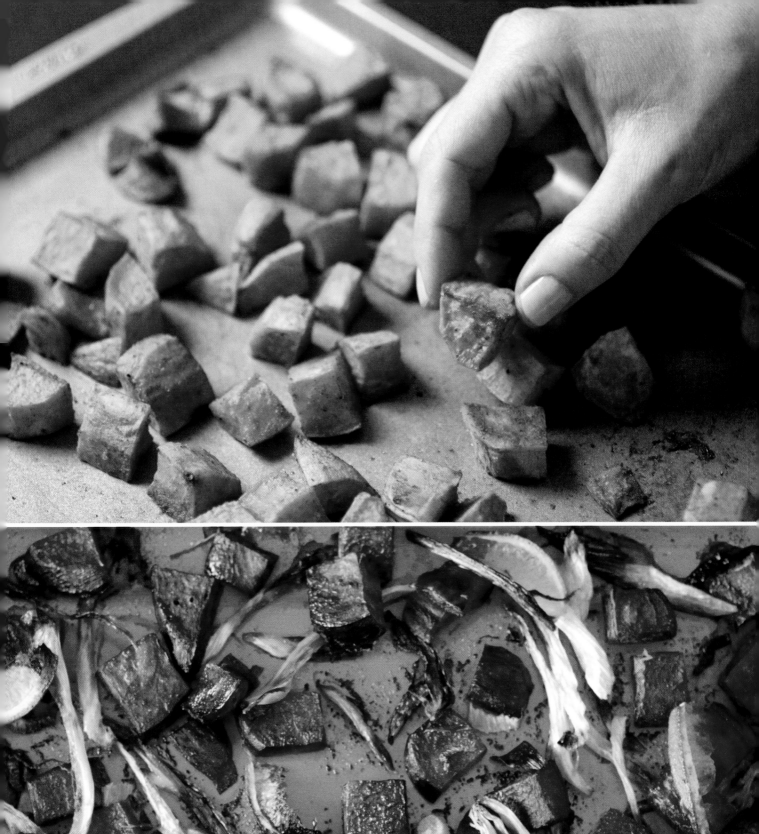

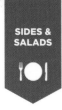
crispy curried
sweet potato coins

PREP TIME
10 minutes

COOKING TIME
20-30 minutes

YIELD
Approximately 4 servings

If you're looking for a "fancier" way to prepare sweet potatoes, this is the recipe for you! By tossing the sliced potatoes in a "breading" of coconut or almond flour and mixing in your favorite spices, you can make this recipe a bit differently every time. Try different cooking fats as well for a varied flavor profile.

2 sweet potatoes, peeled
1/2 cup almond flour or sifted
   coconut flour
2 tablespoons Curry Spice Blend
   or other Spice Blend (recipes on
   page 233)

1-2 eggs, beaten (use 2 if you have
   very large sweet potatoes)
1/4 cup or more of bacon fat,
   coconut oil, or ghee

EGG FREE?
Simply dust the sweet potato coins with a smaller amount of the flour and spice blend, and pan-fry or bake as desired.

Slice the sweet potatoes into 1/4-inch coins. Place them onto a baking sheet, and set aside.

With a fork or whisk, combine almond or sifted coconut flour and the spice blend in a bowl. Set up a "station" and dip the sweet potato coins into the egg, then the flour mixture. After completing each coin, set them back onto the baking sheet.

Place a large skillet over medium heat, and melt the cooking fat. Use enough to cover the bottom of the skillet completely. Place the "breaded" sweet potato coins into the skillet, and allow them to cook for approximately 2-3 minutes per side or until golden brown. Add more fat to the skillet as needed so that the level remains constant.

Remove the potatoes from the skillet as they are finished, and replace them in the skillet with more until the entire batch is done.

CHANGE IT UP
If you prefer to bake your sweet potato coins, combine the egg, flour mixture, and cooking fat together to create a batter. Dip each coin, and then place on a parchment paper-lined baking sheet. Cook in the oven for approximately 20-30 minutes at 350°F or until they are golden brown on the outside and fork-tender.

NUTS
EGGS
NIGHTSHADES
FODMAPS

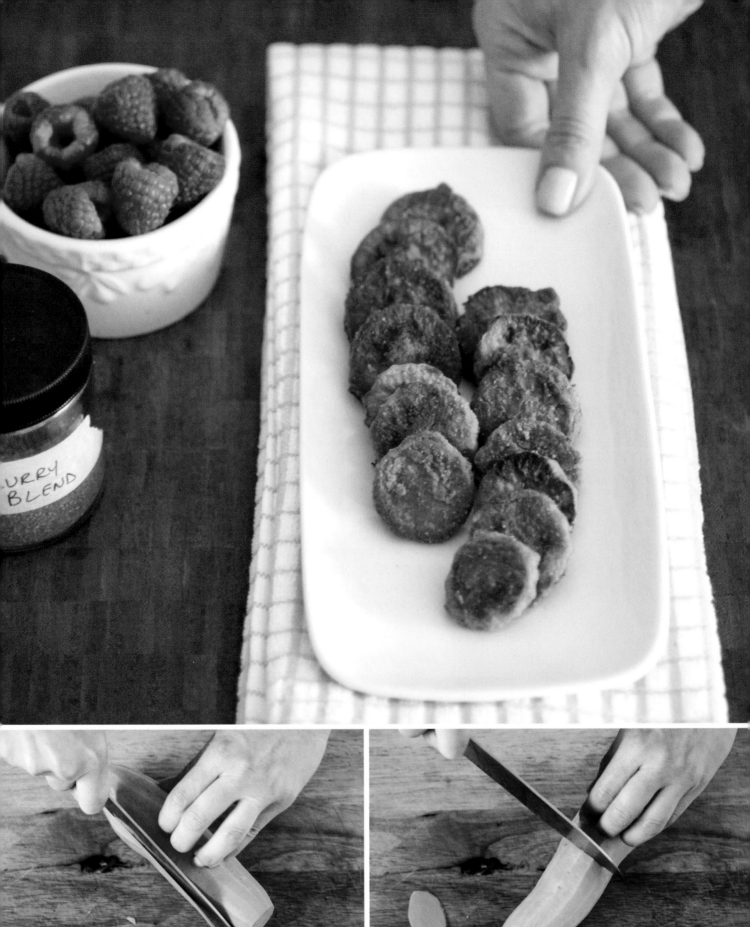

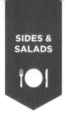
confit cherry tomatoes

Enjoy these tomatoes as a side dish or use the finished dish as a base for creating an easy sauce to pour over spaghetti squash. To make a sauce, puree the tomatoes together with a few basil leaves, a clove of garlic, and some olive oil!

PREP TIME
5 minutes

COOKING TIME
20-25 minutes

YIELD
2 servings

SIDE NOTE
A cast iron skillet makes moving from the stove-top to the oven a cinch!

NUTS

EGGS

NIGHTSHADES

FODMAPS

2 cups cherry tomatoes
1 tablespoon duck fat, bacon fat, or
    coconut oil, melted
Sea salt and black pepper to taste

Preheat oven to 400°F.

Place the tomatoes and the duck fat in an oven-safe dish or pan, and toss to coat. Season with sea salt and black pepper to taste.

Place the dish in the oven, and remove after each 10 minutes to baste the tomatoes with the pan liquid. Roast for a total of 20-25 minutes or until the tomatoes appear soft and begin to burst open.

sautéed spinach with pine nuts & currants

One of my favorite tapas restaurants in San Francisco serves a spinach dish with golden raisins and almonds that's very similar to this one. I put my own twist on it using pignoli (pine) nuts and currants.

PREP TIME
5 minutes

COOKING TIME
10 minutes

YIELD
2 servings

SIDE NOTE
You can make this recipe with raisins and walnuts if you prefer.

NUTS

EGGS

NIGHTSHADES

FODMAPS

2 tablespoons raw pine nuts
    (pignoli nuts)
1 tablespoon butter or coconut oil

4 cups of baby spinach, washed
Sea salt and black pepper to taste
2 tablespoons dried currants

In a large skillet, toast the pine nuts over low heat for approximately 5 minutes, tossing often to prevent burning. Set the toasted pine nuts aside.

Melt the butter in the skillet, add the spinach, sea salt, and black pepper. Cover for about 2 minutes. Stir the spinach, and cook until it is wilted.

Top with toasted pine nuts and currants.

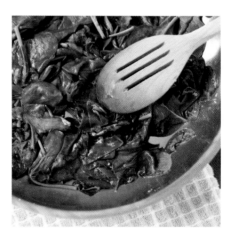

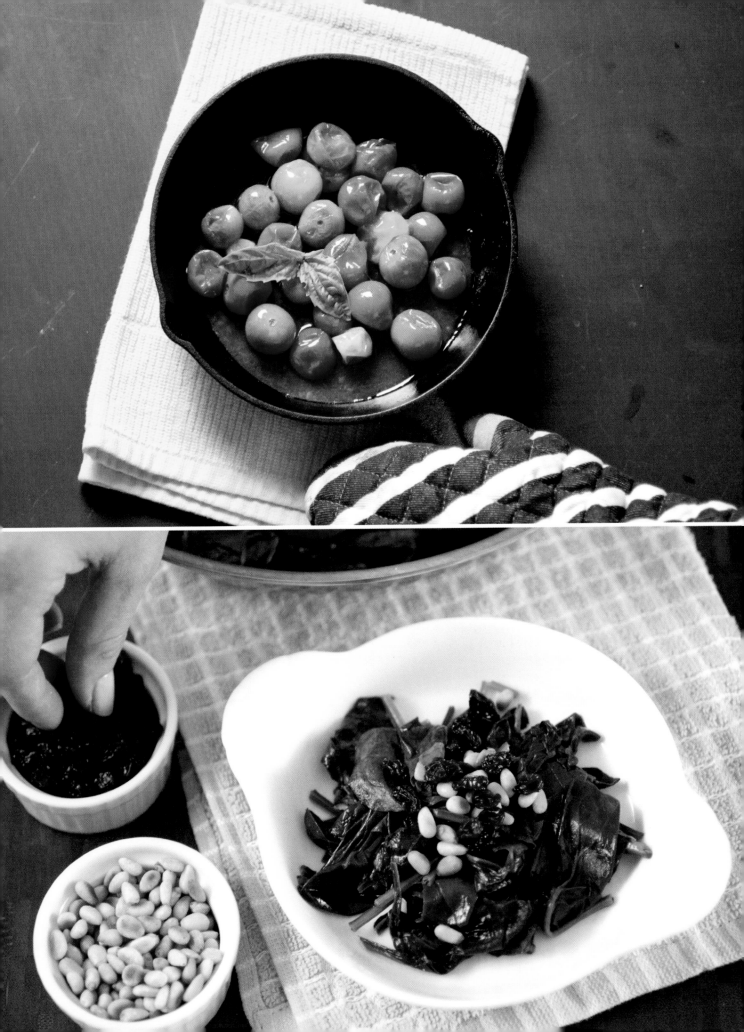

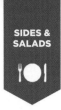
bacon-wrapped
pecan dates & pineapple

PREP TIME
20 minutes

COOKING TIME
20-30 minutes

YIELD
2 dozen pieces,
12 of each kind

If you already follow a Paleo diet, you know that this dish is not only a classic combination, but also a crowd-favorite at parties. If you've never tried these before, watch out—they're addictive! The salty and sweet combination really makes these a fantastic two-bite appetizer or dessert!

12 dried medjool dates
2 dozen pecan halves
12 slices of bacon

1-2 cups fresh pineapple
(to yield 12 chunks, about 1 inch each)

SIDE NOTE
Be very careful when biting into these little treats—right out of the oven, they'll be extremely hot in the center!

Preheat oven to 425°F.

Slice the dates down the center lengthwise; remove and discard the pits. Place 2 pecan halves in the center of each date where the pit had been.

Slice the bacon in half so that you now have 2 pieces from each strip, each approximately 4 inches long. Wrap one piece of bacon around each pecan-stuffed date, and secure with a toothpick. Wrap the remaining bacon, 1 piece each, around the pineapple chunks, and secure with a toothpick.

Place the bacon-wrapped dates and bacon-wrapped pineapple onto a baking sheet, and bake for 20-30 minutes or until the bacon is done to your liking.

CHANGE IT UP
Use walnuts instead of pecans to stuff the dates.

Medjool dates are ideal for this recipe, but if you can only find deglet, they will work but may not be large enough for stuffing with a pecan!

NUTS

EGGS

NIGHTSHADES

FODMAPS

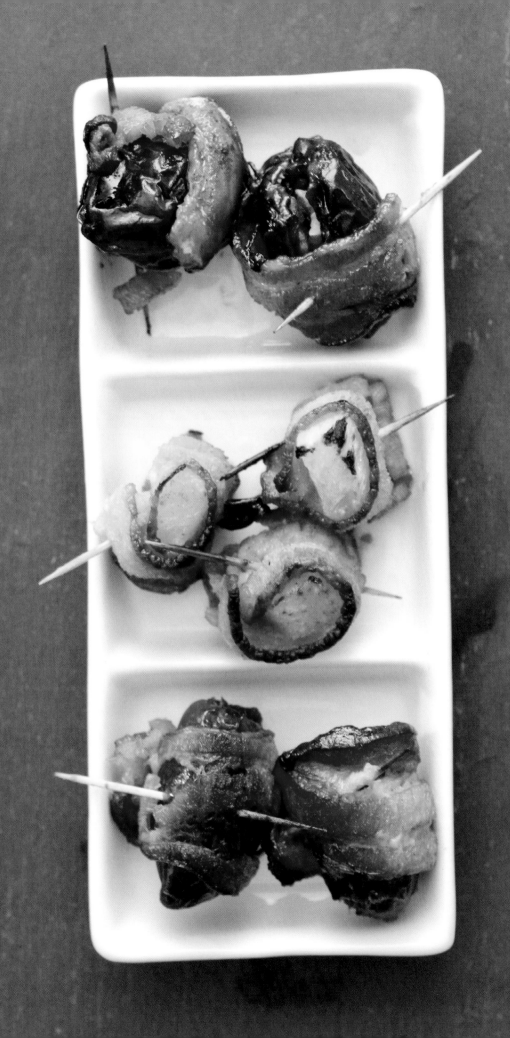

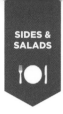

red roasted garlic

Roasted garlic adds a richness and depth of flavor to any dish. To replace fresh garlic with roasted garlic in recipes, use 2-3 cloves of roasted garlic per 1 clove of fresh garlic, as the taste of roasted garlic is very mild.

PREP TIME
5 minutes

COOKING TIME
45 minutes

YIELD
1 bulb (approx. 12 cloves)

SIDE NOTE
Use any cooking fat you like (page 45) in place of the red palm oil.

NUTS

EGGS

NIGHTSHADES

FODMAPS

1 bulb of garlic
1 tablespoon + 1 teaspoon
red palm oil

Preheat oven to 350˚F.

Slice off the top and bottom of the garlic, peeling the outer skin off but leaving most of the skin otherwise intact. Set the garlic on a large sheet of foil, and top it with 1 tablespoon of red palm oil. Wrap the foil around the garlic so that the oil does not drip out while baking.

Bake for 45 minutes. Remove the garlic from the oven and foil, and top it with the remaining 1 teaspoon of red palm oil.

To eat or use the roasted garlic in recipes, allow the garlic to cool slightly before you simply slide the cloves out of the skin.

roasted pearl onions

Roasted onions are a lovely side dish to pair with any meat or to use as a base for a sauce or dressing. Check out the Roasted Allium Spread (recipe on page 388) for one way to turn this simple side into a burger-friendly spread.

PREP TIME
5 minutes

COOKING TIME
30 minutes

YIELD
4 servings

SIDE NOTE
You can also make this recipe with large onions chopped into 1/2 inch pieces.

NUTS

EGGS

NIGHTSHADES

FODMAPS

2 cups pearl onions
2 teaspoons melted duck fat, bacon fat, butter, or coconut oil

Sea salt and black pepper to taste
1 teaspoon of your favorite spice blend (optional)

Preheat oven to 375˚F.

In a medium-sized mixing bowl, toss the onions with the melted duck fat, bacon fat, butter, or coconut oil. Spread the onions evenly on a baking sheet or in a large cast iron skillet.

Sprinkle them with sea salt and black pepper (and additional spices if you like).

Roast for 30 minutes or until the onions appear translucent and have browned a bit on the edges.

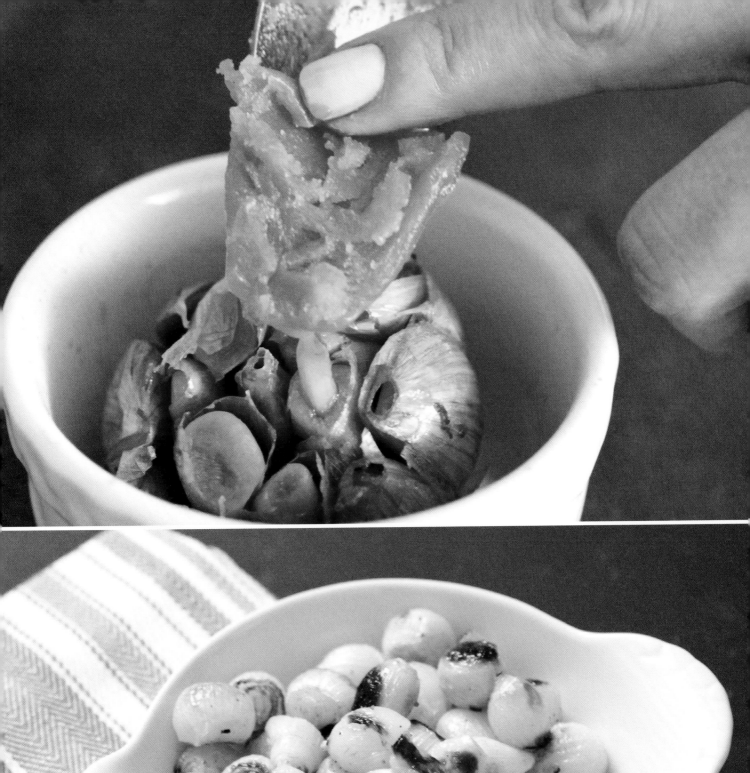
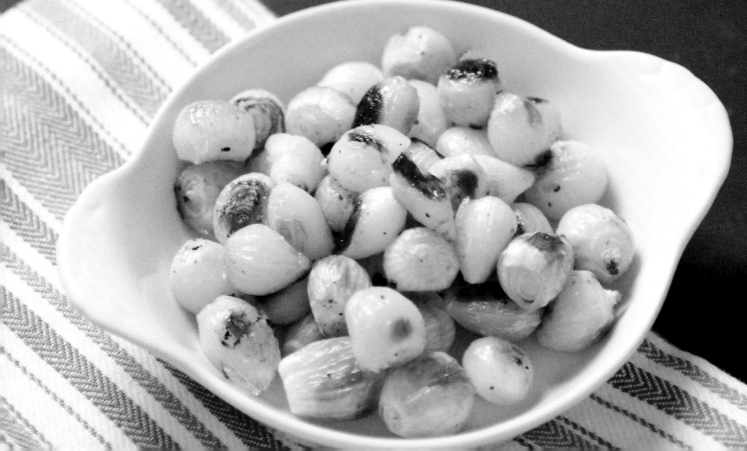

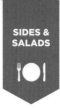
rainbow red cabbage salad

PREP TIME
30 minutes

COOKING TIME
-

YIELD
4-6 servings

SIDE NOTE
If mango isn't in season, fresh apple chunks work nicely.

Bring this bright and crisp salad to a party or barbecue to make a colorful impression! This salad pairs nicely with the Citrus Macadamia Nut Sole on page 314.

1 cup red cabbage, finely sliced
    or shredded
1/2 cup carrot, shredded
1/2 cup broccoli stems, shredded
1/2 mango, finely diced

Juice of 1-2 limes
2 tablespoons macadamia nut oil
Sea salt and black pepper to taste
2 tablespoons macadamia nuts,
    chopped

In a large mixing bowl, combine the red cabbage, carrots, broccoli, and mango.

Top the vegetable mixture with lime juice, macadamia nut oil, sea salt, and black pepper. Toss to coat the mixture well with the dressing.

CHANGE IT UP
If you don't have macadamia nut oil, try extra-virgin olive oil.

Transfer to a serving dish, and garnish with the chopped macadamia nuts.

NUTS
EGGS
NIGHTSHADES
FODMAPS

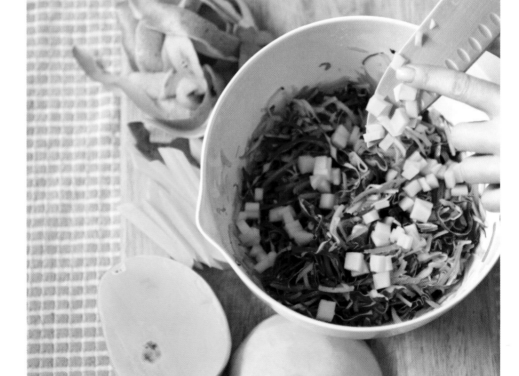

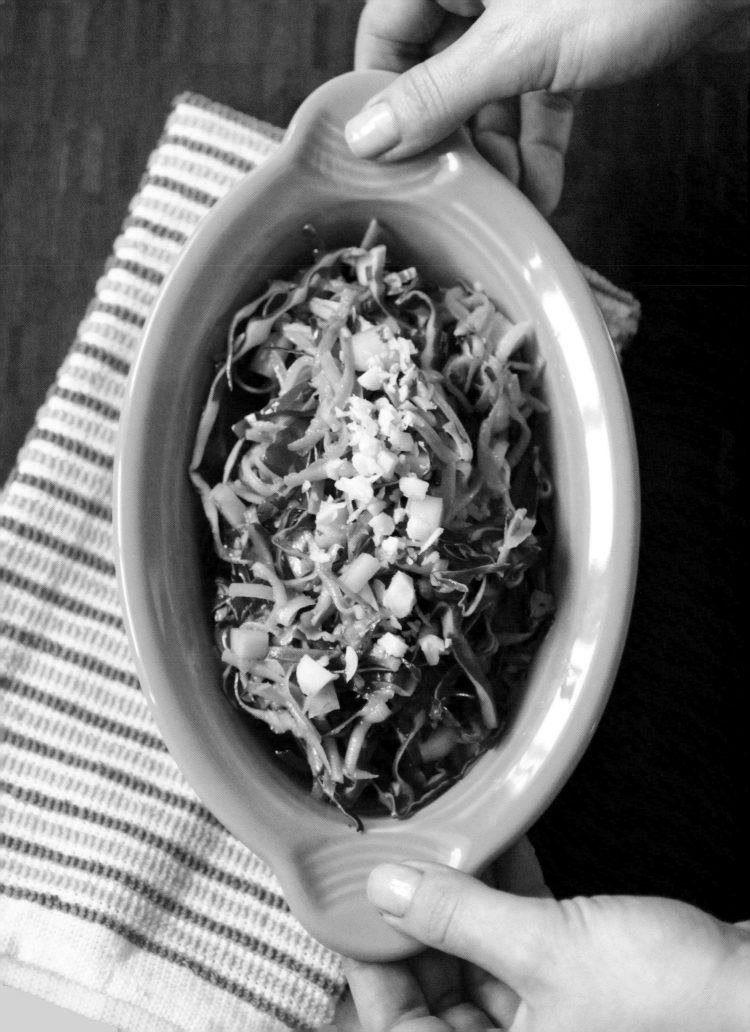

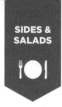
summer squash
caprese noodle salad

If Caprese salad is one of your favorites at Italian restaurants, you'll love this recipe. It's especially great at a summertime cookout.

PREP TIME
30 minutes

COOKING TIME
-

YIELD
4-6 servings

NIGHTSHADE FREE?
Leave out the tomatoes—add shredded carrots for color instead.

NUTS
EGGS
NIGHTSHADES
FODMAPS

4-6 zucchini/yellow squash (to yield 5 cups julienned)
1 cup cherry tomatoes, quartered
1/4 cup basil, thinly sliced

1 clove garlic, grated or finely chopped
1/4 cup extra-virgin olive oil
Sea salt and black pepper to taste

Chop the ends off of the zucchini, and peel down to the center seedy section with a julienne vegetable peeler to make fettuccine-like noodles. (You can use a standard peeler if you don't have a julienne peeler.)

Combine the cherry tomatoes, basil, garlic, extra-virgin olive oil, sea salt, and black pepper in a medium-sized mixing bowl.

Toss the squash with the tomato mixture, and place onto a flat dish or into a bowl to serve.

CHANGE IT UP
For a warm dish, steam the squash "noodles" for approximately 2 minutes. Remove the squash from the steamer pot, and allow it to sit in the basket over a plate to drain for 10 minutes before combining with the tomato mixture.

greek salad
with avo-ziki dressing

The most traditional Greek salads don't include any lettuce, but this is my twist on the classic.

PREP TIME
15 minutes

COOKING TIME
-

YIELD
2 salads

SIDE NOTE
Pair this salad with the lamb chops on page 326.

NUTS
EGGS
NIGHTSHADES
FODMAPS

4 cups romaine lettuce, chopped
1/2 cup cucumber slices
1/2 cup cherry tomatoes, halved
1/4 cup Kalamata olives, halved
2 tablespoons capers

1/4 cup Avo-ziki Sauce (recipe on page 322)
2 tablespoons extra-virgin olive oil
1/2 teaspoon dried oregano

Plate the romaine lettuce and top it with the cucumbers, cherry tomatoes, Kalamata olives, and capers.

In a small mixing bowl, combine the Avo-ziki Sauce and extra-virgin olive oil.

Top the salad with the dressing and sprinkle with the dried oregano.

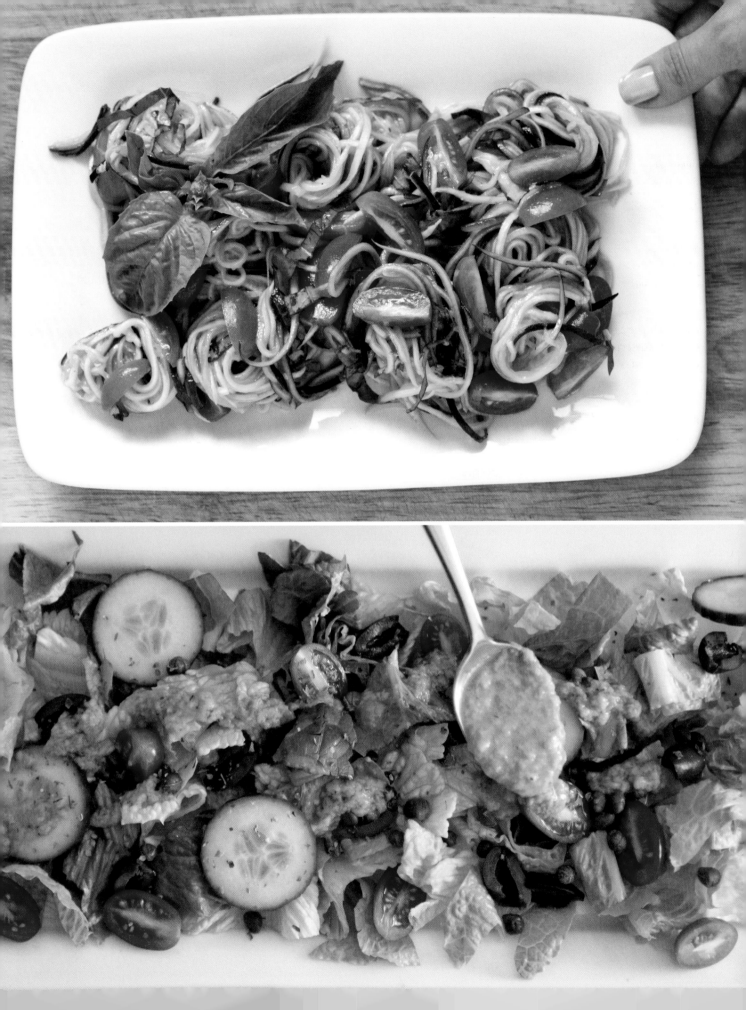

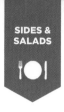

kale & carrot salad with lemon-tahini dressing

Raw kale can be tough to handle on its own, but by bruising it and combining it with lettuce, you can tastily add the nutrient-dense green to salads.

PREP TIME
10 minutes

COOKING TIME
-

YIELD
2 salads

FODMAP FREE?
Leave off the avocado and the garlic from the dressing.

NUTS
EGGS
NIGHTSHADES
FODMAPS

2 cups kale, chopped
2 cups mixed greens
1 cup carrot, shredded/grated
1 cup cucumber slices
1/2 avocado, sliced

LEMON TAHINI DRESSING
1 tablespoon tahini
1 tablespoon extra-virgin olive oil
Juice of 1 lemon
Pinch of garlic powder
Sea salt and black pepper to taste

Place the kale in a large mixing bowl, and massage it with your hands, squeezing and "bruising" it until the color changes from a dull green to a brighter shade. Add the mixed greens and shredded carrots, and gently toss to combine.

In a small mixing bowl, make the dressing by whisking together the tahini, extra-virgin olive oil, lemon juice, garlic powder, sea salt, and black pepper.

Pour the dressing over the lettuce, kale, and carrots, and toss together to evenly disperse the dressing. Top with sliced cucumber and avocado, and serve.

mixed greens salad with beets & blood oranges

The combination of the fresh citrus with the bite of the red onion makes this salad a delicious accompaniment to any fish or poultry dish. Try it alongside the Citrus Macadamia Nut Sole (recipe on page 314) or Savory Baked Chicken Legs (recipe on page 264).

PREP TIME
10 minutes

COOKING TIME
-

YIELD
2 salads

FODMAP FREE?
Leave out the mushrooms and onions.

NUTS
EGGS
NIGHTSHADES
FODMAPS

4 cups mixed greens
1/2 cup cooked beets, sliced into matchstick-sized pieces
1/2 of a blood orange, segmented, or other citrus
4 mushrooms, sliced

2 thin slices of red onion
2 tablespoons sliced almonds (optional)
Juice of 1 orange
2 tablespoons extra-virgin olive oil
Sea salt and black pepper to taste

Place mixed greens on a large salad plate.

Top the mixed greens with the beets, blood orange segments, white button mushrooms, red onion, and sliced almonds.

Squeeze the orange over the salad, and top with extra-virgin olive oil, sea salt, and black pepper to taste.

CHANGE IT UP
Use any kind of fruit to pair with this salad. Blood oranges were in season when I created it, but apples or berries would work well too!

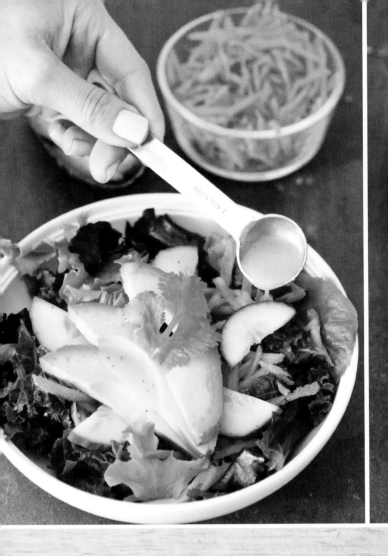

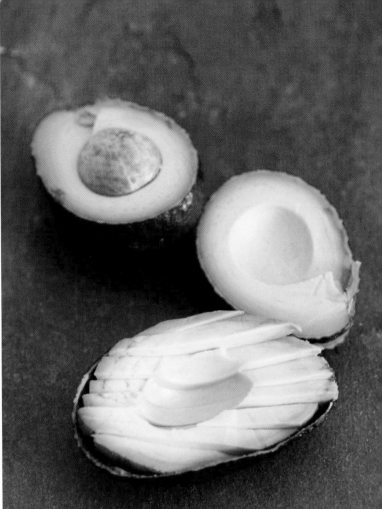

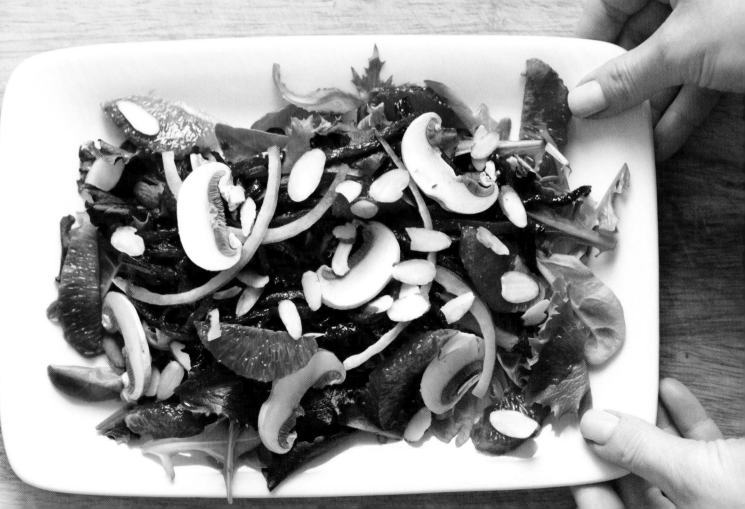

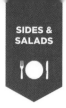

flank steak salad with fruit & balsamic vinaigrette

PREP TIME
10 minutes

COOKING TIME
-

YIELD
1 meal-sized salad
1 cup dressing/16 servings

FODMAP FREE?
Omit the apple and mushrooms; add grated carrots instead.

Grilled flank steak is a fantastic protein to cook up and have on-hand to use in a variety of ways. Use the recipe on page 294 to prepare the steak, then use leftovers to make this salad for lunch the next day.

2 cups baby spinach or mixed
   greens
4-8 ounces Garlic Flank Steak
   (recipe on page 294)
1/4 cup Granny Smith apple, sliced
2 button or baby bella
   mushrooms, sliced
2 tablespoons raspberries
1 tablespoon raw almonds, sliced

BALSAMIC VINAIGRETTE
1/3 cup balsamic vinegar
1 teaspoon Dijon mustard
   (gluten-free)
1/2 teaspoon anchovy paste
Sea salt and black pepper to taste
2/3 cup extra-virgin olive oil

Plate the spinach or mixed greens, and top with the flank steak, apple, mushrooms, raspberries, almonds, and Balsamic Vinaigrette.

For the Balsamic Vinaigrette:

In a small mixing bowl, whisk the balsamic vinegar, Dijon mustard, anchovy paste, sea salt, and black pepper together. Slowly drizzle in the extra-virgin olive oil, and continue whisking until well combined.

Store extra dressing in a glass bottle in the refrigerator for up to two weeks.

CHANGE IT UP
Use walnuts, macadamia nuts, or pecans instead of almonds.

Use any fruit that is in season.

NUTS
EGGS
NIGHTSHADES
FODMAPS

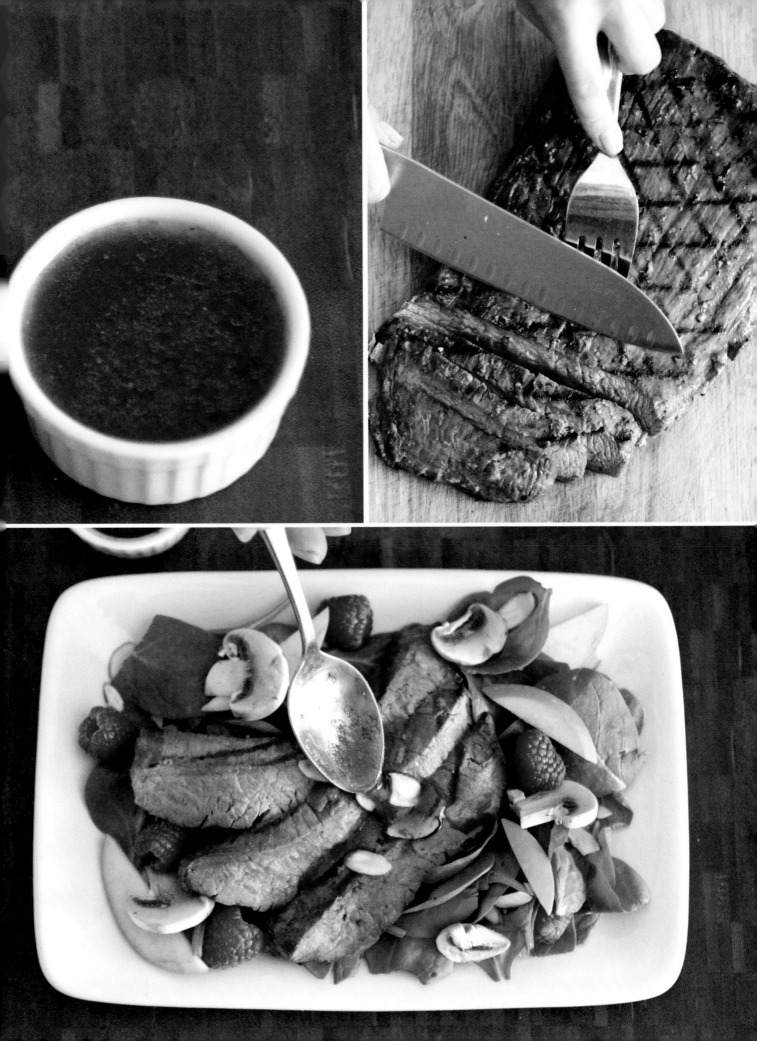

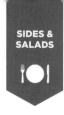
spinach salad
with walnuts & artichokes

The combination of the crunchy walnuts and the creamy artichoke hearts pairs well with the crisp spinach.

PREP TIME
10 minutes

COOKING TIME
-

YIELD
2 servings

SIDE NOTE
Top this with grilled chicken or steak for a complete meal.

NUTS
EGGS
NIGHTSHADES
FODMAPS

4 cups of baby spinach
1/2 cup raw beets, sliced into matchstick-sized pieces (optional)

1/2 of an orange, segmented
1/2 cup artichoke hearts
16 walnut halves

Place the baby spinach on a large salad plate. Top the spinach with the beets, orange segments, artichoke hearts, and walnut halves.

Dress with 2 tablespoons per serving of Balsamic Vinaigrette (recipe on page 378).

mixed greens salad with
persimmons, asparagus & fennel

Persimmons are one of my favorite fall and winter fruits. While seasonally available only for a short time, their flavor is worth the wait. Replace persimmons with apples other times of year.

PREP TIME
10 minutes

COOKING TIME
-

YIELD
2 servings

SIDE NOTE
Top this with grilled chicken or fish for a complete meal.

NUTS
EGGS
NIGHTSHADES
FODMAPS

4 cups mixed greens
1/2 cup raw asparagus, chopped

1 persimmon, thinly sliced
1/4 cup fennel, thinly sliced

Place the mixed greens on a large salad plate. Top the mixed greens with the asparagus, persimmon, and fennel.

Dress with 2 tablespoons per serving of Orange Vinaigrette (recipe on page 382).

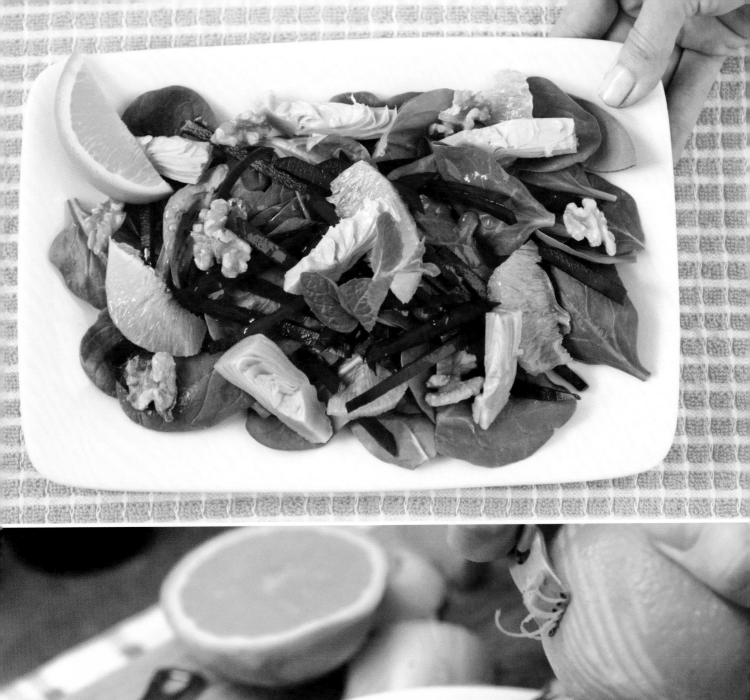
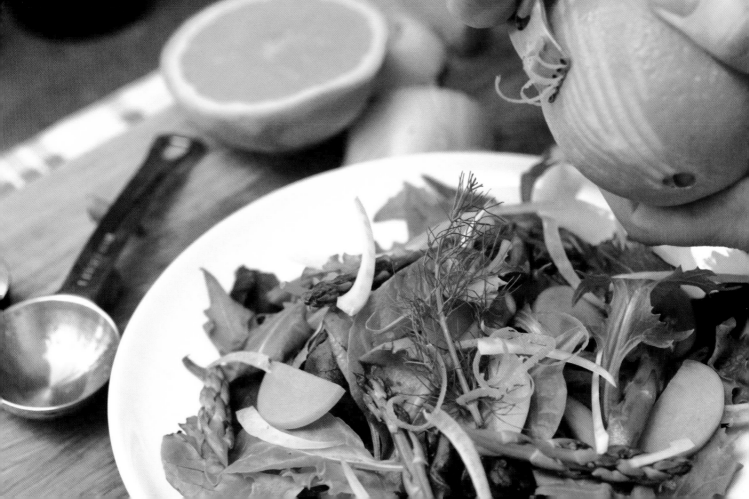

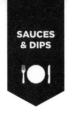
creamy cauliflower hummus

This twist on the traditional Mediterranean favorite tastes exactly the same as the chickpea (garbanzo bean) variety.

PREP TIME
15 minutes

COOKING TIME
-

YIELD
Approximately 2 cups

CHANGE IT UP

Substitute zucchini for the cauliflower, but shred and strain it first to remove most of its water content.

NUTS
EGGS
NIGHTSHADES
FODMAPS

4 cups cauliflower, steamed
2 tablespoons tahini (sesame paste)
1/4 cup + 1 tablespoon extra-virgin olive oil
1 lemon, juice and zest for garnish

Pinch of cumin
Sea salt and black pepper to taste
Pinch of paprika (optional, as garnish)

In a food processor, combine the cauliflower, tahini, extra-virgin olive oil, lemon juice, and cumin until smooth. Add more tahini or extra-virgin olive oil to-taste.

Scoop out the hummus from the food processor, and garnish with lemon zest, the additional tablespoon of extra-virgin olive oil, and paprika.

Serve with your choice of fresh, sliced vegetables and olives.

Note: I used an orange cauliflower for this recipe. If you spot one in your store or market, use it instead of the white variety for a deeper colored dip.

orange vinaigrette

This dressing pairs perfectly with the Persimmon Salad (recipe on page 380), but it's also delicious over any salad, especially in winter when oranges are in season.

PREP TIME
10 minutes

COOKING TIME
-

YIELD
3 servings of dressing
(6 Tablespoon total)

DRESS IT UP

Save time and make extra of this dressing to pour over salads in the near future.

FODMAP FREE?

Leave out the garlic powder.

NUTS
EGGS
NIGHTSHADES
FODMAPS

2 tablespoons fresh orange juice (about half an orange)
1 tablespoon unfiltered apple cider vinegar
1 teaspoon Dijon mustard (gluten-free)

Sea salt and black pepper to taste
Pinch of garlic powder (optional)
Ground fennel seeds (optional)
3 tablespoons extra-virgin olive oil
1 teaspoon orange zest (optional)

In a small mixing bowl, whisk the orange juice, apple cider vinegar, Dijon mustard, sea salt, black pepper, garlic powder, and fennel seeds together.

Slowly drizzle in the extra-virgin olive oil, and continue whisking until well combined.

Garnish with orange zest.

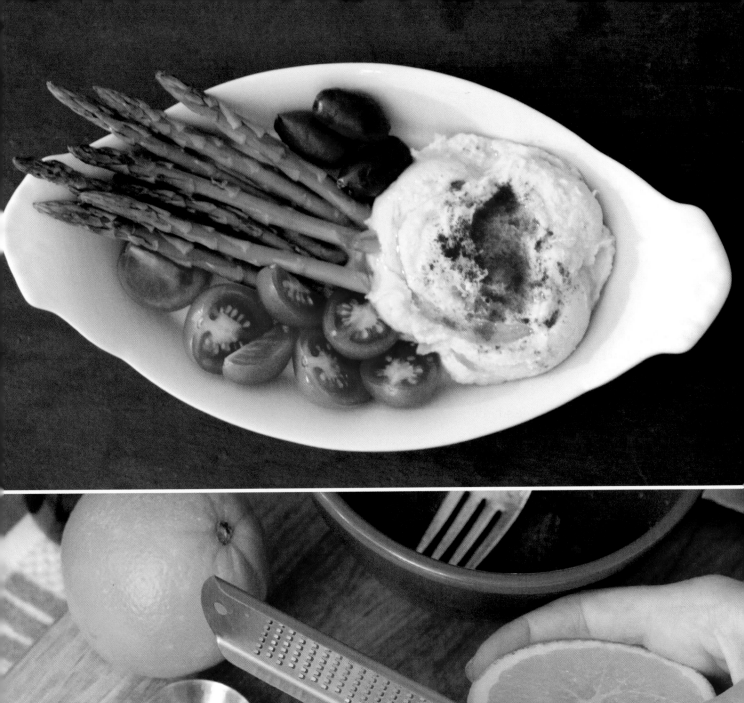
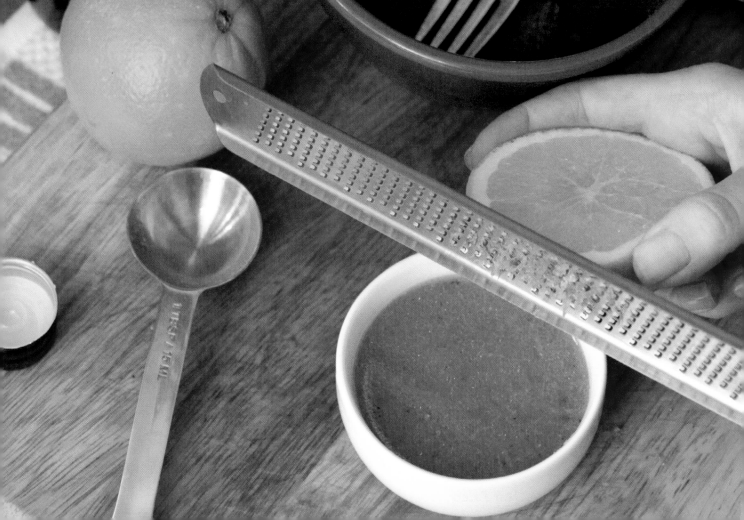

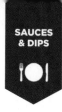
chicken liver pâté

One bite of this recipe and I'm brought back to the age of twelve. More specifically, I'm brought back to the table in my great grandmother's Upper West Side apartment in New York City. It tastes exactly like the authentic pâté I ate back then, surrounded by my mother, grandmother, and great aunts.

PREP TIME
15 minutes

COOKING TIME
30 minutes

YIELD
16 ounces
(4-8 servings)

CHANGE IT UP
Substitute apple cider vinegar or balsamic vinegar for the red wine.

1 lb chicken livers
    (or other kind, if you like)
1 small onion or 1/2 large onion, chopped
2 tablespoons + 1/2 cup butter or bacon fat
1/2 cup red wine
2-4 cloves garlic, crushed

1 teaspoon Dijon mustard
    (gluten-free)
1 sprig fresh rosemary
2 sprigs fresh thyme
1 tablespoon fresh lemon juice
Sea salt and black pepper to taste

In a large pot, sauté the chicken liver and onions in 2 tablespoons of the butter until the livers are browned and the onions are tender. Add the wine, garlic, mustard, rosemary, thyme, and lemon juice, and cook uncovered until most of the liquid is gone.

Transfer the mixture into a food processor, and blend to a smooth paste along with the rest of the butter (1 tablespoon at a time) until it reaches a smooth, creamy consistency. Add sea salt and black pepper to taste.

Put pâté in a shallow dish to refrigerate before serving.

Enjoy this spread on celery, carrots, cucumbers, peppers, or any other veggies you want to dip.

NUTS
EGGS
NIGHTSHADES
FODMAPS

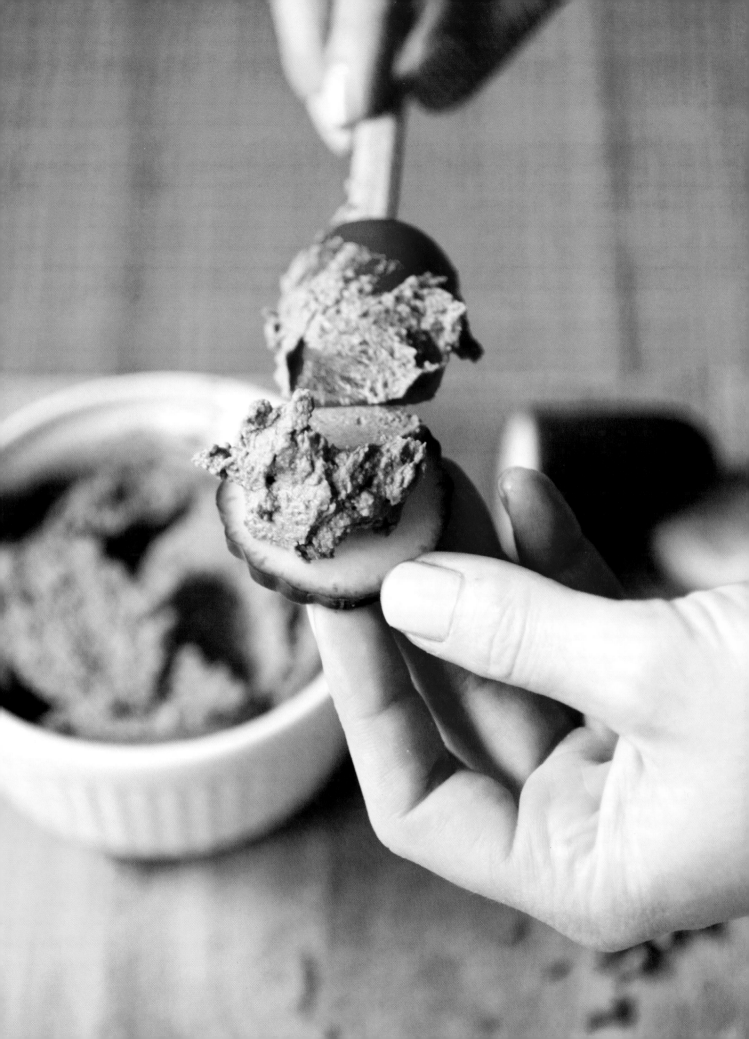

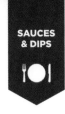

taramasalata

If you are a very active person, this salty, traditional Greek dip is a perfect way to replenish your body with sodium and starch. Taramasalata pairs nicely with Lemony Lamb Dolmas (recipe on page 318).

PREP TIME
10 minutes

COOKING TIME
30 minutes

YIELD
8 servings

1 1/2 cups white potatoes, peeled
4 ounces carp roe (fish eggs)
　　(it may be labeled as Tarama)

Juice of 2 lemons
1/4 onion, minced
1/2 cup extra-virgin olive oil

SIDE NOTE

This dip is traditionally made using bread as the thickener—be aware of this fact if you see it on a restaurant menu and are interested in trying it.

Since carp roe tends to be naturally quite salty, this recipe does not call for adding any salt, but adjust to your taste if you use a less-salty roe.

Boil the potatoes in a large pot of water for approximately 30 minutes or until tender.

Place the potato, carp roe, lemon juice, onion, and extra-virgin olive oil in a food processor, and blend until smooth. Add more extra-virgin olive oil if you like. Add sea salt and black pepper to taste.

Tastes great with cucumbers, carrot slices, or any other vegetables you like.

WHITE POTATOES?

This recipe incorporates the flesh of white potatoes, which is not traditionally a "Paleo" ingredient, but once the skin is removed, potatoes are nearly pure starch and okay to eat on occasion.

NUTS

EGGS

NIGHTSHADES

FODMAPS

roasted garlic tahini sauce

This simple sauce is delicious for dipping Lemony Lamb Dolmas (recipe on page 318), and it makes a nice burger topping or fresh vegetable dip.

PREP TIME
10 minutes

COOKING TIME
-

YIELD
3/4 cup,
approximately 6 servings

1/4 cup tahini
1/2 cup extra-virgin olive oil
4 cloves roasted garlic (recipe on
　　page 370)

Juice of 1 lemon
Sea salt and black pepper to taste

CHANGE IT UP

Substitute fresh garlic for the roasted garlic. Simply use 1 finely grated clove, adding it little by little to taste.

Whisk all ingredients together, or combine them in a small blender.

NUTS

EGGS

NIGHTSHADES

FODMAPS

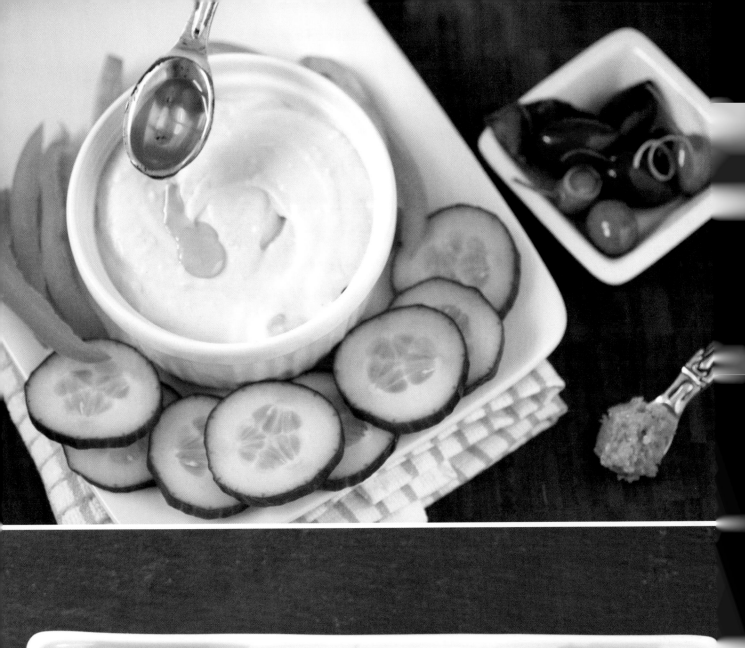
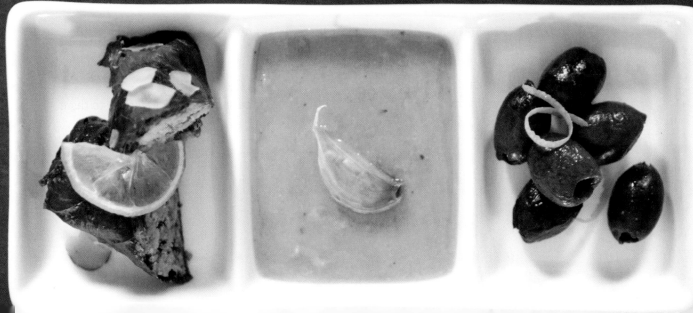

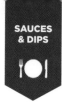
simple cranberry sauce

Pair this sauce with Thanksgiving Stuffing Meatballs (recipe on page 334), use it in Mom's Stuffed Cabbage recipe (recipe on page 290), or simply add it to your own holiday recipes list.

PREP TIME
5 minutes

COOKING TIME
15 minutes

YIELD
2 cups

SIDE NOTE
Spread this sauce over the Pumpkin Cranberry Muffins on page 246.

NUTS
EGGS
NIGHTSHADES
FODMAPS

15-16 ounces fresh cranberries
Organic honey or maple syrup to
taste (about 1-4 tablespoons)

Juice + zest of one orange (optional; do not include if you are adding this recipe to Mom's Stuffed Cabbage)

In a medium-sized sauce pot, simmer the cranberries with the water/juice until all berries have "popped" open, and the texture is gelatinous. Add the honey or maple syrup to taste.

Remove the mixture from the heat, and allow it to come to room temperature before refrigerating for later use.

CHANGE IT UP
To make a chunky cranberry sauce, add 1 cup mandarin orange segments, drained; 1 cup pineapple (fresh is ideal; check canned for additives, and get one without added sugar); 1/2 cup raw walnuts, chopped (soaked/dehydrated raw nuts are ideal).

roasted allium spread

Spread this on any kind of meat, or mix a spoon-full into any salad dressing to add depth and flavor.

PREP TIME
10 minutes

COOKING TIME
-

YIELD
1 cup of spread

CHANGE IT UP
Add roasted peppers or olives to give this spread more of a kick.

NUTS
EGGS
NIGHTSHADES
FODMAPS

1 cup Roasted Pearl Onions
    (recipe on page 370)
1 head of Red Roasted Garlic
    (recipe on page 370)

1-2 tablespoons extra-virgin olive oil
Sea salt and black pepper to taste

Blend onions and garlic in a food processor, adding the olive oil until you have reached your preferred consistency.

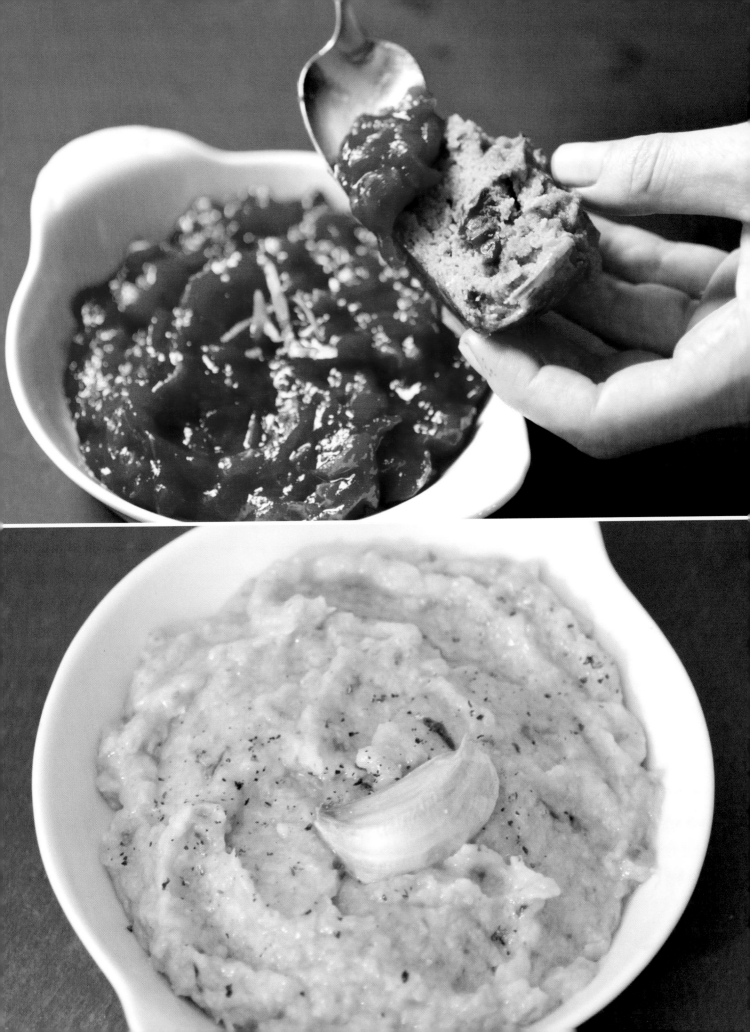

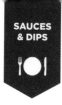
baconnaise

If you make a lot of Perfectly Baked Bacon (recipe on page 236), you have plenty of bacon fat sitting in the refrigerator. When you make the effort to procure pasture-raised pork, you should absolutely save the fat that drips off during the baking process.

PREP TIME
15 minutes

COOKING TIME
-

YIELD
3/4 cup

2 egg yolks
1 tablespoon lemon juice
1 teaspoon Dijon mustard (gluten-
   free)

3/4 cup bacon fat, melted and
   cooled to room temperature

SIDE NOTE

Use this Baconnaise to make Bacon & Egg Salad (recipe on page 248).

In a medium-sized mixing bowl, whisk together the egg yolk, lemon juice, and mustard until blended and bright yellow (about 30 seconds). Add 1/4 cup bacon fat to the yolk mixture a few drops at a time, whisking constantly. Gradually add the remaining bacon fat in a slow, thin stream, whisking constantly, until the mayonnaise is thick and lighter in color.

CHANGE IT UP

You can also make Baconnaise in a small blender, and you can double the recipe to make blending easier. Use the opening at the top of your blender to slowly stream in the bacon fat.

NUTS

EGGS

NIGHTSHADES

FODMAPS

Store in a glass jar in the refrigerator for up to a week.

---

pineapple (or mango) teriyaki

This is a delicious, soy-free sauce to use as a dip or to top meats with while grilling.

PREP TIME
15 minutes

COOKING TIME
15 minutes

YIELD
1 cup

1/2 cup water
1 cup chopped pineapple
   (or mango)
1/4 teaspoon ground ginger
1/4 teaspoon garlic powder

1 tablespoon coconut aminos
1 tablespoon cold-pressed
   sesame oil
1 teaspoon white and/or black
   sesame seeds as garnish

SIDE NOTE

This sauce is perfect for dipping with Chicken Wings, page 258.

In a small sauce pan, simmer the water, pineapple, ginger, garlic powder, and coconut aminos over medium-low heat for about 10 minutes or until the liquid reduces a bit and the pineapple is cooked through.

Place the cooked pineapple mixture in a blender, and blend until smooth. Add the sesame oil at the very end, and pulse the blender a couple of times to incorporate it.

NUTS

EGGS

NIGHTSHADES

FODMAPS

Garnish with sesame seeds.

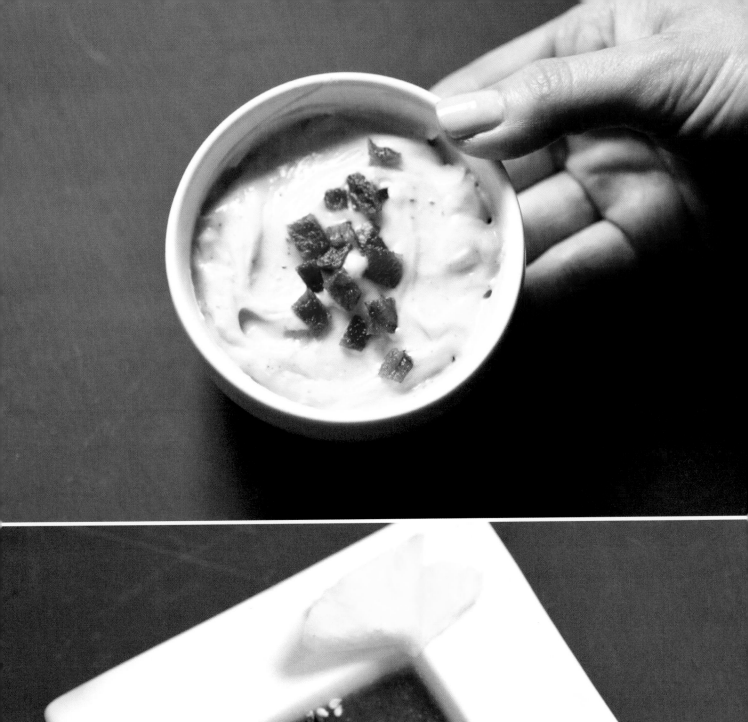
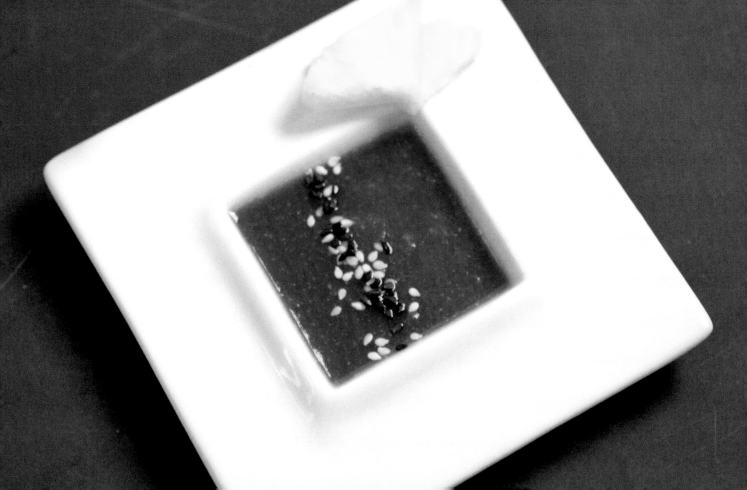

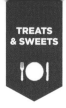
chocolate orange
& mint chip truffles

*Impress guests with these super-simple truffles that look elegant but use
ingredients you probably have lying around in your pantry.*

PREP TIME
25 minutes

COOKING TIME
-

YIELD
1 dozen truffles

SPICE IT UP
*Add a pinch of cayenne
pepper to the chocolate
orange flavor to give
them a kick!*

2-WAYS
*To make both flavors,
either split the base and
use 1/2 of the flavoring
ingredients, or double the
base and make one batch
of each!*

NUTS
EGGS
NIGHTSHADES
FODMAPS

BASE FOR ONE FLAVOR
2 tablespoons coconut oil
3 tablespoons coconut butter or
    coconut manna (cream concen-
    trate)
2 tablespoons almond butter
1/4 teaspoon pure vanilla extract

MINT CHIP FLAVOR
2 teaspoons mint extract
1 teaspoon pure maple syrup
1 tablespoon cacao nibs
2 tablespoons unsweetened cacao
    powder for the coating

CHOCOLATE ORANGE FLAVOR
2 tablespoons unsweetened cocoa
    powder
2 teaspoons pure maple syrup
Zest of one orange (1 teaspoon set
    aside for the coating)
2 tablespoons shredded coconut
    for the coating

*Make double the base if you want
to make both flavors at once!*

Place the coconut oil, coconut butter, almond butter, and pure vanilla extract
into a bowl, and combine until smooth. Add your selected flavor ingredients.
Mix thoroughly.

The mixture will be soft, so place it in the freezer for about 10 minutes or until
you can form the batter into 1-inch balls with your hands. Roll each ball in the
coating for your flavor.

Set the truffles on a plate, and refrigerate to solidify.

Serve chilled.

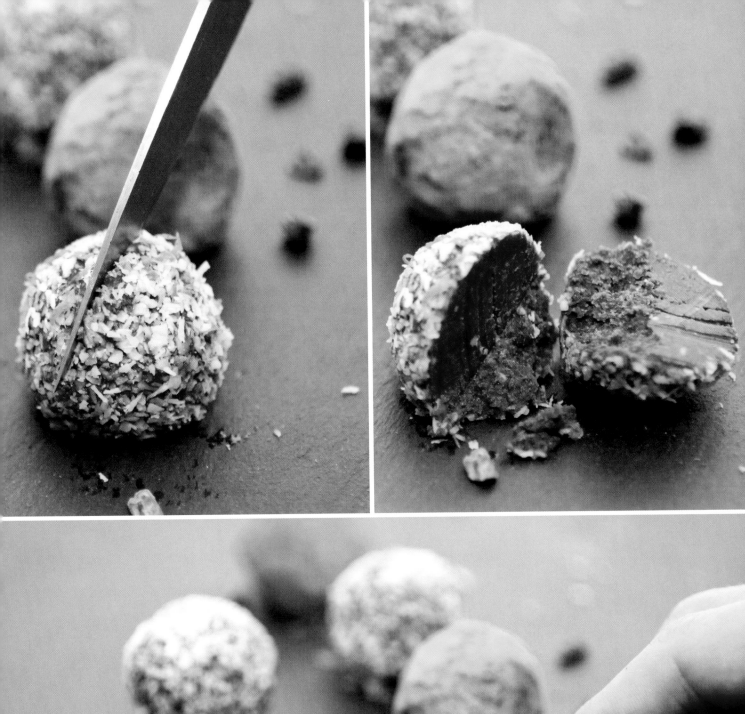
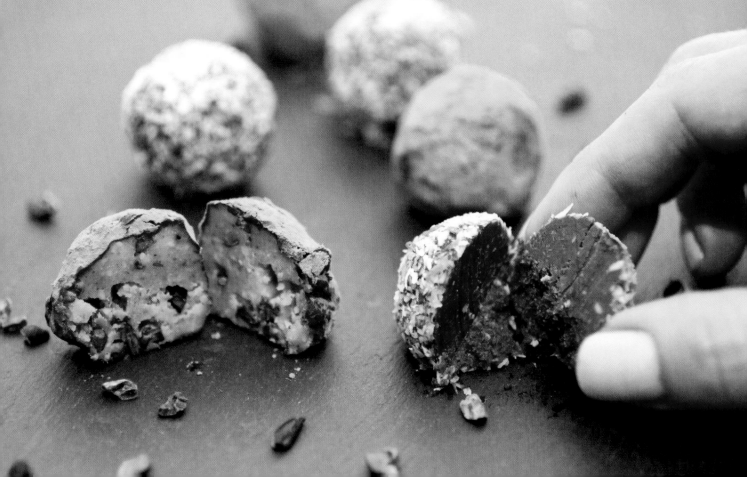

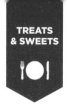
orange cream and mint melt-aways

Whip these delicious treats up any weeknight to enjoy, or bring them to a party. No one will ever guess that they're as simple to make as they are!

PREP TIME
15 minutes

COOKING TIME
-

YIELD
24 melt-aways

SIDE NOTE
Try adding your own favorite flavors to the base ingredients!

NUTS
EGGS
NIGHTSHADES
FODMAPS

BASE FOR ONE FLAVOR
1/2 cup coconut oil
1/2 cup coconut cream or coconut manna (cream concentrate)

Make double the base if you want to make both flavors at once!

FOR THE ORANGE CREAM
1/2 teaspoon pure vanilla extract
Zest of 1 orange
2 teaspoons pure maple syrup

FOR THE MINT
2 teaspoons fresh mint, chopped
2 teaspoons mint extract oil
2 teaspoons pure maple syrup

Combine base plus flavor ingredients in a small mixing bowl until smooth. Place paper liners in a 24-mini-muffin pan, and spoon the mixture evenly into each section.

Place the pan in the refrigerator or freezer to set, and serve cold.

chocolate coconut cookies

This cookie recipe is so easy that you can make it "to-order" after dinner and enjoy them warm from the oven.

PREP TIME
10 minutes

COOKING TIME
20-30 minutes

YIELD
1 dozen cookies

SIDE NOTE
Add walnuts and chocolate chips for added texture and some crunch!

NUTS
EGGS
NIGHTSHADES
FODMAPS

2 eggs
2 tablespoons butter, melted and cooled
2 tablespoons maple syrup (or more for sweeter cookies)
1/2 teaspoon vanilla extract
1 cup shredded coconut

2 tablespoons unsweetened cocoa powder
1 pinch baking soda
1/4 cup sliced almonds or 1/2 cup fresh raspberries (optional)

Preheat oven to 350°F.

In a medium-sized mixing bowl, whisk the eggs, melted butter, maple syrup, and vanilla. Mix in the unsweetened cocoa powder, baking soda, and shredded coconut until well combined. Fold in the almonds, if desired.

Divide into 12 dollops on a parchment paper-lined cookie sheet, and flatten them with a fork. Bake for 20-30 minutes or until slightly firm to the touch.

If you wish to add raspberries, add one to the center of each cookie after baking and before eating.

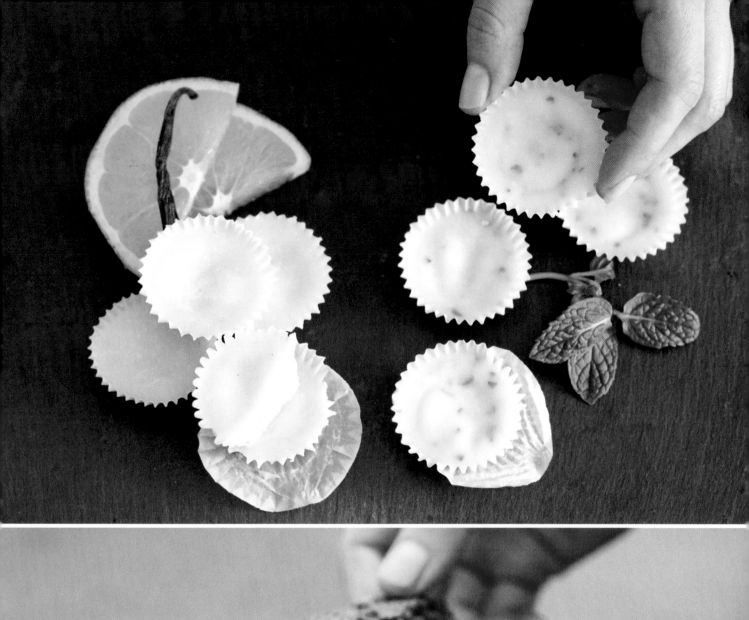

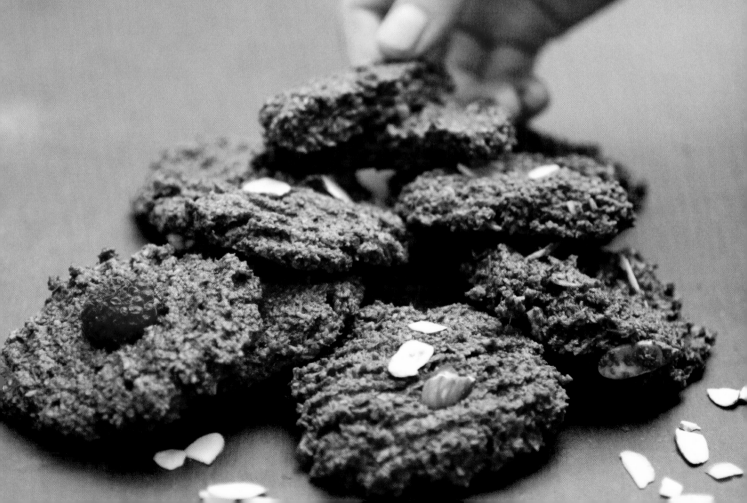

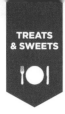
vanilla bean tahini truffles

PREP TIME
25 minutes

COOKING TIME
-

YIELD
1 dozen

If you can't have nuts around your house due to allergies, this sesame seed-based recipe is a great option. These are perfect for finishing off an Asian flavored meal like scallops (recipe on page 304) or stir fry (recipe on page 286).

CHANGE IT UP
1-2 tablespoons of any or both of the following may be used as a coating: unsweetened shredded coconut; white or black sesame seeds.

2 tablespoons raw tahini
   (sesame paste)
4 tablespoons coconut butter,
   coconut manna, or coconut
   cream concentrate
1 tablespoon unsweetened shredded coconut
1-2 teaspoons pure maple syrup

1/4 teaspoon cinnamon
Pinch of sea salt
Seeds from 1/2 vanilla bean pod
   or 1/2 teaspoon pure vanilla
   extract
2 tablespoons sesame seeds for
   coating

In a mixing bowl, combine tahini, softened coconut butter, shredded coconut, maple syrup, cinnamon, sea salt, and vanilla bean or extract until smooth. (If you're using a vanilla bean, slice it down the center and run the back of your knife along the inside edges of the pod to scrape out the seeds.)

Form the mixture into 1-inch balls, and roll each one in the sesame seeds or your choice of coating (see Change It Up). Set the truffles on a plate, and refrigerate to solidify.

NUTS

EGGS

NIGHTSHADES

FODMAPS

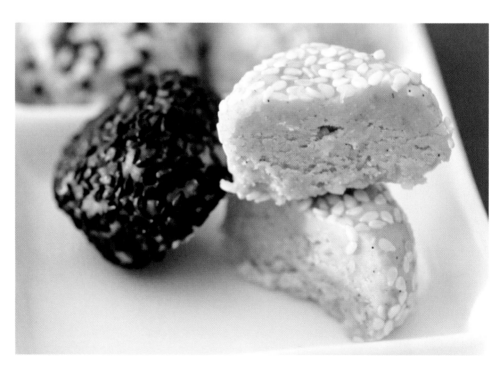

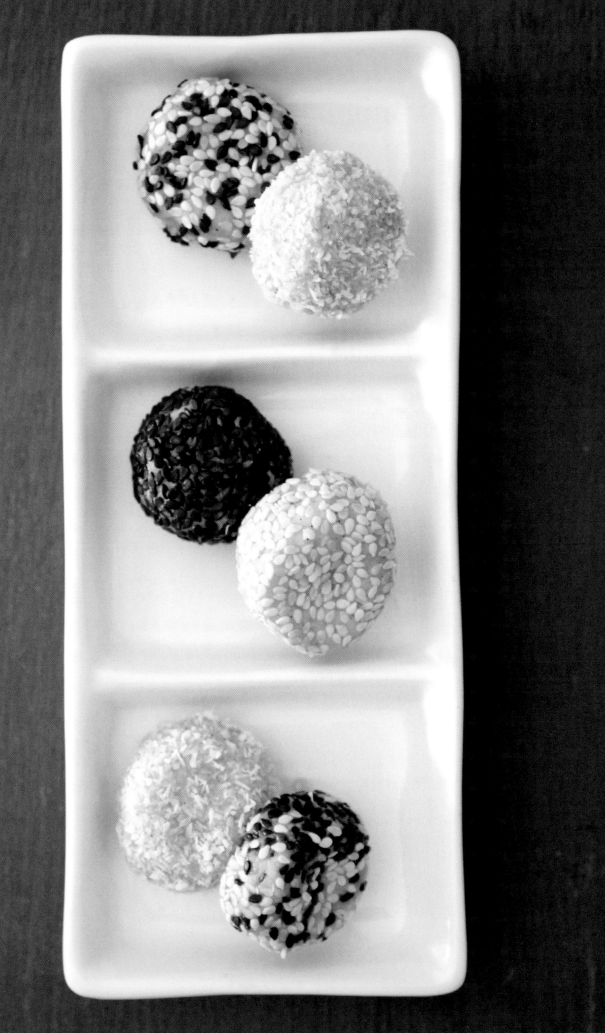

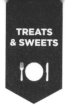
almond butter cups, dark and light

PREP TIME
40 minutes

COOKING TIME
Less than 5 minutes

YIELD
24 almond butter cups

CHANGE IT UP
Use walnut or pecan butter for the filling if you don't want to use almond butter.

NUTS
EGGS
NIGHTSHADES
FODMAPS

Peanut butter cups were a favorite of mine for many years. This updated version uses very little sweetener and more wholesome/natural ingredients.

FOR DARK SHELLS
2 tablespoons coconut oil, melted
2 tablespoons coconut butter, coconut manna, or coconut cream concentrate, softened
1/4 cup unsweetened cocoa powder
1 teaspoon pure maple syrup
1/4 teaspoon pure vanilla extract
Pinch of sea salt
Pinch of cinnamon

FOR LIGHT SHELLS
3 tablespoons coconut oil, melted
3 tablespoons coconut butter or coconut manna (cream concentrate), softened
1 teaspoon pure maple syrup
1/4 teaspoon pure vanilla extract
Vanilla "flecks" from 1/2 a vanilla bean pod (to remove the vanilla "flecks" from the vanilla bean pod, slice it down the middle and scrape with the back of your knife)
1 tablespoon shredded coconut

FOR THE FILLING
3 tablespoons almond butter (or other nut butter)
1 tablespoon coconut oil
1 teaspoon pure maple syrup
Pinch of sea salt

In a medium-sized mixing bowl, whisk together all of the ingredients for the Dark Shells. In another medium-sized mixing bowl, whisk together all of the ingredients for the Light Shells.

Place paper liners in a 24-mini-muffin baking tin (or 2 12-muffin tins), and spoon a 1/8-inch layer (approximately 1 teaspoon) of the Dark Shell mixture in the bottom of 12 of the muffin spaces and the Light Shell mixture in the remaining 12.

Place the trays in the refrigerator or freezer to set/solidify. While the first layer of the shells is setting, combine all of the ingredients for the filling in a small mixing bowl. Next, place the filling mixture into a quart-sized plastic bag or a pastry bag. Snip a tiny corner off of the bag with scissors.

Take the shells from the refrigerator or freezer, and begin to pipe a small amount (about 1/2 teaspoon) of the filling into the center of each one, leaving some of the edge visible. Once all of the shells have been filled, add the remaining Dark or Light Shell mixture until the filling is covered.

Place the tray back in the refrigerator or freezer to set, and serve cold or at room temperature.

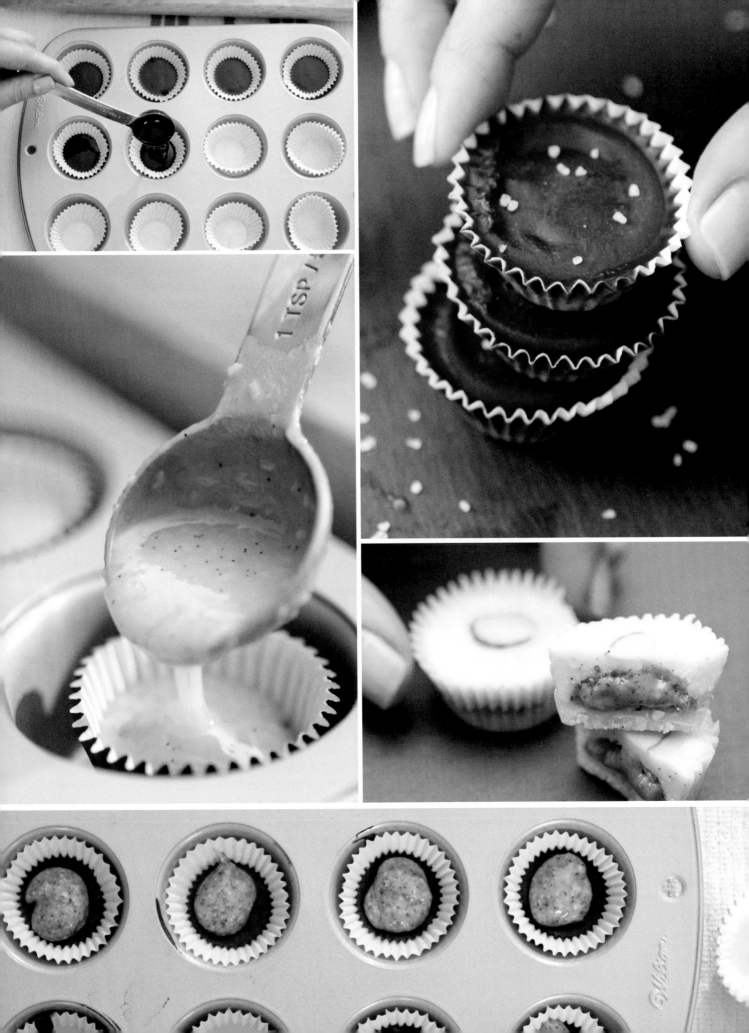

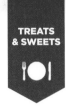
pepita goji berry bark

Dark chocolate bark can be made with almost any combination of nuts and dried fruit. What I love about this recipe are the bright colors that pop within the rich, dark chocolate.

PREP TIME
15 minutes

COOKING TIME
Less than 5 minutes

YIELD
10-12 pieces

NIGHTSHADE FREE?
Swap out the goji berries for cranberries or cherries.

NUTS

EGGS

NIGHTSHADES

FODMAPS

1 cup dark chocolate chips
1 teaspoon bacon grease or coconut oil
2 tablespoons goji berries, roughly chopped

2 tablespoons pepitas (pumpkin seeds), roughly chopped
2 tablespoons walnuts, roughly chopped
Pinch of coarse sea salt

Melt the chocolate chips with the bacon grease over a double-boiler on low heat or in the microwave for 30 seconds. Stir vigorously before adding more chocolate chips. Add microwave time only in 10-second increments to prevent burning the chocolate.

Stir in the goji berries, pepitas, walnuts, and sea salt, and spread the mixture on parchment paper over a cookie sheet. Place in the refrigerator to cool. After it has set, chop the chocolate roughly.

nutty bacon bark

There are few better ways to enjoy bacon than when it's combined with chocolate. This is a quick way to impress your guests with a delicious treat.

PREP TIME
10 minutes

COOKING TIME
Less than 5 minutes

YIELD
10-12 pieces

MIXED NUTS
Use two or three kinds of nuts in this recipe—live on the edge!

NUTS

EGGS

NIGHTSHADES

FODMAPS

1 cup dark chocolate chips
1 teaspoon bacon grease or coconut oil
1/4 cup toasted hazelnuts (or any other nut)

4 strips bacon, cooked & chopped
1/2 teaspoon sea salt (smoked sea salt is ideal)

Melt the chocolate chips with the bacon grease over a double-boiler on low heat or in the microwave for 30 seconds. Stir vigorously before adding more chocolate chips. Add microwave time only in 10-second increments to prevent burning the chocolate.

Spread the melted chocolate on parchment paper over a cookie sheet, and set aside to cool. Once the chocolate is nearly set but not entirely, sprinkle the hazelnuts, bacon, and sea salt evenly over the top. Chop roughly before serving.

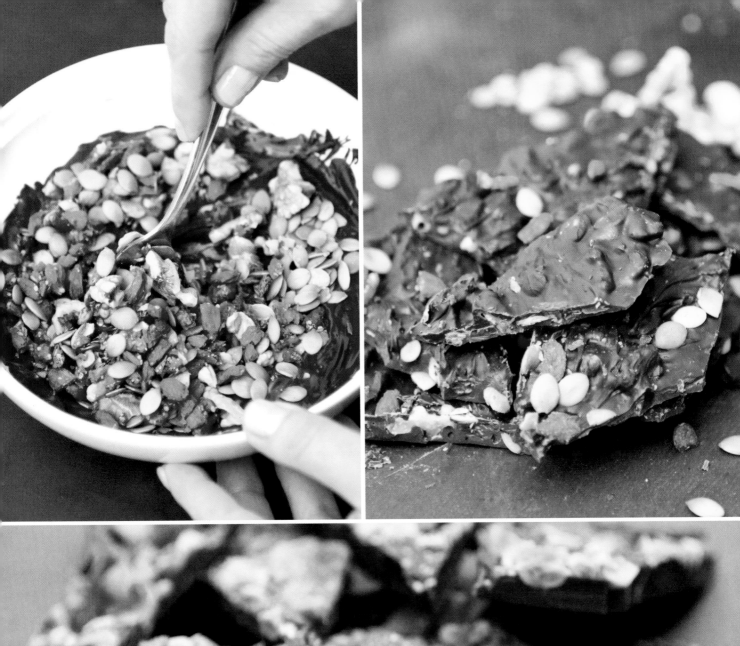

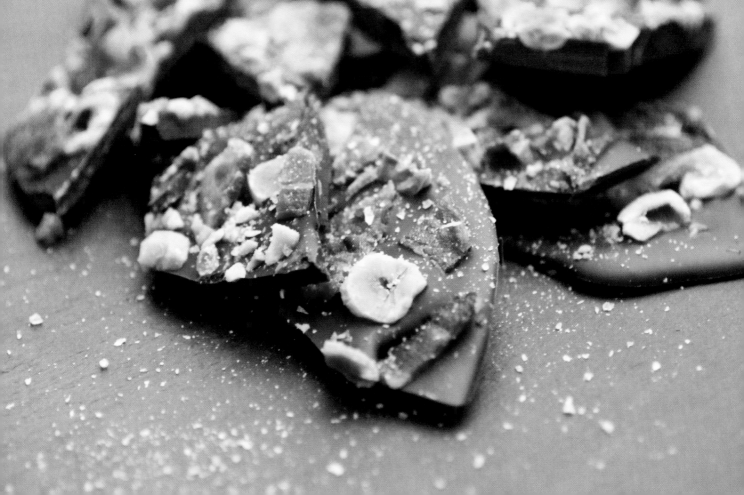

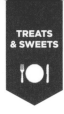
moo-less chocolate mousse

Eliminating dairy products can feel daunting when making desserts, but this avocado-based mousse is surprisingly delicious.

PREP TIME
10 minutes

COOKING TIME
-

YIELD
2 servings

NUTS
EGGS
NIGHTSHADES
FODMAPS

2 ripe avocados
1/4 cup unsweetened cacao powder
2-4 tablespoons coconut milk
1 ripe banana (optional)
1-4 tablespoons maple syrup or softened honey (optional to taste and may not be necessary if the banana is sweet enough)

1/2 teaspoon pure vanilla extract
Pinch of cinnamon
Pinch of sea salt

Scoop out the flesh of the avocados into a small food processor, or mash them by hand. Add the cacao powder, coconut milk, ripe banana, maple syrup, vanilla extract, cinnamon, and sea salt, and process until creamy, whipped, and well blended. You may whisk the ingredients together as well, if necessary.

Serve in individual dishes or bowls. Garnish with with cacao nibs (pictured), toasted hazelnuts, or coconut.

moo-less pistachio mousse

A twist on the classic chocolate mouse, this recipe uses the natural color of the avocado for an entirely different taste combination.

PREP TIME
10 minutes

COOKING TIME
-

YIELD
2 servings

NUTS
EGGS
NIGHTSHADES
FODMAPS

2 ripe avocados
1-2 teaspoon pistachio or almond extract (use 1 if the extract has an alcohol base; use 2 if it has an oil base)
1/4 cup coconut milk
1 large or 2 small bananas

1 tablespoon maple syrup or softened honey (optional to taste and may not be necessary if bananas are sweet enough)
Pinch of sea salt
2 tablespoons chopped pistachios

Scoop out the flesh of the avocados into a small food processor, or mash them by hand. Add the pistachio extract, coconut milk, bananas, maple syrup, and sea salt, and process until creamy, whipped, and well blended. You may whisk the ingredients together as well, if necessary.

Serve in individual dishes or bowls. Garnish with chopped pistachios.

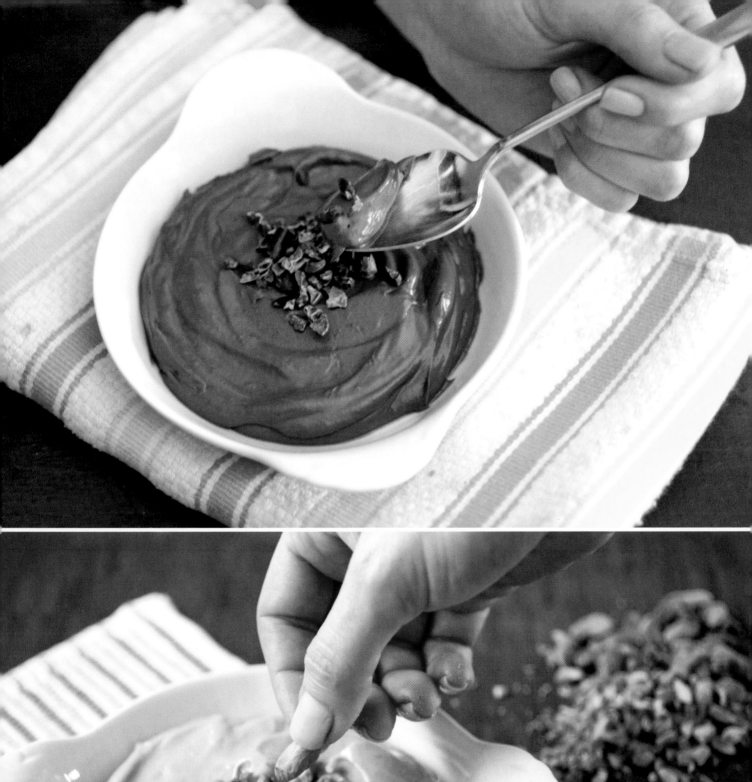
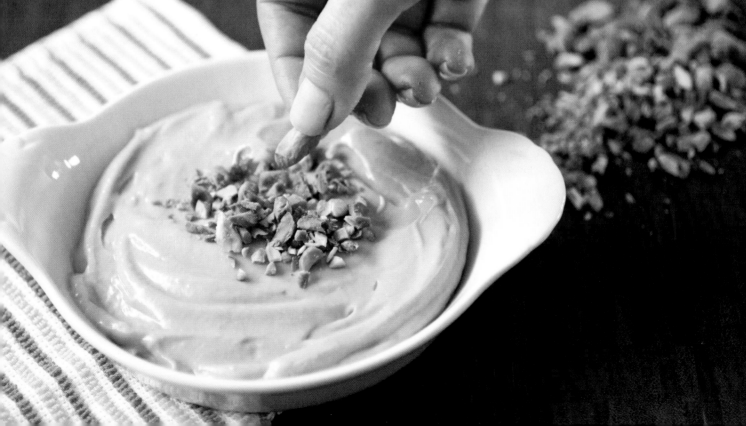

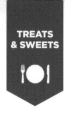

pumpkin-pie custard

PREP TIME
10 minutes

COOKING TIME
45-60 minutes

YIELD
4 servings

CHANGE IT UP
You can make this into a savory side dish by leaving out the cinnamon, maple syrup, and vanilla and substituting onion powder. Garnish with fresh sage leaves pan-fried in butter (instructions accompany the Butternut Sage Soup recipe on page 348).

NUTS
EGGS
NIGHTSHADES
FODMAPS

If you have a nut allergy, and a grain-free pumpkin pie is out of the question, try this custard. It's delicious enough that everyone will enjoy it and not miss the crust one bit.

1 teaspoon cinnamon
1/4 teaspoon ground ginger
2 pinches of grated nutmeg
Pinch of sea salt
1 cup canned pumpkin puree (or made from fresh pumpkin and strained)

2 eggs, beaten
1/4 cup maple syrup
1 teaspoon vanilla extract
1 cup full-fat coconut milk

Preheat oven to 350°F.

Boil a pot of water (enough water to fill the baking pan as directed below).

In a small mixing bowl, combine the cinnamon, ginger, nutmeg, and sea salt. In a medium-sized mixing bowl, combine the pumpkin puree, eggs, maple syrup, vanilla extract, and coconut milk. Whisk the dry ingredients into the liquid mixture until well combined.

Pour the custard into small ramekins (oven-safe ceramic or glass dishes). Place the ramekins in a baking pan and add enough boiling water to the dish to come up halfway to the top of the ramekins. Carefully place the dish with the ramekins and water in the oven.

Bake for 45-60 minutes or until a knife inserted into the center of the custard comes out clean.

Serve warm or chilled.

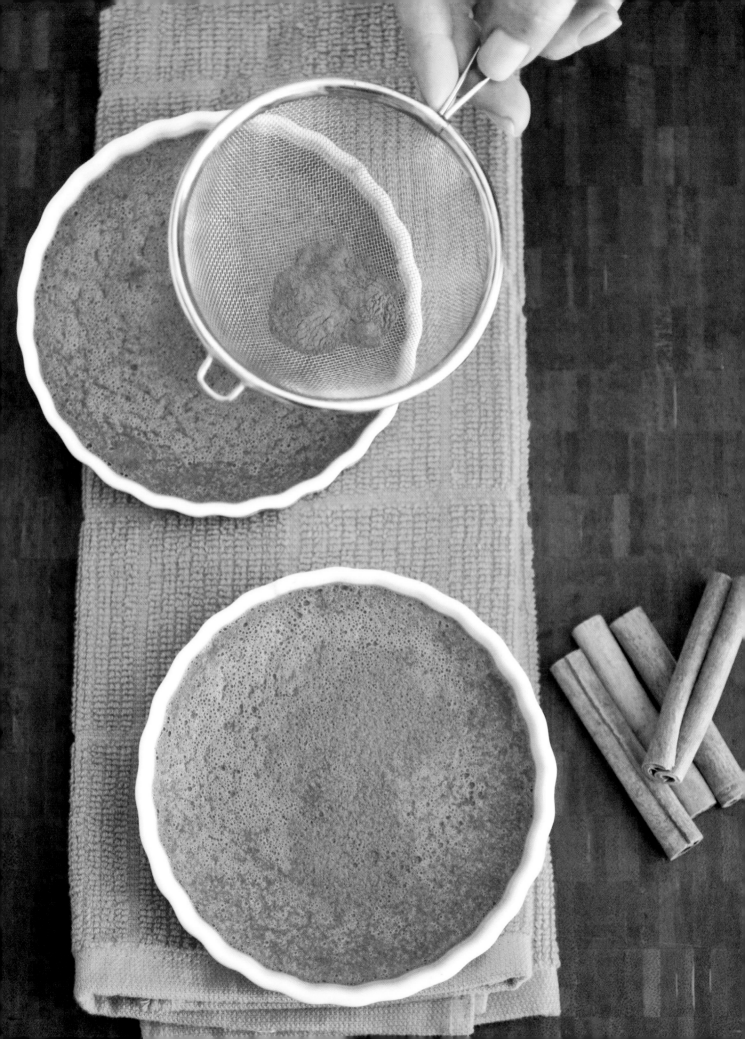

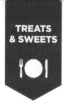
fresh blueberry crumble

PREP TIME
15 minutes

COOKING TIME
30-40 minutes

YIELD
6 servings

CHANGE IT UP
Use any fruit you like, just bake long enough to see the fruit juices bubbling and the top becoming golden brown.

When you're looking for a quick and easy dessert, baking fruit with a nutty topping is probably the easiest thing you can do.

2 pints of fresh blueberries
Juice of 1 lemon
1 cup almond meal/almond flour
1/4 cup chopped macadamia
    or walnuts

1/4 cup melted butter
    or coconut oil
2 tablespoons maple syrup
1/4 teaspoon cinnamon
2 pinches of sea salt

Preheat oven to 375°F.

Place the blueberries in a 9 inch x 9 inch baking dish, and squeeze the juice from half of the lemon over them. Toss slightly to coat the blueberries with the juice.

In a mixing bowl, combine the almond meal or flour, macadamia nuts, melted butter, remaining lemon juice, maple syrup, cinnamon, and salt.

Spread the nut topping evenly over the blueberries, and bake until the fruit is well cooked/bubbly and the topping is golden brown (approximately 30-40 minutes).

NUTS

EGGS

NIGHTSHADES

FODMAPS

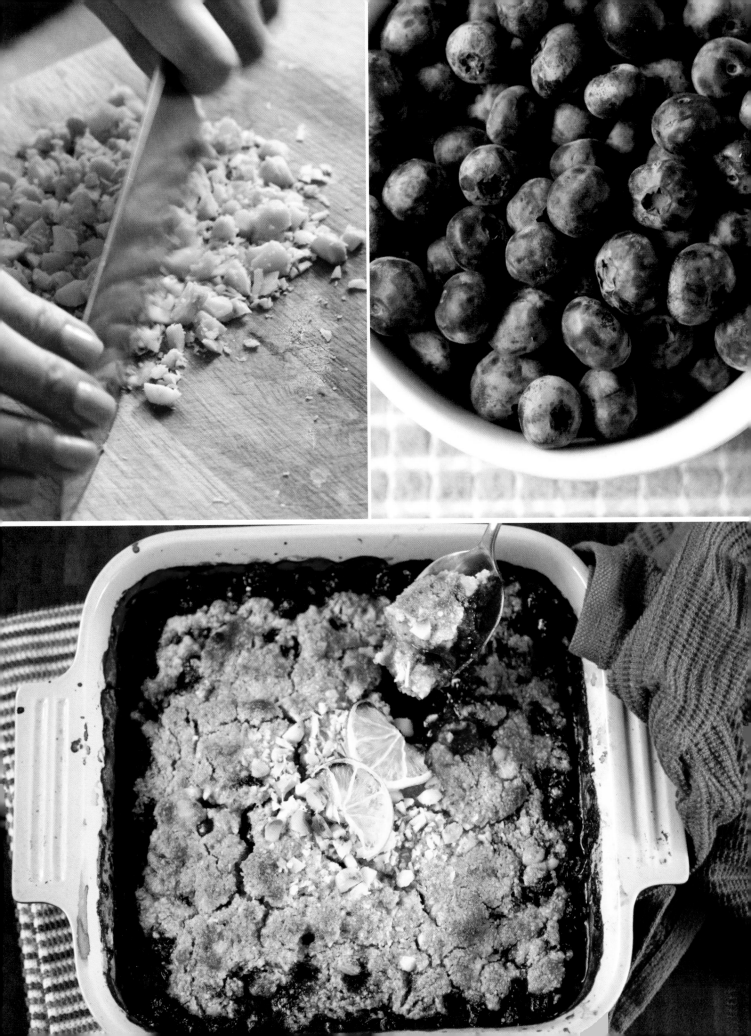

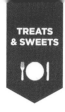
frozen raspberry torte

PREP TIME
40 minutes

FREEZE TIME
2-3 hours

YIELD
1 pie

This raw recipe is fantastic for impressing dinner party guests or to serve after a barbecue. It's the perfect summertime treat since there's no need to turn on the oven and heat up your house.

CRUST
1 cup macadamia nuts
1 cup walnuts
4-6 medjool dates

FILLING
12 ounces fresh raspberries (or other berries of your choice)
1/2 lemon, juice and zest
2 tablespoons coconut butter
1 tablespoon coconut oil
6 medjool dates (more or less to taste depending on the sweetness of your berries)

SIDE NOTE
If you change the type of fruit you use for the filling, adjust the amount of coconut butter. The amount of coconut butter will depend on the type of fruit, so there will be a learning curve. Keep track of what you use for future reference.

Place the macadamia nuts and walnuts in a food processor, and process until they are a very fine consistency, almost like nut flour. Add the dates until the mixture becomes sticky and forms a giant "ball" in the processor.

Press the crust mixture into a 9-inch round pie pan (lined with parchment paper if you have it), and place it in the freezer to set.

Place the raspberries, lemon juice, coconut butter, coconut oil, and dates in the food processor, and process until smooth. Taste it to make sure you have added enough dates for your desired sweetness.

Remove the crust from the freezer, and fill the pan with the berry mixture. Place the pie back in the freezer, and chill it for at least 2-3 hours.

Remove from the freezer before serving to soften it slightly.

CHANGE IT UP
Use smaller dishes if you'd like to make individual pies. Substitute blueberries or strawberries for a different flavor. If you can't eat berries, use 12 ounces of mashed banana.

NUTS
EGGS
NIGHTSHADES
FODMAPS

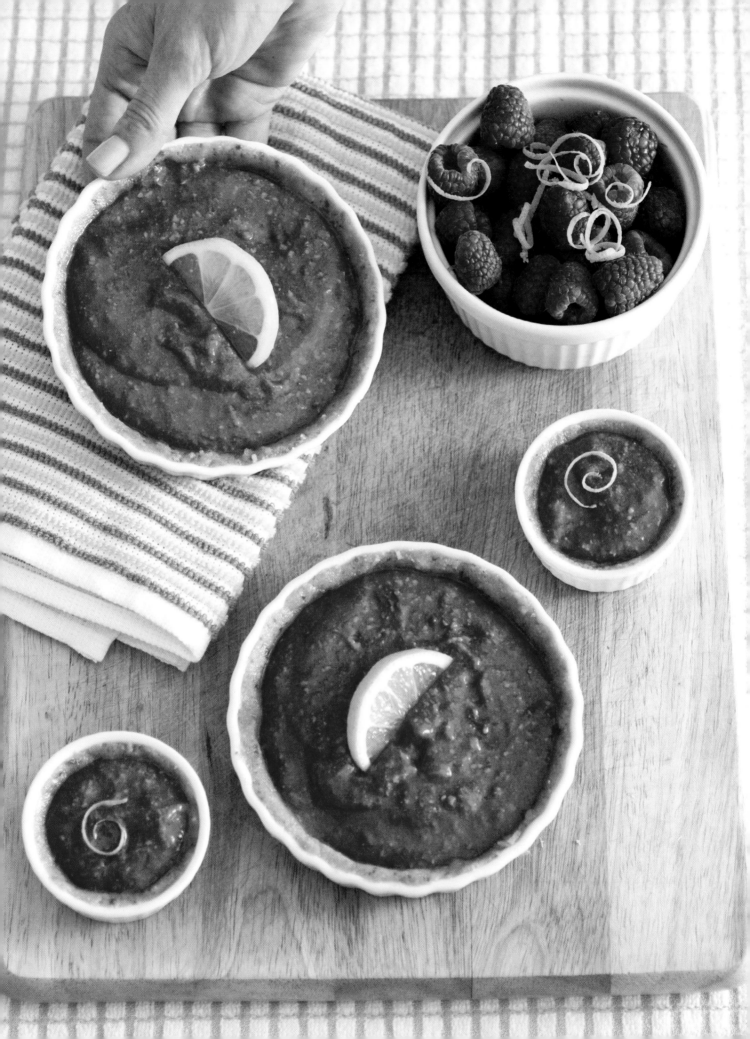

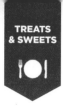
flourless mocha-bacon brownies

PREP TIME
20 minutes

COOKING TIME
30 minutes

YIELD
9-12 brownies

Who needs flour when you can use cocoa, eggs, and butter to make brownies? Okay, it's a few more ingredients than that, but these are a very simple way to make a rich and delicious treat without the grains!

4 ounces dark chocolate,
    melted and cooled
1/2 cup butter or coconut oil,
    melted and cooled
1/2 cup pure maple syrup
3 eggs

1/2 cup + 2 tablespoons
    unsweetened cocoa powder
2 tablespoons very strong coffee
2 tablespoons fine coffee grinds
2 slices baked bacon, chopped

SIDE NOTE

This recipe is much easier and more economical than a lot of other grain-free brownie recipes that call for a lot of almond butter!

Preheat oven to 375˚F.

In a medium-sized mixing bowl, combine the melted dark chocolate, butter or oil, pure maple syrup, and eggs. Slowly sift the cocoa powder over the wet ingredients, whisking it evenly. Add the strong coffee and the coffee grinds, and stir until well combined.

Line a 9 inch x 9 inch square pan with parchment paper, and fill the pan with the brownie batter. Top the batter with the chopped bacon pieces, and bake for approximately 30 minutes or until a toothpick inserted in the center comes out completely clean.

Dust with sifted cocoa powder as garnish.

CHANGE IT UP

For extra bacon-y brownies, use 1/4 cup bacon fat in place of half of the butter or coconut oil.

NUTS
EGGS
NIGHTSHADES
FODMAPS

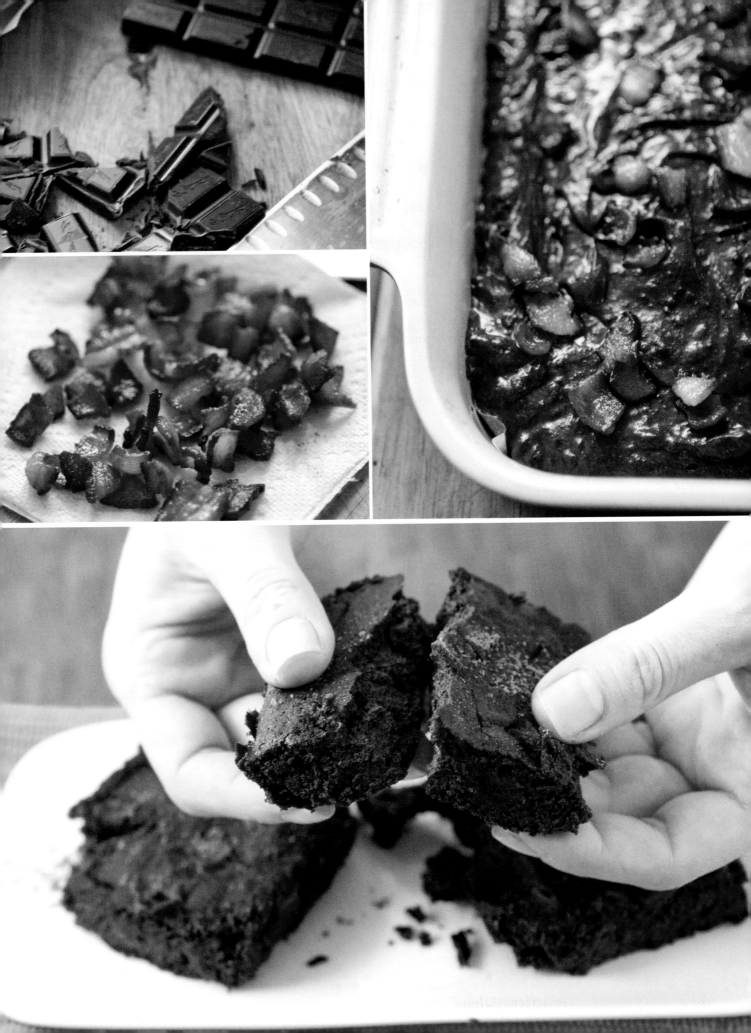

INDEX

INGREDIENT INDEX

guide to: paleo foods

Eat whole foods. Avoid foods that are modern, processed, and refined. Eat as close to nature as possible, and avoid foods that cause stress for the body (blood sugar, digestion, etc.). Eat nutrient-dense foods to maintain energy levels. Enjoy your food, and hold positive thoughts while you consume it.

meat, seafood & eggs

INCLUDING BUT NOT LIMITED TO:

- Beef
- Bison
- Boar
- Buffalo
- Chicken
- Duck
- Eggs
- Game meats
- Goat
- Goose

- Lamb
- Mutton
- Ostrich
- Pork
- Quail
- Rabbit
- Squab
- Turkey
- Veal
- Venison
- Catfish

- Carp
- Clams
- Grouper
- Halibut
- Herring
- Lobster
- Mackerel
- Mahi mahi
- Mussels
- Oysters
- Salmon

- Sardines
- Scallops
- Shrimp
- Prawns
- Snails
- Snapper
- Sword-fish
- Trout
- Tuna

fats & oils

- Avocado oil
- Bacon fat/lard
- Butter
- Coconut milk
- Coconut oil

- Duck fat
- Ghee
- Macadamia oil
- Olive oil: CP
- Palm oil

- Schmaltz
- Sesame oil: CP
- Suet
- Tallow
- Walnut oil

nuts & seeds

- Almonds
- Brazil nuts
- Chestnuts
- Hazelnuts

- Macadamia
- Pecans
- Pine nuts
- Pistachios*

- Pumpkin seeds
- Sesame seeds
- Sunflower seeds
- Walnuts

liquids

- Almond Milk, fresh
- Coconut Milk
- Coconut water

- Herbal tea
- Mineral water
- Water

superfoods

GRASS-FED DAIRY:
- butter, ghee,

ORGAN MEATS:
- Liver, kidneys, heart, etc.

SEA VEGETABLES:
- Dulse, kelp, seaweed
- Herbs & spices

BONE BROTH:
- Homemade, not canned or boxed

FERMENTED FOODS:
- *Sauerkraut*, carrots, beets, high-quality yogurt, kefir, kombucha

NOTES
CP = cold-pressed
Bold = nightshades
Italics = goitrogenic

* = FODMAPs (p. 115)
^ = buy organic

vegetables

INCLUDING BUT NOT LIMITED TO:

- Artichokes*
- Asparagus*
- Arugula
- Bamboo shoots
- Beets*
- *Bok choy*
- *Broccoli**
- *Brussels sprouts**
- *Cabbage**
- Carrots
- Cassava
- *Cauliflower**
- Celery^
- Chard

- *Collard greens^*
- Cucumbers
- Daikon
- Dandelion greens*
- **Eggplant***
- Endive
- Fennel*
- Garlic*
- Green beans
- Green onions*
- Jicama*
- *Kale^*
- *Kohlrabi*
- Leeks*

- Lettuce^
- Lotus roots
- Mushrooms*
- Mustard greens*
- Okra*
- Onions*
- Parsley
- Parsnips
- **Peppers*^**
- Purslane
- Radicchio
- *Radishes*
- *Rapini*
- Rutabagas
- Seaweed

- Shallots*
- Snap peas
- *Spinach^*
- Squash
- Sugar snaps
- Sunchokes*
- *Sweet potatoes*
- Taro
- **Tomatillos**
- **Tomatoes**
- Turnip greens
- Turnips
- *Watercress*
- Yams
- Yuccas

fruits

INCLUDING BUT NOT LIMITED TO

- Apples*^
- Apricots*
- Avocados*
- Bananas
- Blackberries*
- Blueberries^
- Cherries*
- Cranberries
- Figs*

- Grapefruit
- Grapes^
- Guavas
- Kiwis
- Lemons
- Limes
- Lychees*
- Mangoes*
- Melons

- Nectarines*^
- Oranges
- Papayas
- Passionfruit
- *Peaches*^*
- *Pears**
- Persimmons*
- Pineapples
- Plantains

- Plums*
- Pome-granates
- Raspberries
- Rhubarb
- Star fruit
- *Strawberries^*
- Tangerines
- Watermelon*

herbs & spices

INCLUDING BUT NOT LIMITED TO

- Anise
- Annatto
- Basil
- Bay leaf
- Caraway
- Cardamom
- Carob
- **Cayenne pepper**
- Celery seed
- Chervil
- Chicory*
- **Chili pepper**
- **Chipotle powder**
- Chives
- Cilantro
- Cinnamon
- Clove
- Coriander

- Cumin
- Curry
- Dill
- Fennel*
- Fenugreek
- Galangal
- Garlic
- Ginger
- Horseradish*
- Juniper berry
- Kaffir lime leaves
- Lavender
- Lemongrass
- Lemon verbena
- Licorice
- Mace
- Marjoram
- Mint

- Mustard
- Oregano
- **Paprika**
- Parsley
- Pepper, black
- Peppermint
- Rosemary
- Saffron
- Spearmint
- Star anise
- Tarragon
- Thyme
- Turmeric
- Vanilla
- *Wasabi**
- Za'atar

PRACTICAL PALEO

guide to: stocking a paleo pantry

Fresh is best. Shopping the perimeter of the grocery store is ideal for the bulk of your foods, but you will want to add spices and some pantry items to your arsenal to cook up some tasty dishes and have some stand-by foods on-hand. Some of these foods are sold in cold sections of the store and need to be kept cold despite being packaged items.

herbs & spices

SOME HERBS CAN BE FOUND IN BOTH FRESH AND DRIED FORMS. INCLUDING BUT NOT LIMITED TO

- Anise
- Annatto
- Basil
- Bay leaf
- Caraway
- Cardamom
- **Cayenne**
- Celery seed
- Chervil
- Chicory*
- **Chili powder**
- **Chipotle**
- Chives
- Cilantro
- Cinnamon
- Clove
- Coriander
- Cumin
- Curry
- Dill
- Fennel
- Fenugreek
- Galangal
- Garlic
- Ginger
- *Horseradish*
- Juniper berry
- Kaffir lime leaves
- Lavender
- Lemongrass
- Lemon verbena
- Licorice
- Mace
- Marjoram
- Mint
- *Mustard*
- Nutmeg
- Onion powder*
- Oregano
- **Paprika**
- Parsley
- Pepper, black
- Peppercorns, whole black
- Peppermint
- Pumpkin pie spice
- Rosemary
- Saffron
- Sage
- Sea salt
- Spearmint
- Star anise
- Tarragon
- Thyme
- Turmeric
- Vanilla
- *Wasabi*
- Za'atar

canned & jarred

INCLUDING BUT NOT LIMITED TO

- Anchovy paste
- Applesauce*
- Capers
- Coconut milk*
- Coconut water/ Juice*
- Fish roe
- Herring - wild
- Olives
- Oysters
- Pickles
- Pumpkin
- Salmon - wild
- Sardines - wild
- **Sun-dried tomatoes**
- *Sweet potato*
- Tahini
- **Tomato paste**
- **Tomato sauce**
- Tuna - wild

nuts, seeds & dried fruit

- Almonds
- Almond butter
- Almond flour
- Banana chips (check ingredients)
- Brazil nuts
- Chestnuts
- Coconut butter*
- Coconut*: shredded, flakes
- Dates
- Dried apples*
- Dried apricots*
- Dried blueberries
- Dried cranberries
- Dried currants
- Dried figs*
- Dried mango*
- Dried pineapple
- Dried raspberries
- Hazelnuts
- Macadamia nuts
- Pecans
- Pine nuts
- Pistachios*
- Pumpkin seeds
- Sesame seeds
- Sunflower seeds
- Walnuts

add your own!

MAYBE YOU HAVE FAVORITE ITEMS NOT LISTED ABOVE THAT YOU KNOW ARE PALEO-FRIENDLY; WRITE THEM IN TO USE THIS AS A SHOPPING LIST

fats & oils

SEE THE FATS & OILS GUIDE FOR DETAILS

- Avocado oil: CP
- Bacon fat
- Ghee
- Coconut oil
- Macadamia oil: CP
- Extra-virgin olive oil
- Palm oil
- Palm shortening
- Sesame oil: CP
- Walnut oil: CP

sauces

- Coconut aminos* (soy-replacement)
- Fish sauce (Red Boat brand)
- **Hot sauce (gluten-free)**
- *Mustard (gluten-free)*
- Vinegars: apple cider*, red wine, distilled, rice and balsamic (avoid malt vinegar)

beverages

- Green tea
- Herbal tea
- Mineral water
- White tea
- Organic coffee

treats & sweets

FOR OCCASIONAL USE

- Carob powder
- Cocoa powder
- Honey
- Maple syrup
- Molasses
- Dark chocolate

NOTES
CP = cold-pressed
bold = nightshades
italics = goitrogenic
* = FODMAPs (p.115)

Buy as many of your pantry items as possible in organic form.

PRACTICAL PALEO

guide to: food quality

Seek out as much real, whole food as possible. This includes foods without health claims on the packages or, better yet, not in packages at all. Think produce and butcher counter meats and seafood. After you've mastered making proper food choices, it's important to begin looking at the quality of the items. While buying the best quality is ideal in a perfect world, don't let those "best" labels keep you from doing the best you can within your means.

meat, eggs & dairy

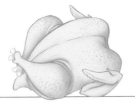

beef & lamb
Best! 100% grass-fed and finished, pasture-raised, local
Better: grass-fed, pasture-raised
Good: organic
Baseline: commercial (hormone/antibiotic-free)

pork
Best! pasture-raised, local
Better: free-range, organic
Good: organic
Baseline: commercial

eggs & poultry
Best! pasture-raised, local
Better: free range, organic
Good: cage-free, organic
Baseline: commercial

dairy
ALWAYS BUY FULL-FAT
Best! grass-fed, raw/unpasteurized
Better: raw/unpasteurized
Good: grass-fed
Baseline: commercial or organic —*not recommended*

seafood

Best! wild fish
Better: wild-caught
Good: humanely harvested, non-grain-fed
Baseline: farm-raised—*not recommended*

WILD FISH/ WILD-CAUGHT FISH
"Wild fish" indicates that the fish was spawned, lived in, and was caught in the wild. "Wild-caught fish" may have been spawned or lived some part of their lives in a fish farm before being returned to the wild and eventually caught. The Monterey Bay Aquarium maintains a free list of the most sustainable seafood choices on their website.

WHAT THE LABELS ON MEAT, EGGS & DAIRY MEAN

pasture-raised
Animals can roam freely in their natural environment where they are able to eat nutritious grasses and other plants or bugs/grubs that are part of their natural diet. There is no specific pasture-raised certification, though certified organic meat must come from animals that have continuous access to pasture regardless of use.

cage-free
"Cage-Free" means uncaged inside barns or warehouses, but they generally do not have access to the outdoors. Beak cutting is permitted. There is no third party auditing.

organic
Animals may not receive hormones/antibiotics unless in the case of illness. They consume organic feed and have outdoor access but may not use it. Animals are not necessarily grass-fed. Certification is costly and some reputable farms are forced to forego it. Compliance is verified through third party auditing.

natural
"Natural" means "minimally processed," and companies use this word deceivingly. All cuts are, by definition, minimally processed and free of flavorings and chemicals.

free-range/roaming
Poultry must have access to the outdoors at least 51% of the time, and ruminants may not be in feedlots. There are no restrictions regarding what the birds can be fed. Beak cutting and forced molting through starvation are permitted. There is no third party auditing.

naturally raised
"Naturally Raised," is a USDA verified term. It generally means raised without growth-promoters or unnecessary antibiotics. It does not indicate welfare or diet.

no added hormones
It is illegal to use hormones in raising poultry or pork; therefore, the use of this phrase on poultry or pork is a marketing ploy.

vegetarian-fed
"Vegetarian Fed" implies that the animal feed is free of animal by-products but isn't federally inspected. Chickens are not vegetarians, so this label on chicken or eggs only serves to indicate that the chickens were not eating their natural diet.

produce

Best! local, organic, and seasonal
Better: local and organic
Good: organic or local
Baseline: conventional

WHEN TO BUY ORGANIC:
Buy organic as often as possible, prioritize buying the Environmental Working Group's "The Dirty Dozen" as organic versus "The Clean Thirteen" - visit: www.ewg.org for details

PRODUCE SKUs:
Starts with 9 = organic - ideal
Starts with 3 or 4 = conventionally grown
Starts with 8 = genetically modified (GMO) or irradiated - avoid

fats & oils

SEE THE FATS & OILS GUIDE FOR DETAILS.
Best! organic, cold-pressed, and from well-raised animal sources
Better: organic, cold-pressed
Good: organic or conventional

nuts & seeds

KEEP NUTS & SEEDS COLD FOR FRESHNESS
Best! local, organic, kept cold
Better: local, organic
Good: organic
Baseline: conventional

sources: www.humanesociety.org, www.ewg.org, www.sustainabletable.org

PRACTICAL PALEO

guide to: fats & oils

Cleaning up your diet by using the right fats and oils is essential to improving your health from the inside out. Changing the fats and oils you use at home is the first step toward creating dishes from nutrient-dense, whole foods based on what you have on hand. Avoid overly processed and refined forms of fats and oils. Opt for organic whenever possible. Refer to the "Guide to Cooking Fats" for more details.

eat these: HEALTHY, NATURALLY OCCURRING, MINIMALLY PROCESSED FATS

saturated: FOR HOT USES

BUY ORGANIC, UNREFINED FORMS

· Coconut oil
· Palm oil

IDEALLY FROM PASTURE-RAISED, GRASS-FED, ORGANIC SOURCES

· Butter
· Ghee, clarified butter
· Lard, bacon grease (pork fat)
· Tallow (beef fat)
· Duck fat
· Schmaltz (chicken fat)
· Lamb fat
· Full-fat dairy
· Eggs, meat, and seafood

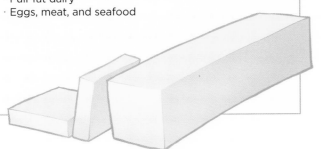

unsaturated: FOR COLD USES

BUY ORGANIC, EXTRA-VIRGIN, AND COLD-PRESSED FORMS

· Olive oil
· Sesame oil
· Macadamia nut oil
· Walnut oil
· Avocado oil
· Nuts & seeds (including nut & seed butters)
· Flaxseed oil**

NOTE: Unsaturated fats (typically liquid at 68 degrees room temperature) are easily damaged/oxidized when heat is applied to them. Do not consume damaged fats.

Cold-pressed flaxseed oil is okay for occasional use but supplementing with it or doses of 1-2 tablespoons per day is ***not* recommended as overall PUFA (polyunsaturated fatty acid) intake should remain minimal.

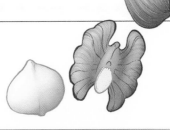

ditch these: UNHEALTHY, MAN-MADE FATS & REFINED SEED OILS ARE NOT RECOMMENDED

Hydrogenated or partially hydrogenated oils, as well as manmade trans-fats or "buttery spreads" like Earth Balance, Benecol, and I Can't Believe It's Not Butter are not healthy. These oils are highly processed and oxidize easily via one or more of the following: light, air, or heat.

· Margarine/buttery spreads
· Canola oil (also known as rapeseed oil)
· Corn oil
· Vegetable oil
· Soybean oil
· Grapeseed oil
· Sunflower oil
· Safflower oil
· Rice bran oil
· Shortening made from one or more of the above-listed "ditch" oils

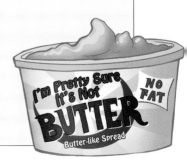

PRACTICAL PALEO

guide to: cooking fats

Choose fats and oils based on: 1. How they're made—choose naturally occurring, minimally processed options first; 2. Their fatty acid composition—the more saturated they are, the more stable/less likely to be damaged or oxidized; 3. Smoke point—this tells you how hot is too hot before you will damage the fats, though it should be considered a secondary factor to fatty acid profile.

culinary whizzes, listen up: COOK WITH GOOD FATS!

ITEM NAME	% SFA	%MUFA	% PUFA	SMOKE POINT UNREFINED/REFINED
best bets - recommended for high-heat cooking THE MOST STABLE FATS				
Coconut oil	86	6	2	350/450
Butter/ghee	63	26	.03	300/480
Cocoa butter	60	35	5	370
Tallow/suet (beef fat)	55	34	.03	400
Palm oil	54	42	.10	455
Lard/bacon fat (pork fat)	39	45	11	375
Duck fat	37	50	13	375
okay - for very low-heat cooking MODERATELY STABLE FATS				
Avocado oil*	20	70	10	520
Macadamia nut oil*	16	80	4	410
Olive oil*	14	73	11	375
Peanut oil**	17	46	32	320/450
Rice Bran Oil**	25	38	37	415
not recommended for cooking VERY UNSTABLE FATS				
Safflower oil**	8	76	13	225/510
Sesame seed oil*	14	40	46	450
Canola oil**	8	64	28	400
Sunflower oil**	10	45	40	225/440
Vegetable shortening**	34	11	52	330
Corn oil	15	30	55	445
Soybean oil	16	23	58	495
Walnut oil*	14	19	67	400
Grapeseed oil	12	17	71	420

SFA - saturated fatty acid   MUFA - monounsaturated fatty acid   PUFA - polyunsaturated fatty acid

* While not recommended for cooking, cold-pressed nut and seed oils that are stored in the refrigerator may be used to finish recipes or after cooking is completed—for flavor purposes.

** While the fatty acid profile of these oils may seem appropriate at first glance, the processing method by which they are made negates their healthfulness—they are not recommended for consumption, neither hot nor cold.

Practical Paleo

PRACTICAL PALEO

guide to: dense sources of paleo carbs

Removing grains, legumes, and refined foods from your diet doesn't mean that carbohydrates need to all disappear! Check out this list of dense sources of carbohydrates while eating a Paleo diet. While fruits and nuts are all fairly high in carbohydrates, this list is a guide to starchy vegetables to eat. Remember, these are some of your "good carbs!"

there *are* carbs beyond bread EAT UP

ITEM NAME	CARBS PER 100G	FIBER PER 100G	CARBS PER 1 CUP	OTHER NOTABLE NUTRIENTS
Cassava (raw)	38g	2g	78g	Vit C, Thiamin, Folate, Potassium, Manganese
Taro root	35g	5g	46g, sliced	B6, Vitamin E, Potassium, Manganese
Plantain	31g	2g	62g, mashed	Vitamin A (beta carotene), Vitamin C, B6, Magnesium, Potassium
Yam	27g	4g	37g, cubed	Vit C, Vitamin B6, Manganese, Potassium
White potato	22g	1g	27g, peeled	Trace Vitamin C
Sweet potato	21g	3g	58g, mashed	Vit A (beta carotene), Vit C, B6, Potassium, Manganese, Magnesium, Iron, Vitamin E
Parsnips	17g	4g	27g, sliced	Vitamin C, Manganese
Lotus root	16g	3g	19g, sliced	Vitamin C, B6, Potassium, Copper, Manganese
Winter squash	15g	4g	30g, cubed	Vitamin C, Thiamin, B6
Onion	10g	1g	21g, chopped	Vitamin C, Potassium
Beets	10g	2g	17g, sliced	Folate, Manganese
Carrots	10g	3g	13g, chopped	Vitamin A (beta carotene), Vitamin K1
Butternut squash	10g	-	22g	Vitamin A (beta carotene), Vitamin C
Rutabaga	9g	2g	21g, mashed	Vitamin C, Potassium, Manganese,
Jicama (raw)	9g	5g	12g, sliced	Vitamin C
Kohlrabi	7g	1g	11g, sliced	Vit C, B6, Potassium, Copper, Manganese
Spaghetti squash	6g	1g	9g	Trace
Turnips	5g	2g	12g, mashed	Vitamin C, Potassium, Calcium, B6, Folate, Manganese
Pumpkin	5g	1g	12g, mashed	Vitamin C, Vitamin E, Potassium

source: nutritiondata.com
Practical Paleo

PRACTICAL PALEO

guide to: sweeteners

How many of these sweeteners do you use or find in your favorite packaged foods? Perhaps it's time for a change! Artificial sweeteners are never recommended, while the limited use of selected, more naturally derived options can be okay for treats and special occasions. Sweeteners should not be considered "food" or nourishment.

natural USE SPARINGLY

PREFERRED CHOICES ARE IN BOLD. USE ORGANIC FORMS WHENEVER POSSIBLE

- Brown sugar
- **Dates (whole)**
- Date sugar
- Date syrup
- Cane sugar
- Raw sugar
- Turbinado

- Cane juice
- Cane juice crystals
- Coconut nectar
- Coconut sugar/crystals
- **Fruit juice (real, fresh)**
- **Fruit juice concentrate**
- **Honey (raw)**

- **Maple syrup (grade b)**
- **Molasses**
- Palm sugar
- **Stevia (green leaf or extract)**

natural BUT NOT RECOMMENDED

- Agave
- Agave nectar
- Barley malt
- Beet sugar
- Brown rice syrup
- Buttered syrup
- Caramel
- Carob syrup
- Corn syrup
- Corn syrup solids
- Demerara sugar
- Dextran
- Dextrose
- Diastatic malt

- Diastase
- Ethyl maltol
- Fructose
- Glucose / glucose solids
- Golden sugar
- Golden syrup
- Grape sugar
- High fructose corn syrup
- Invert sugar
- Lactose
- Levulose
- Light brown sugar
- Maltitol
- Malt syrup

- Maltodextrin
- Maltose
- Mannitol
- Muscovado
- Refiner's syrup
- Sorbitol
- Sorghum syrup
- Sucrose
- Treacle
- Yellow sugar
- Xylitol (or other sugar alcohols, typically they end in "-ose")

artificial NEVER CONSUME

- Acesulfame K (Sweet One)
- Aspartame (Equal, Nutra-Sweet)
- Saccharin (Sweet'N Low)
- Stevia: white/bleached (Truvia, Sun Crystals)
- Sucralose (Splenda)
- Tagatose

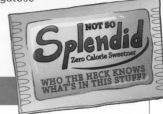

sugar is sugar BUT NOT REALLY

IT DOES MAKE A DIFFERENCE WHICH SWEETENERS YOU SELECT, CONTRARY TO POPULAR BELIEF AND THE MAINSTREAM MEDIA. WHILE ALL CALORIC SWEETENERS HAVE THE SAME NUMBER OF CALORIES (16 PER TEASPOON), EVALUATING THEIR PLACE IN YOUR DIET MAY BE DONE BY CONSIDERING A FEW FACTORS.

HOW IT'S MADE

The more highly refined a sweetener is, the worse it is for your body. For example, high fructose corn syrup (HFCS) and artificial sweeteners are all very modern, factory-made products. Honey, maple syrup, green leaf stevia (dried leaves made into powder), and molasses are all much less processed and have been made for hundreds of years. In the case of honey, almost no processing is necessary. As a result, I vote for raw, organic, local honey as the ideal natural sweetener.

WHERE IT'S USED

This is a reality check. When you read the ingredients in packaged, processed foods, it becomes obvious how most of them use highly-refined, low-quality sweeteners. Food manufacturers often even hide sugar in foods that you didn't think were sweets! Many foods that have been made low or non-fat have added sweeteners or artificial sweeteners—avoid these products!

HOW YOUR BODY PROCESSES IT

Here's where the HFCS commercials really get things wrong: your body actually does not metabolize all sugar the same way.

Interestingly enough, sweeteners like HFCS and agave nectar were viewed as better options for diabetics for quite some time since the high fructose content of both requires processing by the liver before the sugar hits your blood stream. This yielded a seemingly favorable result on blood sugar levels after consuming said sweeteners. However, it's now understood that isolated fructose metabolism is a complicated issue and that taxing the liver excessively with such sweeteners can be quite harmful to our health.

Fructose is the primary sugar in all fruit. When eating whole fruit, the micronutrients and fiber content of the fruit actually support proper metabolism and assimilation of the fruit sugar. Whole foods for the win!

PRACTICAL PALEO

guide to: gluten

What is it? Gluten is a protein found in wheat, rye oats, and barley. Gluten is the composite of a prolamin and a glutelin, which exist, conjoined with starch, in the endosperm of various grass-related grains. Gliadin, a water-soluble, and glutenin, a water-insoluble, (the prolamin and glutelin from wheat) compose about 80% of the protein contained in wheat seed. Being insoluble in water, they can be purified by washing away the associated starch. Worldwide, gluten is a source of protein, both in foods prepared directly from sources containing it, and as an additive to foods otherwise low in protein.

sources of gluten OR ITEMS THAT MAY CONTAIN HIDDEN GLUTEN

- Ales
- Barley
- Barley malt/ extract
- Beer & lagers
- Bran
- Breading
- Broth
- Brown rice syrup
- Bulgur
- Candy coating
- Communion "wafers"
- Couscous
- Croutons
- Durum
- Einkorn
- Emmer
- Farina
- Farro
- Gloss & balms
- Graham flour
- Herbal blends
- Imitation
- Imitation seafood
- Kamut
- Lipstick
- Luncheon meats
- Malt
- Makeup
- Marinades
- Matzo flour/meal
- Meat/sausages
- Medications
- Orzo
- Panko
- Pasta
- Play dough
- Roux
- Rye
- Sauces
- Seitan
- Self-basting poultry
- Semolina
- Soup base
- Soy sauce
- Spelt
- Spice blends
- Stuffing
- Supplements
- Thickeners
- Triticale
- Udon
- Vinegar (malt only)
- Vital wheat gluten
- Vitamins
- Wafers
- Wheat
- Wheat bran
- Wheat germ
- Wheat starch

gluten-free* (BUT STILL NOT RECOMMENDED)

*Nearly all processed foods and grains carry some risk of cross-contamination. For the safest approach to a gluten-free diet, eat only whole, unprocessed foods.

- Amaranth
- Arrowroot
- Buckwheat
- Corn
- Flax
- Millet
- Montina™
- Nut flour
- Bean flour
- Potato flour
- Potato starch
- Quinoa
- Rice
- Rice bran
- Sago
- Seed flour
- Sorghum
- Soy (soya)
- Tapioca
- Teff

signs of gluten EXPOSURE

- Abdominal bloating
- Fatigue
- Skin problems or rashes
- Diarrhea or constipation
- Irritable, moody
- Change in energy levels
- Unexpected weight loss, mouth ulcers, depression, and even Crohn's disease are all more severe gluten allergy symptoms that you may experience.
- Consult with your nutritionist or physician if you experience symptoms of a gluten exposure that result in prolonged discomfort.

most common sources of HIDDEN GLUTEN

Alcohol:
Beer, malt beverages, grain alcohols

Cosmetics:
Check ingredients on makeup, shampoo, and other personal care items

Dressings:
Thickened with flour or other additives

Fried foods:
Cross contamination with breaded items in fryers

Vinegar: Malt varieties

Medications, vitamins, and supplements:
ask the pharmacist and read the labels closely

Processed / packaged foods:
Additives often contain gluten

Sauces, soups, and stews: Thickened with flour

Soy, Teriyaki, and Hoisin sauces:
Fermented with wheat

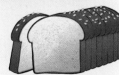

gluten-free BOOZE**

- Brandy
- Bourbon
- Cognac
- Gin
- Grappa
- Rum
- Sake
- Scotch
- Sherry
- Tequila
- Vermouth
- Vodka
- Whiskey
- Wine
- Champagne
- Mead
- Hard cider
- Gluten-free beers

i am allergic TO GLUTEN

I have a severe allergy and have to follow a STRICT gluten-free diet.

I may become very ill if I eat food containing flours or grains of wheat, rye, barley, or oats.

Does this food contain flour or grains of wheat, barley rye, or oats? If you or the chef/kitchen staff are uncertain about what the food contains, please tell me.

I CAN eat food containing rice, maize, potatoes, vegetables, fruit, eggs, cheese, milk, meat, and fish as long as they are NOT cooked with wheat flour, batter, breadcrumbs, or sauce containing any of those ingredients.

Thank you for your help!

For more gluten-guides, visit: www.celiactravel.com

for more information ON GLUTEN

These sites are not necessarily "Paleo" but will give ample information for those who need to be 100% strictly gluten-free

- celiac.com
- celiac.org
- celiaccentral.org
- celiaclife.com
- celiactravel.com
- celiacsolution.com
- elanaspantry.com
- glutenfreegirl.com
- surefoodsliving.com

^ Cut me out and take me with you

***According to celiac.com, all distilled alcohols are gluten-free but for someone with overt Celiac Disease, avoiding alcohols made from wheat, barley, and rye is still recommended.

PRACTICAL PALEO